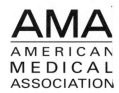

Understanding Medicare's NCCI Edits:

Logic and Interpretation of the Edits

Susan E. Garrison, CHCA, CHC, PCS, FCS, CCS-P, CPAR, CPC, CPC-H

Library of Congress Cataloging-in-Publication Data

Garrison, Susan E.
  Understanding Medicare's NCCI edits: logic and interpretation of the edits / Susan E. Garrison.
    p.;cm.
  Includes bibliographical references.
  Summary: "The purpose of this book is to help readers navigate the NCCI edits in order to code correctly. The book also helps readers understand the the NCCI and CPT coding guidelines"--Provided by publisher.
  ISBN 978-1-60359-196-6 (alk. paper)
  1. Operations, Surgical--Code numbers. 2. Medicare. I. American Medical Association. II. Title.
  [DNLM: 1. Forms and Records Control--classification--United States. 2. Medicare--classification. 3. Chronic Disease--classification--United States. 4. Insurance Claim Reporting--classification--United States. 5. Insurance, Health, Reimbursement--economics--United States. 6. Medical Records--classification--United States.
W 80 G242u 2010]

RD16.G37 2010
368.4'2600973--dc22

                    2009028822

ISBN 978-1-60359-196-6
AC44: 09-P-041:11/09

Dedication

This book is dedicated to all those who strive to understand the complex demands of documenting, coding, and billing correctly. With your devotion to "getting it right," you are helping providers, payers, and patients. Thank you for investing the time to better understand the National Correct Coding Initiative (NCCI) Edits.

About the Author

Susan Garrison, CHCA, CHC, PCS, CCS-P, CPAR, CPC, CPC-H, FCS, is one of those rare people who is adeptly qualified as a consultant, speaker, auditor, educator, and author. As Executive V.P. for Med Law Advisors and Magnus Confidential, her clients include solo practicing physicians, large teaching facilities, free-standing Ambulatory Surgery Centers, hospitals, national associations, law firms, publishers, and over 100 other leading facilities and affiliated organizations. Susan serves on the boards of directors of the Association of Health Care Auditors and Educators (AHCAE) and the American College of Medical Coding Specialists (ACMCS). She is also past president of the American Academy of Professional Coders.

Susan's speaking and educating typically includes 10 keynotes a year at major national conferences, and dozens of seminars and workshops for providers, payors, and member organizations. She has taught courses on advanced topics for documentation, coding, billing, and reimbursement issues for physicians and hospitals. Whether to audiences of 1 or 1,000, Susan capably relays her message while inspiring the audience to action. She is also interviewed and quoted frequently in the health care management media.

Susan is a member of the Association of Health Care Auditors and Educators, the American College of Medical Coding Specialists, the American Health Information Management Association, the Health Care Compliance Association, and the American Academy of Professional Coders. She holds credentials for each of these associations as well as being credentialed in Patient Accounting by the Healthcare Financial Management Association. Susan especially enjoys sharing her knowledge through newsletters, books, hundreds of industry-related articles, and other published works.

Acknowledgements

I wish to thank four very special individuals, who, by their unique strengths helped this book idea become reality. Elizabeth Kennedy, Developmental Editor, whose patience and diligence in editing this work were always much appreciated. Elise Schumacher, Senior Acquisitions Editor, who grasped the concept immediately and honed it so well, Karen O'Hara, CPT Specialist whose review of CPT-related content is accurate, and Stephen Garrison, husband and believer, who gave up many weekends, offered sound counsel, and helped me "think outside the code" when writing this book.

Each of these individuals is dedicated, intelligent, and pure magic—my many thanks.

Table of Contents

Preface

"How do I work?...I grope."

Albert Einstein

Writing this book on the National Correct Coding Initiative (NCCI) edits represented the opportunity to share ideas of how professionals involved in coding, billing, and paying health care claims can more effectively understand and address bundling edits. The goal of this book is to help improve the accuracy and completeness of medical encounter documentation, coding, billing, and reimbursement, specifically as it relates to the NCCI edits.

Like Einstein's method, this was a process of groping—I groped to determine what the most essential elements for coders, providers, payers, and auditors were in understanding the NCCI process. Those essential elements are the focus of this book.

The essential elements were gathered through hundreds of chart audits, coder and physician education sessions, and general brainstorming with coding and auditing colleagues. The elements that we will expand on in this book are the links between the edits, the guidelines, and the gray areas of deciding when to bypass an edit.

Building an understanding of the logic behind all of the edits is clearly more important than focusing on specific edits. There are several reasons for this:

- History shows that the specific NCCI edits change more often than their guidelines.
- Because *Current Procedural Terminology (CPT®)* codes are subject to annual updates, memorizing code-specific edits is not helpful in the long-term.
- The more someone understands the rationale, the easier correct coding becomes.

This is akin to teaching someone to fish rather than giving her a fish. We want to feed your coding intellect so that you will know how to make good decisions on bundling edits.

This book does not review every edit of the NCCI, because that would not be practical or particularly helpful, and it would require too many updates. Rather, we are going to delve into the guidelines in detail and review the logic of the system. The purpose of this book is to teach you how to determine appropriate coding when faced with bundling edits.

People make choices using many different methodologies: There's the "rock, paper, scissor" decision-making process or perhaps "Close enough is good enough" or, worse yet, "How do I code it to get higher reimbursement?"

A better method of decision making with the NCCI edits is to work toward understanding the NCCI and CPT coding guidelines. With a solid understanding of the guidelines and with substantial case-specific documentation, you should be able to make the right decision and be able to defend that decision. This book prepares those new to the NCCI edits as well as experienced coding professionals to grasp why edits exist, the logic of the edits, and how to appropriately code the claim (whether to bundle or unbundle). You will be learning the basic conventions for NCCI edits, but, more importantly, you will be learning the appropriate handling of these edits.

The NCCI edits pair the Healthcare Common Procedure Coding System (HCPCS) codes that *potentially* should not be coded together when provided:

- for a single patient
- on a single date of service
- by a single provider (or same specialty provider within the same group practice)

The word *potentially* is important here and is a key to the purpose of this book. To know the edit is one piece of understanding NCCI guidelines, but it certainly does not complete the picture of how to code correctly within the NCCI guidelines.

For a quick summary of NCCI guidelines, there are three different types of NCCI edits:

Column 1/Column 2 codes

Mutually exclusive codes

Medically unlikely edits (MUEs)

In both Column 1/Column 2 edits and mutually exclusive edits, payment will be made for only one set of codes. Column 1/Column 2 code pair edits include related services. When coding, do not fragment or separate a single service into that service's component parts. This could be perceived as attempting to maximize reimbursement.

Mutually exclusive code pair edits are those codes for services that cannot reasonably be performed at the same anatomic site or in the same patient encounter. If, based on the code descriptors, multiple services billed together appear to be medically impossible or improbable to have been performed at the same patient encounter, one will be denied.

MUEs are different in that two codes are not edited against each other. Instead, the units of service for a single code are edited to control the units of service being billed.

The edits in many cases can be overridden by appending a modifier, but to do so correctly, you must:

1. know that the edit exists;
2. understand the guideline behind the edit;
3. review the documentation to see if both services are appropriate to code and the edit appropriate to bypass;
4. track the edits to determine patterns within your practice;
5. notify the practice clinical and management staff with a trend report (on a quarterly basis);
6. track reimbursement to see if both services are, indeed, paid when a modifier is appended to bypass the edit; and
7. educate the clinicians, coders, billers, accounts receivable staff if errors or insufficiencies are found when cases are analyzed.

Learning Break

For MUE edits, each line of a claim is adjudicated separately against the MUE value on that line. In order to bypass the edits (when appropriate and allowed), modifiers may be used to report the same code on separate lines of a claim. CPT modifiers such as -76 (repeat procedure by same physician), -77 (repeat procedure by another physician), anatomic modifiers (eg, RT, LT, F1, F2), -91 (repeat clinical diagnostic laboratory test), and -59 (distinct procedural service) are options—always choose the most appropriate modifier that reflects the scenario correctly.

In Closing

Our goal for this book was to open up a window into the NCCI edit guidelines to help providers, payers, coders, and other related professionals better understand the appropriate coding of multiple services when provided. Often in this profession we are heavily reliant on resources and research, and we hope this becomes a great resource for you.

Some additional thoughts to help the book be a practical resource for you are offered here along with all the tools provided throughout this book.

When working with NCCI edits, we recommend that you:

Keep a List

Keep a list of edits that your practice commonly encounters. Tracking and trending are very important to understand where insufficiencies in coding, documentation, billing, or accounts receivable management might exist. Do not stop with a list of edits that your practice encounters, add to the list how you handled the edit, and be detailed here. This is one of the best ways to ensure you can make positive changes.

Finish What You Start

This will require working with coding throughout the revenue cycle—from clinical encounter to payment. If a procedure is not understood, ask the clinician. If you file again for payment, ask accounts receivable if the correct payment was obtained. Make sure the patient was not billed if the edit was properly applied.

Ask Around

Network with others in other practices (within and outside your same specialty) to see if they encounter the same edits and how they handle them and their thoughts on the edits, and so forth. Research the Medicare Web site to see if there is any additional information (frequently asked questions, memos). Go to the source! Even if I am not sure of exactly how an edit should be handled, odds are, someone I know has an opinion. I might not necessarily agree with their "take" on the edit, but at least it gives me something to think about and loosens up my own block about the edit.

Be Patient and Think

Change takes time, learning the process takes time, correcting deficiencies takes time and thinking. Do not short-cut either...you will get that "Aha" moment of clarity if you work through the process.

Layer

Take what you learn from one scenario to the next one. Coding is very much a building process. If you can break down the edits into smaller parts and really work on understanding the parts, that will often impact the next edit quandary.

You will gain knowledge and learn new skills to become a more effective coder or auditor for your organization. Not only will you be learning new skills in coding, you can also use these skills in other job responsibilities, be able to think through complex coding issues, and improve your everyday understanding of claims processing and billing oversight.

This book provides the fundamentals of critical thinking for NCCI edits. Whether you are a coder, practice manager, accounts receivables representative, or clinician, I think you'll find some useful tips in these pages.

Good luck and happy coding!

Susan Garrison, CHCA, CHC, PCS, FCS, CCS-P, CPC, CPC-H, CPAR

Note for the reader:
This book uses references from both NCCI policy and the *CPT Assistant* newsletter. Although the codes may have changed or have been deleted, the concept or policy still applies.

Introduction: Overview of Medicare's National Correct Coding Initiative Edits

Chapter 1 introduces the Centers for Medicare and Medicaid Services National Correct Coding Initiative (NCCI) and reviews our recommendation for the decision-making matrix with NCCI edits. This chapter also addresses some of the overarching NCCI guidelines and logic seen in later chapters. There is also a brief explanation of the recommended procedures for making sound coding decisions.

Later chapters introduce more specific NCCI guidelines. This book analyzes and interprets those guidelines and provides case examples reflective of common scenarios for the specific area of coding. Such scenarios will provide insight for determining whether or not a particular bundle is appropriate or whether the use of a modifier is warranted. Each chapter concludes with a summary of issues for reflection and discussion.

Each step in this NCCI book details the key concepts and the practical skills that should be understood and mastered for effectively and accurately coding within the NCCI structure. Today, almost every health care organization is seeking to ensure that its coding is correct and optimal while making the most efficient use of available resources.

The History and Rationale Behind the NCCI Edits[1]

The Centers for Medicare and Medicaid Services (CMS) is the department of the federal government under the Department of Health and Human Services (HHS) that oversees the health care programs supported by the government. This includes the federal program for Medicare insurance and state programs for Medicaid insurance.

CMS developed the NCCI for implementation January 1, 1996, to promote correct coding by physicians and facilities and to ensure that appropriate payments are made for health care services. This chapter explains and illustrates how to locate the guidelines on the CMS web site.

NCCI edits apply to claims that contain *all* of the following:
- Multiple services reported
- Same beneficiary
- Same date of service
- Same provider

Remember, all of these conditions must be met before an NCCI edit would apply. NCCI edits will not review across service dates, for example.

The goals of the NCCI are to promote *national* correct coding and to control improper coding that could lead to inappropriate payments. The fact that the edits are national edits is important, as this helps ensure that different jurisdictions are bundling services consistently. The NCCI manual produced by CMS includes important instructions that every coder should understand. This book will walk through those instructions provided in the NCCI manual and provide additional insight into how to grasp the concepts completely.

Coding represents every aspect of a patient's health history; therefore, accuracy is critically important. If incorrectly coded, a patient's diagnoses and procedures can be misstated, which could affect the patient's future insurability or quality of health care. Additionally, accurate coding is necessary to help ensure that the facility's reimbursement is appropriate and that no compliance risks (from overcoding) exist.

CMS Tip: *In your facility, do you know what is being denied because of failure to meet NCCI? How do you know this?*

Data mining (ie, the gathering of data to determine problem areas) is important. Accounts receivable management personnel also need to be involved in the process of capturing correct reimbursement and determining when services have been denied. There should be a direct link throughout the revenue cycle in communicating how claims are processed.

NCCI edits are one of the biggest challenges providers (and payers) face today. The edits are challenging for two reasons:

- Not all code combinations are included in the edits. This means a solid foundation in understanding coding guidelines is necessary because one cannot rely solely on the edits to drive coding decisions.
- Knowing specific edits (or code combinations) is only one step in the process. It is important to know when a combination of codes creates a bundling edit; however, it is equally important to know when it is appropriate to bypass the edit. Understanding the rationale behind these edits, therefore, allows users to make the right decision on coding cases.

The principles of NCCI edit decisions can be summarized as follows:

1. Determine whether an NCCI edit exists. Resources are provided to access the edits.
2. If an edit exists within the codes selected for the encounter, verify the accuracy of the original coding.
3. If original coding is incorrect, re-code as appropriate.
4. If original coding is correct, research the edit's logic. This book will work through that process.
5. Once the logic is understood, documentation of the encounter should be reviewed to determine whether or not the edit should be bypassed.
   If the decision is to bypass the edit, the appropriate modifier(s) should be appended, as shown later in this book. If the edit is bypassed, payment of the claim should be followed to ensure appropriate processing.
6. If the decision is to not bypass the edit, the claim must be re-coded. If the original coding is being changed, the individual(s) who made the original coding decision should be educated so that the same issue does not recur.
7. Findings and decisions should be tracked for future education.

Figure 1-1 shows these steps and can be used as a guide for decision making when NCCI edits occur. This matrix can aid in remembering the process steps for making NCCI decisions. The process of determining accuracy of code edits can vary from simple, quick checks and verifications to complex decisions about which the physician or others must be consulted.

NCCI edits are usually seen as a big challenge for providers, but why? The challenge is not so much the existence of an edit—the challenge comes in knowing how to handle the edit. By and large, the edits are based on well-established coding guidelines, and the edits can help highlight the nuances that are necessary for correct coding. This is why personnel need to completely understand the edits, the rationale behind the edits, and how to determine the best possible coding on cases.

Rather than settling for doing mediocre coding, coders should embrace researching, learning, and moving beyond the quick answer into the deeper thought process of analysis. To become an expert in this element of coding and adding significant value to the facility takes time devoted to understanding the logic of NCCI edits.

Walking through the process of decision making in coding is important. The best way to understand coding is to understand the process of coding rather than memorizing codes. Coders cannot make the right decisions without good documentation within the medical record. This book will repeatedly share examples of what *should* be in the documentation in order to bypass an edit. So, clinicians might need to improve the quality of their documentation. Coders, payers, or auditors involved in the decision-making process might need to work with their clinicians to help them understand what information is necessary within the medical record. This is a team effort.

Coding is a process, and working through NCCI edits is also a process. Learn the process, and one step in correct coding has been completed.

FIGURE 1-1 *Decision Matrix for NCCI Edits*

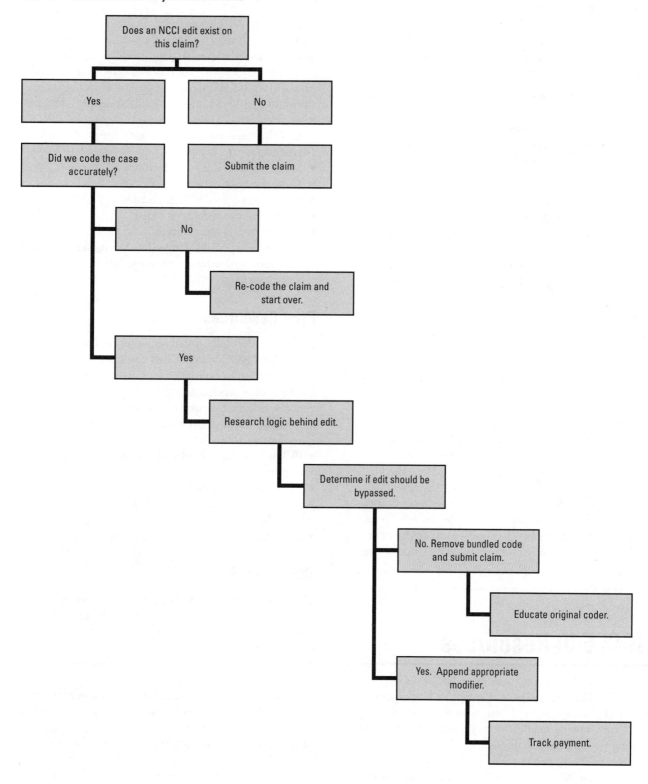

Would you code all of these services if they were performed on the same patient during the same encounter by the same provider?

99213 **Office or other outpatient visit** for the evaluation and management of an established patient, which requires at least 2 of these 3 key components:

- **An expanded, problem focused history;**
- **An expanded, problem focused examination;**
- **Medical decision making of low complexity.**

Counseling and coordination of care with other providers or agencies are provided consistent with the nature of the problem(s) and the patient's and family's needs.[2]

Usually, the presenting problems are of low to moderate severity. Physicians typically spend 15 minutes face-to-face with the patient and/or family.

20610 Arthrocentesis, aspiration and/or injection; major joint or bursa (eg, shoulder, hip, knee joint, subacromial bursa)

29881 Arthroscopy, knee, surgical; with meniscectomy (medial OR lateral, including any meniscal shaving)

If you would, why?

If not, why?

If you would, are there any modifiers you would append? Which modifiers and on which codes?

The answers are usually something along the lines of "Yes, why not?" or something like "No, never." Think about that for a moment—these answers are completely opposite, yet these are the answers I hear. That is one reason for this book—to teach the right decision process to help coders avoid making a wrong coding decision.

NCCI Edit Resources

It is helpful to have access to as many NCCI resources as possible. Because this book does not include all of the NCCI edits, the resources listed in this book should be considered integral to effectively understanding the edits. The experienced coder will understand the value and necessity of good, current resources. It is extremely unwise to code a claim for services rendered today using last year's CPT codebook. The same is true for NCCI edits. Because the edits change quarterly, current resources are critical. In addition to suggested resources, checklists are provided to help a facility ensure that its resources are current and optimized.

Software

Some facilities employ software that includes all of the NCCI edits. In such facilities, the software should be updated quarterly. Current data should always be used.

The American Medical Association includes NCCI edits within its *CodeManager* software. CodeManager allows for easy searching of 11 medical coding reference books and includes pop-up tips and other tools.

It is also important to track your software. Questions to ask include:

- What software does your facility use?
- Is the contract current?
- Does the contract include updates?
- How often are updates provided?
- Are the NCCI edits current?
- Do those responsible for coding, billing, and accounts receivable understand how to use the software effectively?

Print Resources

Several vendors sell printed resources (ie, books and manuals) with all NCCI edits. When a practice uses a print resource, it must ensure that staff use the correct set of data for the date of service in question. It is best to check with vendors to learn how quarterly updates are dispersed.

It is also important to track your print resources. Questions to ask include:

- What manuals or books related to NCCI does your facility use?
- How are updates provided?
- How often are updates provided?
- Are these resources current?
- Are any of these resources duplicative?

CMS Web Site

CMS, the official overseer for NCCI, has a wealth of information on its Web site. As shown in Figure 1-2 the following four steps explain how to access the NCCI edits on the CMS web site:

Step 1. Visit www.cms.hhs.gov[3] and select the Medicare category.

Step 2. Scroll down to the Provider Type category and select Physician Center. For hospital edits, select Hospital Center.

Step 3. For physicians, once you enter the Physician Center, scroll down to the Billing/Payment or Coding category and select National Correct Coding. For hospitals, scroll down to the Coding category for Physicians. For hospitals, select Hospital.

Step 4. Review all the appropriate information in this section. This will show where to look for additional

FIGURE 1-2 *Four Steps to Accessing NCCI Information on the CMS Web Site*[3]

Step 1

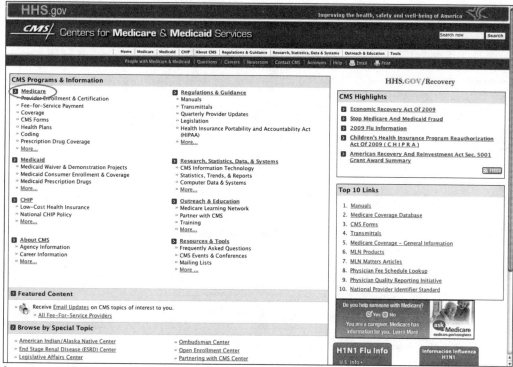

Source: www.cms.hhs.gov/

Step 2

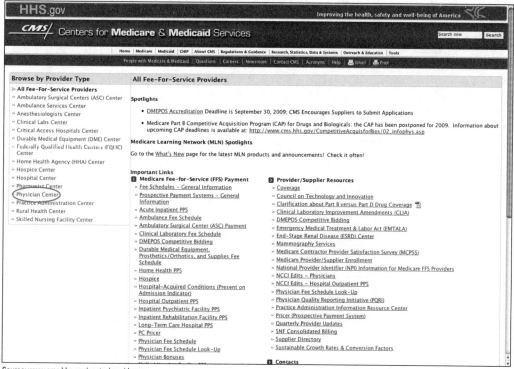

Source: www.cms.hhs.gov/center/provider.asp

FIGURE 1-2 *(continued)*

Step 3

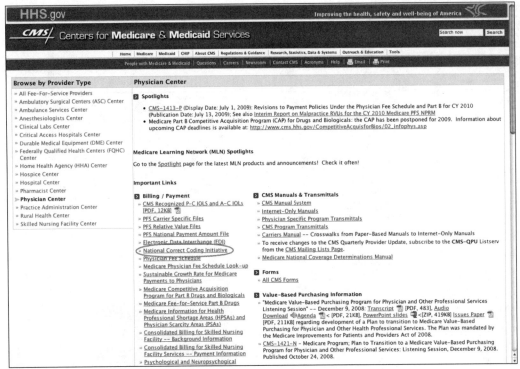

Source: www.cms.hhs.gov/center/physician.asp

Step 4

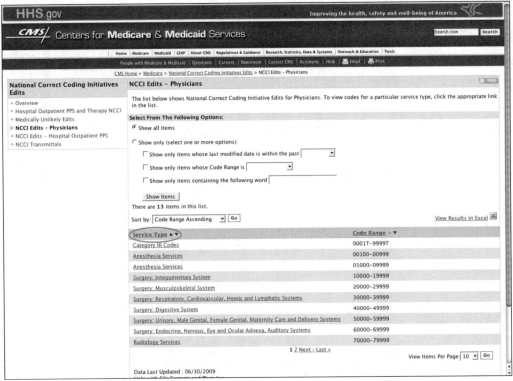

Source: www.cms.hhs.gov/NationalCorrectCodInitEd/NCCIEP/list.asp#TopOfPage

FIGURE 1-3 *Example of FAQs on the CMS Web Site*[4]

	ID ▼▲	Summary ▼
1	3373	What is the column 1/column 2 correct coding edit table?
2	3517	How should modifier -59 be reported under the CCI?
3	3510	What modifiers are allowed with the CCI edits?
4	2435	How often will the Correct Coding Initiative (CCI) edits be updated for FIs?
5	3365	If I want to determine what codes/procedures are paired with a certain code, how can I find this out?
6	2392	Do the critical care Correct Coding Initiative (CCI) edits apply to hospitals?
7	3356	How do I obtain the CCI Edits Manual?
8	3367	What are Correct Coding Initiative (CCI) edits?
9	3369	What exactly does "column 1" mean in the column 1/column 2 correct coding edits table and in the mutually exclusive edits table?
10	3366	If I receive a denial for a procedure bundled into another service, and I cannot find this code pair in the column 1/column 2 correct coding list of edits, where else should I look?
11	3372	What is the mutually exclusive edit table?
12	3368	What does it mean when codes are considered "mutually exclusive" of each other?
13	3516	How should modifier "-25" be reported under the CCI?

59 Answers Available

instruction. Look at the Overview section first, which provides the background for the NCCI edits as well as several downloadable transmittals, the policy manual (a must-read), the section of the Medicare manual addressing NCCI edits, articles, and frequently asked questions (FAQs) relative to the NCCI. Most of these topics are discussed in this book, but it is helpful to know where the resource is accessed.

Those edits important to each claim should be accessed. Billing for a physician's service would require accessing the NCCI Edits for Physicians, billing for outpatient hospital services would require review of those edits, and so on. Medically unlikely edits (MUEs) are discussed later in this chapter.

As mentioned before, additional resources on the CMS web site include the following:
- An NCCI manual, which provides further instructions and background on NCCI edits
- FAQs about the NCCI with Medicare responses (see Figure 1-3)
- Memorandums
- Transmittals
- Articles

Learning Break Tip: The FAQs on the CMS Web site are key to better understanding Medicare's thought process for the NCCI edits. Also, the FAQs are updated on an as-needed basis (there is no regularly scheduled update), which means users should check the site at least quarterly for new information.

Questions that will help in the tracking of Web sites include:
- Which NCCI Web sites do you access?
- Have you bookmarked these on your computer?
- How often do you check for updates?
- Do you look closely to determine any pertinent changes?
- Are any of these resources duplicative?

The NCCI Policy Manual Format[5]

The NCCI policy manual contains a table of contents, introduction, and instructional chapters. The chapters correspond to the sections of the CPT codebook and the Health Care Common Procedure Coding System (HCPCS) codebook. Each section of NCCI is broken down into two procedures tables titled *Column 1/Column 2* and *Mutually Exclusive*. In each table, there are two columns of codes that represent services that should not be coded together. If an encounter has codes from both columns, this creates an edit pair. If both codes of an edit pair are billed for the same beneficiary, on the same date of service, by the same performing provider, the Column 1 code is eligible for payment, and the Column 2 code is subject to denial.

Figure 1-4 is a screen shot of the CMS Web site containing specific NCCI edits.

When a category is selected from the Downloads section, a spreadsheet provides the code edit combinations as shown in Figure 1-5.

Tables 1-1 and 1-2 provide examples of the column layout for both tables.

FIGURE 1-4 *NCCI Edits Page on the CMS Web Site*[1]

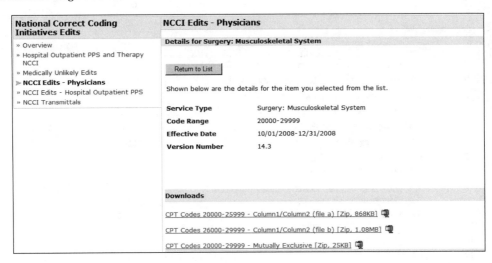

FIGURE 1-5 *NCCI Edits Excel Spreadsheet Example from the CMS Web Site*[6]

	A	B	C	D	E	F
1			Column1/Column 2 Edits			
2	Column 1	Column 2	existence prior to 1996	Effective Date	Deletion Date *=no data	0=not allowed 1=allowed 9=not applicable
3	20000	G0345		20050101	20051231	1
4	20000	G0347		20050101	20051231	1
5	20000	G0351		20050701	20051231	1
6	20000	G0353		20050701	20051231	1
7	20000	G0354		20050701	20051231	1
8	20000	J2001		20040701	*	1
9	20000	20500		19970101	*	1
10	20000	29580		19990101	*	1
11	20000	36000		20021001	*	1
12	20000	36410		20021001	*	1
13	20000	37202		20021001	*	1
14	20000	51701		20071001	*	1
15	20000	51702		20071001	*	1
16	20000	51703		20071001	*	1
17	20000	62318		20021001	*	1
18	20000	62319		20021001	*	1
19	20000	64415		20021001	*	1
20	20000	64416		20030101	*	1
21	20000	64417		20021001	*	1
22	20000	64450		20021001	*	1
23	20000	64470		20021001	*	1
24	20000	64475		20021001	*	1
25	20000	69990		20000605	*	0

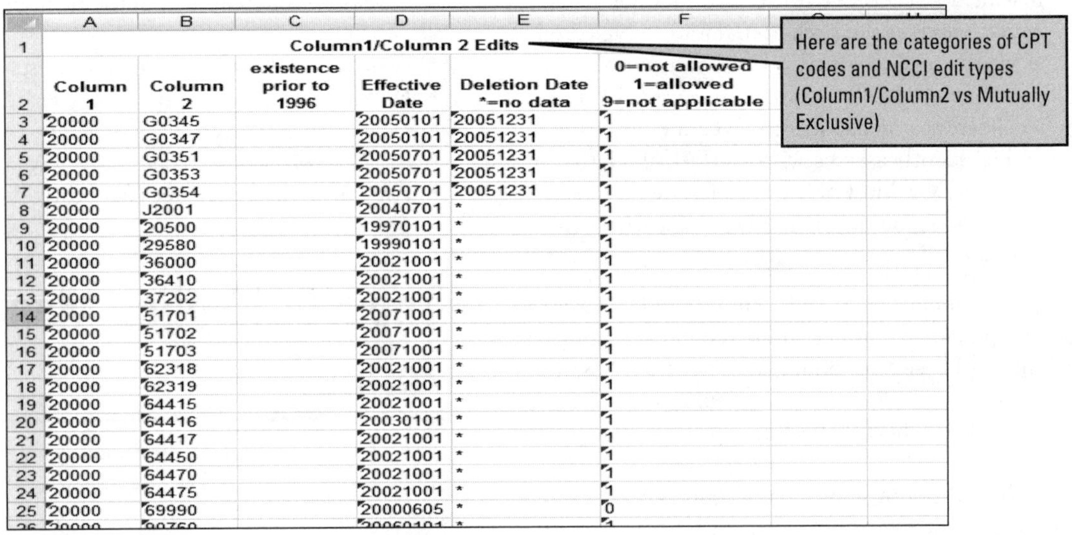

Codes from Column 2 are not payable when billed for the same encounter as the Column 1 code. Therefore, when the Column 2 code is billed, it will be denied as not separately payable unless a modifier is appended to bypass the edit.

Mutually exclusive edits represent codes that most likely should not be reported together. Basically, the mutually exclusive edits include code pairs that are highly unlikely of being performed during the same session. An example would be of a screening colonoscopy (HCPCS G0105) and a diagnostic colonoscopy (CPT 45378) being coded together for a single patient during one encounter. Because it is highly unlikely that two colonoscopies are actually performed, these codes are listed as a mutually exclusive edit.

Column 1/Column 2 edits include edits not classified as mutually exclusive. Many, but not all, of the edits within this category are for codes in Column 2 that are components of the Column 1 code. An example would be billing a hysteroscopy that includes a dilation and curettage (D&C) (CPT 58558) and adding another code for the D&C (CPT 58120). Because the hysteroscopy code includes the D&C, billing the D&C separately would generate an edit because it is a component of the comprehensive code.

Also, the NCCI format includes a correct coding modifier (CCM) indicator. This indicator (seen in the third column of Tables 1-1 and 1-2) simply represents whether a modifier will bypass the bundling edit. A CCM of 1 indicates that, when appropriate, the edit may be bypassed with

TABLE 1-1 *Column 1/Column 2 Edits*

Column 1	Column 2	Modifier 0 = not allowed 1 = allowed 9 = not applicable
20000	C8950	1
20000	C8952	1
20000	G0345	1
20000	G0347	1
20000	G0351	1
20000	G0353	1
20000	G0354	1
20000	J2001	1
20000	20500	1
20000	29580	1
20000	36000	1
20000	36410	1
20000	37202	1
20000	51701	1
20000	51702	1
20000	51703	1
20000	62318	1
20000	62319	1
20000	64415	1
20000	64416	1

TABLE 1-2 *Mutually Exclusive Edits*

Column 1	Column 2	Modifier 0 = not allowed 1 = allowed 9 = not applicable
20000	10061	1
20500	11010	1
20501	11010	1
20550	11010	1
20550	20551	1
20550	20552	1
20550	20553	1
20551	20552	1
20551	20553	1

a modifier, and both services will be allowed if no other reasons for denial (eg, medical necessity) exist. A CCM of 0 indicates that even when a modifier is appended, no payment will be made for the Column 2 service (ie, the edit cannot be bypassed with a modifier). A CCM of 9 indicates that the bundling edit is not applicable and can be ignored. If a code pair has a deletion date that is the same as the effective date, there will be a 9 indicator. This was implemented to avoid blanks in the CCM indicator field.[2]

Medically Unlikely Edits

Medically unlikely edits (MUEs) represent a different type of NCCI edit. Rather than looking at code combinations and bundling codes together, the MUEs focus on how many units are billed for a single CPT code. The MUE edits began with dates of service beginning January 1, 2007.

Usually, NCCI edits look at the entire claim because they are comparing code combinations, but for MUEs, the edits focus on a single line at a time. They are known as *line item edits* rather than *claim level edits*. Remember, all other NCCI edits are based on code combinations and require at least two codes compared to one another, rather than the units of service for a single code to be scrutinized.

Table 1-3 is from the CMS booklet *Medicare's Claims Review Programs* (including MUEs), which can be downloaded from the CMS web site.[3] This table illustrates how the appealing of edits differs between carriers and fiscal intermediaries.

If the units of service exceed that allowed by the MUEs, the entire line will be denied; all of the services will be denied. In other NCCI edits, one service (in Column 2) is denied, while the other (in Column 1) is paid. Because the entire line will be denied, obviously this is an important edit set. As with the other NCCI edits, the MUE edit may also be bypassed if an appropriate modifier is appended and the service separated on different lines of the claim.

Prior to October 1, 2008,[7] the MUEs were not fully disclosed; however, CMS has stated:

> At the start of each calendar quarter, CMS will publish most MUEs active for that quarter. Although the October 1, 2008, publication will contain most MUEs, additional ones will be published on January 1, 2009. CMS is not able to publish all active MUEs because some are primarily designed to detect and deter questionable payments rather than billing errors. Publishing those MUEs would diminish their effectiveness.[8]

The MUE-assigned units for each code are based on various criteria that will be discussed further throughout this book. The following are a few examples of the criteria CMS indicates:

- Anatomic considerations can determine the MUE edit. The example provided by CMS is for cataract surgery. Obviously, in normal anatomy, there are only two eyes; therefore, the MUE for cataract surgery would be 2.

TABLE 1-3 *Units of Service In Excess of Medically Unlikely Edits Criteria*[9(p3)]

Carriers	Fiscal Intermediaries (FIs)
Physicians/suppliers may appeal a claim line denial due to an MUE if medically reasonable and necessary units of service exceed the MUE value.	An appeal process is not available for providers that receive an RTP as a result of an MUE. If the provider performed medically reasonable and necessary units of service in excess of the MUE value, the provider may use CPT modifiers when resubmitting the claim. See the answer to Question #4 in Table 3 [MUEs Frequently Asked Questions (FAQs)].
Physicians/suppliers may request modification of an MUE value by contacting the NCCI contractor. See the answer to Question #8 in Table 3 (MUEs FAQs).	Physicians/suppliers may request modification of an MUE value by contacting the NCCI contractor. See the answer to Question #8 in Table 3 (MUEs FAQs).

- CPT code descriptors or coding instructions may limit the units of service. For example, a procedure described as the "initial 30 minutes" would have an MUE of 1 because of the use of the term *initial*.
- Edits can be established from CMS policies that limit units of service. For example, the bilateral surgery indicator on the Medicare Physician Fee Schedule Database may limit reporting of bilateral procedures.

General NCCI Guidelines and Supporting Examples

As previously mentioned, the goal of the NCCI is correct coding and payment. Medicare instructs providers that procedures should be reported with the most comprehensive code describing the services and that services included in that comprehensive service code should not be unbundled or coded additionally. The following are five general guidelines CMS shares in the NCCI policy manual:

Guideline   Do not report multiple codes when one single code includes all the components in the single code.

Example   **52601** Transurethral electrosurgical resection of prostate, including control of postoperative bleeding, complete (vasectomy, meatotomy, cystourethroscopy, urethral calibration and/or dilation, and internal urethrotomy are included)

This code clearly includes vasectomy, meatotomy, cystourethroscopy, urethral calibration and/or dilation, and internal urethrotomy. Therefore, it would be incorrect to bill any

of these services in addition to the TURP (CPT 52601):

52000 Cystourethroscopy (separate procedure)

52275 Cystourethroscopy, with internal urethrotomy; male

53020 Meatotomy, cutting of meatus (separate procedure); except infant

55250 Vasectomy, unilateral or bilateral (separate procedure), including postoperative semen examination(s)

Note   The CPT codes provided are examples only. There are additional codes that represent similar services. Services should always be coded based on the individual patient scenario and documentation.

Guideline   Do not fragment one procedure into component parts.

Example   Physician performs a colonoscopy, and during the endoscopic procedure, the physician also removes a polyp via snare technique. The correct, comprehensive code is:

45385 Colonoscopy, flexible, proximal to splenic flexure; with removal of tumor(s), polyp(s), or other lesion(s) by snare technique

This code includes the entire procedure performed: colonoscopy and snare polypectomy. It would be incorrect coding to bill this procedure as:

45378 Colonoscopy, flexible, proximal to splenic flexure; diagnostic, with or without collection of specimen(s) by brushing or washing, with or without colon decompression (separate procedure)

In addition to one of the following CPT codes:

45385 Colonoscopy, flexible, proximal to splenic flexure; with removal of tumor(s), polyp(s), or other lesion(s) by snare technique

or

44110 Excision of one or more lesions of small or large intestine not requiring anastomosis, exteriorization, or fistulization; single enterotomy

Note The CPT codes provided are examples only. There are additional codes that represent similar services. Services should always be coded based on the individual patient scenario and documentation.

Guideline Do not code a bilateral procedure as two unilateral procedures if a bilateral code exists.

Example Physician performs a bilateral TMJ x-ray. The correct code is:

70330 Radiologic examination, temporomandibular joint, open and closed mouth; bilateral

This code includes both temporomandibular joints. It would be incorrect coding to bill this procedure with CPT code 70328 ×2 (or with modifier 50):

70328 Radiologic examination, temporomandibular joint, open and closed mouth; unilateral

Note The CPT codes provided are examples only. There are additional codes that represent similar services. Services should always be coded based on the individual patient scenario and documentation.

Guideline Do not code separately for services that are an inherent part of another procedure even if the CPT code does not explicitly state the integral nature of the service.

Example If a physician performs a level 2 consultation for the patient's primary care provider (PCP) and sends a letter back sharing their opinion with the PCP, the following CPT code correctly reflects this service:

99242 **Office consultation** for a new or established patient, which requires these three key components:
- **An expanded, problem focused history;**
- **An expanded, problem focused examination; and**
- **Straightforward medical decision making.**

Counseling and/or coordination of care with other providers or agencies are provided consistent with the nature of the problem(s) and the patient's and/or family's needs.

Usually, the presenting problem(s) are of low severity. Physicians typically spend 30 minutes face-to-face with the patient and/or family.

This code includes performing the consultation and providing the advice back to the requesting physician. Because the advice back to the requesting provider is an inherent part of the consultation service, it would be incorrect coding to bill the following CPT code in addition to the consultation:

99080 Special reports such as insurance forms, more than the information conveyed in the usual medical communications or standard reporting form

Note The CPT codes provided are examples only. There are additional codes that represent similar services. Services should always be coded based on the individual patient scenario and documentation.

Guideline Do not downcode in order to bill multiple services.

Example If an obstetrician is providing the global maternity care for a patient, the correct code for this entire service is:

59400 Routine obstetric care including antepartum care, vaginal delivery (with or without episiotomy, and/or forceps) and postpartum care

This code includes the antepartum, delivery, and postpartum care if there are no complications and the delivery is vaginal. It would be incorrect coding for this care to code lesser services in order to bill multiple codes as follows:

59409 Vaginal delivery only (with or without episiotomy and/or forceps);

59425 Antepartum care only; 4–6 visits

59430 Postpartum care only (separate procedure)

Note The CPT codes provided are examples only. There are additional codes that represent similar services. Services should always be coded based on the individual patient scenario and documentation.

Modifiers

Modifiers are used for many reasons in coding, but as they relate to NCCI edits, modifiers are important because they serve to bypass the NCCI edits. This means that certain modifiers will allow both the Column 1 and Column 2 codes to be paid when those services are performed during a single encounter. Because the modifiers can increase reimbursement on a claim, it is important to use them correctly. Medicare's *Claims Processing Manual*[9] provides some limited instructions for using modifiers with the NCCI edits.

The following modifiers are used to bypass NCCI edits:

E1   Upper left, eyelid

E2   Lower left, eyelid

E3   Upper right, eyelid

E4   Lower right, eyelid

F1   Left hand, second digit

F2   Left hand, third digit

F3   Left hand, fourth digit

F4   Left hand, fifth digit

F5   Right hand, thumb

F6   Right hand, second digit

F7   Right hand, third digit

F8   Right hand, fourth digit

F9   Right hand, fifth digit

FA   Left hand, thumb

LC   Left circumflex coronary artery

LD   Left anterior descending coronary artery

RC   Right coronary artery

LT   Left side (used to identify procedures performed on the left side of the body)

RT   Right side (used to identify procedures performed on the right side of the body)

T1   Left foot, second digit

T2   Left foot, third digit

T3   Left foot, fourth digit

T4   Left foot, fifth digit

T5   Right foot, great toe

T6   Right foot, second digit

T7   Right foot, third digit

T8   Right foot, fourth digit

T9   Right foot, fifth digit

TA   Left foot, great toe

25   Significant, Separately Identifiable Evaluation and Management Service by the Same Physician on the Same Day of the Procedure or Other Service

58   Staged or Related Procedure or Service by the Same Physician During the Postoperative Period

59   Distinct Procedural Service

78   Unplanned Return to the Operating/Procedure Room by the Same Physician Following Initial Procedure for a Related Procedure During the Postoperative Period

79   Unrelated Procedure or Service by the Same Physician During the Postoperative Period

91   Repeat Clinical Diagnostic Laboratory Test

It is important to remember that not all code combinations allow for modifiers to bypass the edits. Users of the NCCI edits should review the CCM indicators to know which code combinations can be bypassed and which cannot.

Many of the anatomical modifiers will bypass the bundling edits and allow payment for both the Column 1 and Column 2 codes. This makes sense because anatomical modifiers can indicate different body sites that would support both services being paid.

Example

A patient had multiple injuries due to a fall. Included in the injuries were a fracture of the right arm and a complex fracture of the left arm. The right arm was repaired by closed reduction, but the left arm was immobilized by placement of a cast, and the patient was referred to a specialist for care.

Both services (fracture repair of the right arm and casting of the left arm) should be coded, but normally the casting is part of the fracture repair and would be denied when billed as being performed during the same encounter. By using modifiers RT (right side) and LT (left side), both services should be allowed because these modifiers clearly indicate different body sites.

More Important Notes and Guidelines to Consider

There are some additional instructions from the policy manual for NCCI edits that are noteworthy:

- Services being denied based on NCCI bundling edits may NOT be billed to Medicare beneficiaries. The thought here is that the denial is made based on incorrect coding rather than medical necessity issues or benefit exclusion.
- Do not obtain an Advance Beneficiary Notice, and do not bill the patient for the denied (bundled) service.

Page 4 in this chapter presented questions to consider. When such questions are answered, the following factors should be considered:

- Do the codes bundle?
- If they bundle, was the claim coded correctly?
- If the claim was coded correctly, what is the rationale behind the edits?
- Based on the rationale and the record's documentation, should the edit be bypassed?

If the edit should be bypassed, a modifier is appended, and the claim is submitted. If the edit should not be bypassed, the coding is changed, and the claim is submitted. Payment is tracked, and education is provided as appropriate.

So, what these questions to consider demonstrate is that the answers are complex, but with the help of this book, a practice should find that answers to such questions come more easily.

SUMMARY

- Gather current nationally recognized resources.

- Do not memorize edits; learn the guidelines.

- Follow the logic of the NCCI edits when deciding how to code encounters.

- Gather data on the facility as to what is coded and how claims are processed.

Definitions and Acronyms

Advance Beneficiary Notice (ABN): An ABN is a form providers have patients sign if a service is expected to be denied for medical necessity issues related to the specific encounter's circumstances.

Centers for Medicare and Medicaid Services (CMS): This is a branch of the Department of Health and Human Services (HHS) responsible for overseeing the Medicare and Medicaid federal health care programs.

correct coding modifier indicator (CCM indicator): A CCM indicator is found in the National Correct Coding Initiative (NCCI) edit tables and indicates whether the edit can be bypassed with a modifier.

facility: For the purpose of this book, the term *facility* will represent a practice, group, hospital, or office.

medically unlikely edits (MUE): MUEs are edits based on the number of services billed per line item. If, per CMS, the units of service for a particular Current Procedural Terminology (CPT®)[2] code are limited to a certain number, there will be an MUE edit for that CPT code.

National Correct Coding Initiative (NCCI): NCCI represents the CMS policy on CPT code bundling.

units of service: Units of service represent how many services are billed per line item.

REFERENCES

1. Centers for Medicare and Medicaid Services. National Correct Coding Initiative Edits. www.cms.hhs.gov/NationalCorrectCodInitEd/NCCIEP/list.asp. Accessed June 10, 2009.

2. American Medical Association. *Current Procedural Terminology CPT® 2009 Professional Edition*. Chicago, IL: American Medical Association; 2008. All CPT codes and descriptors in this chapter are taken from this publication.

3. Centers for Medicare and Medicaid Services. www.cms.hhs.gov/home/medicare.asp. Accessed June 10, 2009.

4. Centers for Medicare and Medicaid Services. Frequently Asked Questions. https://questions.cms.hhs.gov/cgi-bin/cmshhs.cfg/php/enduser/std_alp.php?p_sid=CoZ3G1Aj. Accessed June 10, 2009.

5. Centers for Medicare and Medicaid Services. NCCI Policy Manual for Medicare Services. www.cms.hhs.gov/NationalCorrectCodInitEd/01_overview.asp#TopOfPage. Accessed June 10, 2009.

6. Centers for Medicare and Medicaid Services. National Correct Coding Initiative Edits for CPT codes 20000–23999. www.cms.hhs.gov/apps/ama/license.asp?file=/NationalCorrectCodInitEd/downloads/ccigrp4a.zip. Accessed June 10, 2009.

7. Centers for Medicare and Medicaid Services. MUE Provider/Supplier Letter. www.cms.hhs.gov/NationalCorrectCodInitEd/Downloads/MUE_Prov_Sup_PUB_LTR_9_2008.pdf. Accessed June 10, 2009.

8. Centers for Medicare and Medicaid Services. *Medicare Claims Processing Manual*, Chapter 23: Fee Schedule Administration and Coding Requirements. www.cms.hhs.gov/manuals/downloads/clm104c23.pdf. Accessed June 10, 2009.

9. Centers for Medicare and Medicaid Services. *Medicare Claim Review Programs: MR, NCCI Edits, MUEs, CERT, and RAC*. www.cms.hhs.gov/MLNProducts/downloads/MCRP_Booklet.pdf. Accessed June 10, 2009.

Chapter 2

General Policies of the National Correct Coding Initiative

Introduction to the General Policies of the NCCI

This section will include those general policies covered within the National Correct Coding Initiative (NCCI) guidelines.

NCCI General Policy Instructions

Healthcare Common Procedure Coding System (HCPCS) and Current Procedural Terminology (CPT®) codes are used on health care bills to represent medical care, surgeries, diagnostic services, supplies, and pharmaceuticals provided to patients. Given that health care services vary in level of complexity and methodology used, there can be several different codes that embody similar or related procedures. When there are multiple codes representing similar procedures, care must be exercised to help ensure the code captured reflects precisely the service provided. The code should embody the work for the service and neither over-represents nor under-represents the service.

Example

Hysterectomy CPT codes: the following lists all the potential codes that represent hysterectomy procedures. When the code descriptions are reviewed, one can see that different codes represent the following:
- Different surgical approaches (eg, open vs laparoscopic, abdominal vs vaginal)
- Associated procedures (eg, removal of ovaries)
- Extensiveness of the surgery (eg, radical vs total)

Choosing the code for an approach different than the actual approach used would misrepresent the procedure and potentially support an incorrect level of reimbursement.

58150[1]	Total abdominal hysterectomy (corpus and cervix), with or without removal of tube(s), with or without removal of ovary(s);
58152	with colpo-urethrocystopexy (eg, Marshall-Marchetti-Krantz, Burch)
58180	Supracervical abdominal hysterectomy (subtotal hysterectomy), with or without removal of tube(s), with or without removal of ovary(s)
58200	Total abdominal hysterectomy, including partial vaginectomy, with para-aortic and pelvic lymph node sampling, with or without removal of tube(s), with or without removal of ovary(s)
58210	Radical abdominal hysterectomy, with bilateral total pelvic lymphadenectomy and para-aortic lymph node sampling (biopsy), with or without removal of tube(s), with or without removal of ovary(s)
58240	Pelvic exenteration for gynecologic malignancy, with total abdominal hysterectomy or cervicectomy, with or without removal of tube(s), with or without removal of ovary(s), with removal of bladder and ureteral transplantations, and/or abdominoperineal resection of rectum and colon and colostomy, or any combination thereof
58260	Vaginal hysterectomy, for uterus 250 g or less;
58262	with removal of tube(s), and/or ovary(s)
58263	with removal of tube(s) and/or ovary(s), with repair of enterocele
58267	with colpo-urethrocystopexy (Marshall-Marchetti-Krantz type, Pereyra type), with or without endoscopic control
58270	with repair of enterocele
58275	Vaginal hysterectomy, with total or partial vaginectomy;
58280	with repair of enterocele
58285	Vaginal hysterectomy, radical (Schauta type operation)
58290	Vaginal hysterectomy, for uterus greater than 250 g;

58291	with removal of tube(s) and/or ovary(s)
58292	with removal of tube(s) and/or ovary(s), with repair of enterocele
58293	with colpo-urethrocystopexy (Marshall-Marchetti-Krantz type, Pereyra type), with or without endoscopic control
58294	with repair of enterocele
58541	Laparoscopy, surgical, supracervical hysterectomy, for uterus 250 g or less;
58542	with removal of tube(s) and/or ovary(s)
58543	Laparoscopy, surgical, supracervical hysterectomy, for uterus greater than 250 g;
58544	with removal of tube(s) and/or ovary(s)
58548	Laparoscopy, surgical, with radical hysterectomy, with bilateral total pelvic lymphadenectomy and para-aortic lymph node sampling (biopsy), with removal of tube(s) and ovary(s), if performed
58550	Laparoscopy, surgical, with vaginal hysterectomy, for uterus 250 g or less;
58552	with removal of tube(s) and/or ovary(s)
58553	Laparoscopy, surgical, with vaginal hysterectomy, for uterus greater than 250 g;
58554	with removal of tube(s) and/or ovary(s)

Excerpt From the General Coding Policies Section of NCCI[2(p2)]

CPT and HCPCS Level II code descriptors usually do not define all services included in a procedure. There are often services inherent in a procedure or group of procedures. For example, anesthesia services include certain preparation and monitoring services.

Interpretation

Even though the CPT codes should reflect the service provided, every element of the service cannot be included in the CPT code description. Therefore, this NCCI concept is to remind us that inherent and integral components to the service represented by a specific CPT code should not be separately coded.

Example

58150	Total abdominal hysterectomy (corpus and cervix), with or without removal of tube(s), with or without removal of ovary(s);

This CPT code represents using an open approach to perform the hysterectomy, meaning that the method the surgeon uses to reach the uterus is through an incision into the abdomen. Because the code represents an "open" hysterectomy, the incision into the abdomen is an inherent part of the work involved in this procedure and would not be coded separately. If the code were for a laparoscopic hysterectomy, the insertion of the laparoscope would be included and not separately billed.

The surgeon closes the incision at the conclusion of the abdominal hysterectomy. Closing an incision created by a surgical approach is a necessary part of most procedures and would not be coded separately even though the CPT code description does not include the type of closure. Because the approach and closure are integral to the performance of an abdominal hysterectomy, it is not necessary for the CPT code descriptor to include those elements specifically.

Excerpt From the General Coding Policies Section of NCCI[2(p2-3)]

CMS developed the NCCI to prevent inappropriate payment of services that should not be reported together. There are two NCCI edit tables: "Column One/Column Two Coding Edit Table" and "Mutually Exclusive Edit Table." Each edit table contains edits, which are pairs of HCPCS/CPT codes that in general should not be reported together. Each edit has a column one and a column two HCPCS/CPT code. If a provider reports the two codes of an edit pair, the column two code is denied, and the column one code is eligible for payment. However, if it is clinically appropriate to utilize an NCCI-associated modifier, both the column one and column two codes are eligible for payment.

Interpretation

There are three primary instructions:
1. The overall goal of the NCCI edits is to help prevent overpayments when multiple codes are billed. By using the NCCI edits to analyze claims where multiple codes are billed, there is no need to perform a manual review of each claim. NCCI edits are automated prepayment edits—the computer programs can review the codes, so an individual is not required to review each claim.
2. The NCCI edits are structured into two columns (Columns 1 and 2). Coders can easily access the edits and understand which codes are edit pairs (edit against each other). If a Column 1 code is billed with a Column 2 code, the Column 1 code is the payable service, and the Column 2 code would be denied unless an NCCI modifier is appended. Note: Edits should be bypassed only when the documentation supports the appropriate billing of both services in the specific clinical

circumstance. This book clarifies those circumstances in which the edits may be bypassed appropriately.

3. An NCCI modifier may be used to bypass the edit when appropriate. CMS clearly instructs that the clinical scenario and medical record documentation must support appending a modifier to bypass the edit. This book reviews all the guidelines to help clarify when a modifier would be appropriate.

 CMS Tip: *The Office of Inspector General (OIG) performed a review of modifier 59, which is used to bypass bundling edits. This review was to determine whether the modifier was used correctly. Although performed in 2006, the report still provides valuable insight into what the OIG considered to be problematic.* Use of Modifier 59 to Bypass Medicare's National Correct Coding Initiative Edits *can be found on the OIG Web site.*[3] *Figure 2-1 shows the report cover.*

Within that review, the OIG found that 40% of the cases in the review did not meet the program guidelines for using modifier 59. The incorrectly coded cases included the following:

- Services that were not distinct from each other and should not have been coded separately
- Coded services that were not well documented and should not have been coded.

Excerpt From the General Coding Policies Section of NCCI[2(p3)]

In this Manual many policies are described utilizing the term "physician." Unless indicated differently the usage of this term does not restrict the policies to physicians only but applies to all practitioners, hospitals, providers, or suppliers eligible to bill the relevant HCPCS/CPT codes... In some sections of this Manual, the term "physician" would not include some of these entities because specific rules do not apply to them. For example, Anesthesia Rules and Global Surgery Rules do not apply to hospitals.

Interpretation

The NCCI guidelines and edits apply to all providers billing HCPCS/CPT codes. Physician practices, outpatient hospitals, and free-standing surgical centers all bill

FIGURE 2-1 *Office of Inspector General Report of Modifier 59, Cover Page*[3]

Department of Health and Human Services
OFFICE OF INSPECTOR GENERAL

USE OF MODIFIER 59 TO BYPASS MEDICARE'S NATIONAL CORRECT CODING INITIATIVE EDITS

Daniel R. Levinson
Inspector General

November 2005
OEI-03-02-00771

Medicare using HCPCS/CPT codes and are subject to the NCCI edits. On the other hand, hospital inpatient facility charges are not subject to NCCI edits because HCPCS/CPT codes are not billed for these services.

 CMS Tip: *CMS guidelines remind us that HCPCS/CPT codes denied for NCCI edits may not be billed to Medicare beneficiaries. Because these denials are designated as incorrectly coded, providers cannot issue an Advance Beneficiary Notice form to pursue payment from a Medicare beneficiary. Neither can the provider seek payment from the beneficiary with or without a Notice of Exclusions From Medicare Benefits form.*

NCCI Edit Principles, Issues, and Policies

This section reviews some of the specific policies applicable throughout NCCI as well as covering the primary principles driving NCCI edits.

Standards of Medical/Surgical Practice

CMS provides information on different categories of principles within the General Policies section of the NCCI guidelines. The first category is the standard of medical/surgical practice.

Excerpt From the General Coding Policies Section of NCCI[2(p4)]

Coding Based on Standards of Medical/Surgical Practice

Most HCPCS/CPT code defined procedures include services that are integral to them. Some of these integral services have specific CPT codes for reporting the service when not performed as an integral part of another procedure. (For example, CPT code 36000 [introduction of needle or intracatheter into a vein] is integral to all nuclear medicine procedures requiring injection of a radiopharmaceutical into a vein. CPT code 36000 is not separately reportable with these types of nuclear medicine procedures. However, CPT code 36000 may be reported alone if the only service provided is the introduction of a needle into a vein.) Other integral services do not have specific CPT codes. (For example, wound irrigation is integral to the treatment of all wounds and does not have a HCPCS/CPT code.) Services integral to HCPCS/CPT code defined procedures are included in those procedures based on the standards of medical/surgical practice. It is inappropriate to separately report services that are integral to another procedure with that procedure.

Interpretation

NCCI instructs that all services *clinically* integral to the performance of a service (CPT code) should not be separately billed, regardless of whether a CPT code exists for the integral service. The hysterectomy CPT code example referenced earlier can be used to clarify this policy. Remember, open abdominal hysterectomies require a laparotomy (incision into the abdominal cavity) in order to access the uterus for removal. Therefore, the laparotomy is *integral* to the open abdominal hysterectomy and should not be billed separately even though there is a CPT code (49000) for the laparotomy.

Excerpt From the General Coding Policies Section of NCCI[2(p4)]

Coding Based on Standards of Medical/Surgical Practice, continued

Services that are integral to another service are component parts of the more comprehensive service. When integral component services have their own HCPCS/CPT codes, NCCI edits place the comprehensive service in column one and the component service in column two.

Interpretation

Services that are clinically integral are considered the lesser or component part of the primary service. The integral services are therefore listed as Column 2 codes, which are thought to be included in the Column 1 service and would be the nonbillable, denied services. Again, using the hysterectomy example, it is evident that the laparotomy is the integral component part and would be the nonbillable service. The laparotomy code (CPT code 49000) would be listed as a Column 2 code, with the hysterectomy as the Column 1 (payable) code.

 CMS Tip: *The above guideline is true for Column 1/Column 2 code edits; however, mutually exclusive codes are usually not considered comprehensive-component services—rather, mutually exclusive services are those that would not be performed together.*

Excerpt From the General Coding Policies Section of NCCI[2(p4-5)]

Coding Based on Standards of Medical/Surgical Practice, continued

Some services are integral to large numbers of procedures. Other services are integral to a more limited number of procedures. Examples of services integral to a large number of procedures include:
- Cleansing, shaving and prepping of skin
- Draping and positioning of patient
- Insertion of intravenous access for medication administration
- Insertion of urinary catheter
- Sedative administration by the physician performing a procedure

(continued)

(continued)

- Local, topical or regional anesthesia administered by the physician performing the procedure
- Surgical approach including identification of anatomical landmarks, incision, evaluation of the surgical field, debridement of traumatized tissue, lysis of adhesions, and isolation of structures limiting access to the surgical field such as bone, blood vessels, nerve, and muscles including stimulation for identification or monitoring
- Surgical cultures
- Wound irrigation
- Insertion and removal of drains, suction devices, and pumps into same site
- Surgical closure and dressings
- Application, management, and removal of postoperative dressings and analgesic devices (peri-incisional)
- TENS unit
- Institution of patient controlled anesthesia
- Preoperative, intraoperative and postoperative documentation, including photographs, drawings, dictation, or transcription as necessary to document the services provided
- Surgical supplies, except for specific situations where CMS policy permits separate payment

Interpretation

CMS provides a reasonably comprehensive list of services that are not to be coded separately from the procedure with which they are performed. Some services on the list are obviously integral (eg, preparation of the patient for a procedure), whereas others are not as apparent (eg, institution of patient controlled anesthesia). This book reviews all the available guidelines to help clarify the services considered to be components. Note that these are merely examples, and this is not an all-inclusive list. Some medical knowledge of the procedures and research should help clarify elements that are integral to procedures but not outlined by the NCCI policies.

 Teamwork Tip: *Physicians and coders should work together to identify those services considered integral to procedures. Physicians should educate the coding staff as to clinically integral services, and coders should query physicians when services seem to be integral but are not on the list CMS identifies.*

Excerpt From the General Coding Policies Section of NCCI[2(p5)]

Coding Based on Standards of Medical/Surgical Practice, continued

There are several general principles that can be applied to the edits as follows:
1. The component service is an accepted standard of care when performing the comprehensive service.
2. The component service is usually necessary to successfully complete the comprehensive service.
3. The component service is not a separately distinguishable procedure when performed with the comprehensive service.

Interpretation

CMS provides the basic principle here as to what types of services are bundled into others.

Standard of care: The standard of care is the recognized usual treatment protocol or process providers follow for specific clinical circumstances. When the standard of care for the primary (or Column 1) procedure indicates that the component (Column 2) service is also usually performed, the component should not be separately coded.

Necessary component: A necessary component reflects when a Column 2 service is a necessary part of a Column 1 service and, therefore, should not be independently coded. If the physician needed to perform the component in order to successfully accomplish the comprehensive service, the component should not be separated from the comprehensive service for coding.

Not separately distinguishable: Services that are not separately distinguishable are those in which the component service is essentially a critical part of the comprehensive procedure, and the component should not be separately coded.

Although these all seem similar in concept, there are subtle differences. Table 2-1 illustrates the overlap.

TABLE 2-1 *Example of the Correct Coding Modifier Indicator*

	Column 1/ Column 2 Edits	
Column 1	Column 2	Modifier 0 = not allowed 1 = allowed 9 = not applicable
62319	51701	1
62319	51702	1
62319	61795	9
62319	62270	1
62319	62272	1
62319	62284	1
62319	62311	1
62319	69990	0
62319	72275	1
62319	76000	1
62319	76001	1
62319	76003	1
62319	77002	1
62319	90760	1
62319	90765	1
62319	90772	1
62319	90774	1

Examples

Standard of care: The following is a common standard of care for a laparoscopic cholecystectomy (CPT code 47562). Boldface type is for emphasis.

Laparoscopic Cholecystectomy

1. Using graspers, the liver is elevated.
2. If the gallbladder is not visible, **adhesions are dissected**.
3. If the gallbladder is inflamed, it is decompressed before grasping it is attempted. Decompressing is performed via a needle stab to suction the gallbladder.
4. Dissection is begun adjacent to the gallbladder. **Any adhesions are sharply taken down to the base of the gallbladder.**
5. The cystic duct is identified where it enters the gallbladder.
6. If a cholangiogram is going to be performed, the cystic duct must be dissected free for at least 1 cm to allow cholangiography.

(continued)

(continued)

7. Two clips are placed side-by-side close to the gallbladder, and two similar clips are placed on the cystic duct.
8. The gallbladder is retracted to expose the cystic artery for dissection.
9. The cystic artery is divided with clips, leaving a minimum of two clips on the stump of the artery.
10. The gallbladder is dissected away from its bed.
11. The surgical site is irrigated with saline.
12. After hemostasis is achieved, the gallbladder is freed from the liver.
13. A grasper is used through one of the trocars to grasp the gallbladder near the cystic duct.
14. The gallbladder is removed. If the gallbladder contains bile or stones, they are aspirated from the gallbladder before it is withdrawn through the trocar.
15. After the gallbladder is removed, the site is inspected for bleeding.
16. The trocars are removed, and the wounds are closed in a normal fashion.

Notice that lysis of adhesions is a standard of care and should not be separately coded unless circumstances (extensive lysis of adhesions) discussed in later chapters of this book are met. The lysis is also not separately distinguishable from the cholecystectomy because it was integral to the approach, or access to the operative site.

Necessary component: In order to successfully accomplish an open heart surgery, it would be necessary to open the chest of the recipient patient; therefore, the thoracotomy is a necessary component to the open heart surgery.

Not separately distinguishable: The CPT codebook instructs that when a lesion is excised, the simple suturing of the wound created by that excision is included in the excision. Although wound repairs are services that may be coded, they are not separately distinguishable when they are the simple closure or dressing of a wound created by the lesion excision. Note: If the closure exceeds simple (non-layered) closure, it may be separately coded. For example, if a lesion was excised, and the closure required a complex repair, the complex repair could be coded in addition to the lesion excision.

Excerpt From the General Coding Policies Section of NCCI[2(p6)]

Coding Based on Standards of Medical/Surgical Practice, continued

Specific examples of services that are not separately reportable because they are components of more comprehensive services follow:

Medical: (refer to NCCI manual for complete examples list)

1. Because interpretation of cardiac rhythm is an integral component of the interpretation of an electrocardiogram, a rhythm strip is not separately reportable.

Surgical:

1. Because a myringotomy requires access to the tympanic membrane through the external auditory canal, removal of impacted cerumen from the external auditory canal is not separately reportable.
2. A "scout" bronchoscopy to assess the surgical field, anatomic landmarks, extent of disease, etc. is not separately reportable with an open pulmonary procedure such as a pulmonary lobectomy. By contrast, an initial diagnostic bronchoscopy is separately reportable. If the diagnostic bronchoscopy is performed at the same patient encounter as the open pulmonary procedure and does not duplicate an earlier diagnostic bronchoscopy by the same or another physician, the diagnostic bronchoscopy may be reported with modifier 58 to indicate a staged procedure. A cursory examination of the upper airway during a bronchoscopy with the bronchoscope should not be reported separately as a laryngoscopy. However, separate endoscopies of anatomically distinct areas with different endoscopes may be reported separately (e.g., thoracoscopy and mediastinoscopy).

Interpretation

NCCI guidelines provide a limited list of examples of the comprehensive and component code pairs. Although the guidelines are not a comprehensive list, there are some practical scenarios.

Example

In the medical example of the rhythm strip and electrocardiogram (EKG), the guideline notes that the rhythm strip data are already a part of the EKG data and, therefore, no separate code for the rhythm strip should be used. The rhythm strip is not separately distinguishable. If, however,

a rhythm strip was performed at a different time on the same day as the EKG and was medically necessary, it could be potentially coded, if it was medically necessary and the procedure was clearly documented by appending a modifier to the rhythm strip service.

Special Note

The medical necessity here could be supported if an EKG was first performed and then the physician performed treatment (eg, pharmaceuticals) to manage the patient's condition, then later that same day, a portion of the test (the strip) was repeated to determine if the patient's condition changed.

Example

In the myringotomy example, the guidelines point out that, in order to perform the myringotomy, the provider must reach the tympanic membrane. For a patient who has impacted cerumen, the removal of the cerumen becomes a part of the myringotomy approach and would not be separately reported when performed on the same ear during the same operative session. The cerumen removal is a necessary component of the myringotomy. This is akin to the lysis of adhesions example in that access through abnormal tissue is inherent in the approach to the primary procedure and not separately coded.

Example

For the bronchoscopy example, NCCI includes identification of landmarks as a part of the surgical approach (as noted in the standards of medical/surgical practice). A "scout" scope is for landmark identification (looking at the lay of the land) and not for diagnosing or treating. It is a complementary component of the primary procedure. CMS distinguishes a scout scope from a diagnostic scope, which is an important principle in NCCI. If a truly diagnostic scope is necessary before an open therapeutic procedure, the diagnostic scope may be separately coded, as long as the scope is truly diagnostic (the decision for the therapeutic open procedure is made based on the findings of the scope procedure). The physician's documentation must be very clear that the service is diagnostic. The scope procedure is not separately coded if the following apply:

- The physician knows prior to the scope procedure what therapeutic open procedure is going to be performed.
- The physician has already performed a diagnostic scope.
- The physician goes on to perform a therapeutic scope procedure.

NCCI edits state that when the diagnostic scope is performed prior to an open procedure, both procedures may be coded, and modifier 58 (staged procedure) should be appended to the diagnostic scope code. CPT guidelines for modifier 58 indicate that this modifier should be appended to the second (or later) procedure performed, rather than to the first procedure, which would be the open procedure. Because modifier 58 is appended to the second or staged/related procedure, this modifier should be appended to the later performed procedure. Accurate coding indicates appending modifier 58 to the second procedure. However, if by appending modifier 58 to the second procedure prevents the claim from being correctly reimbursed, modifier 58 may be appended to the diagnostic scope code. The NCCI edits serve as a reimbursement policy, and the instructions may differ from the CPT codebook instructions.

Medical/Surgical Package

The second category of NCCI edit principles is the medical/surgical package. Although there is overlap with the first section (standard of medical/surgical practice), this category is driven by Medicare reimbursement policies rather than standards of clinical practice.

Excerpt From the General Coding Policies Section of NCCI[2(p7)]

Most medical and surgical procedures include preprocedure, intraprocedure, and postprocedure work. When multiple procedures are performed at the same patient encounter, there is often overlap of the preprocedure and postprocedure work. Payment methodologies for surgical procedures account for the overlap of the preprocedure and postprocedure work.

Interpretation

Preprocedure and postprocedure services (patient preparation, anesthesia, recovery, etc) overlap when multiple procedures are performed during the same patient encounter. Two separate recovery sessions or anesthesia inductions are unnecessary if multiple surgeries are performed during the operative session. Medicare often reduces payment for secondary procedures performed during the same encounter as other procedures to allow for any consolidation of services.

Chapter 12, Physicians/Nonphysician Practitioners (Section 40.6) of the *Medicare Claims Processing Manual*[4] discusses the multiple surgery payment guidelines as follows.

CMS Multiple Surgery Payment Guidelines

(Rev. 1, 10-01-03)
B3-4826, B3-15038, B3-15056

A. General

Multiple surgeries are separate procedures performed by a single physician or physicians in the same group practice on the same patient at the same operative session or on the same day for which separate payment may be allowed. Co-surgeons, surgical teams, or assistants-at-surgery may participate in performing multiple surgeries on the same patient on the same day.

Multiple surgeries are distinguished from procedures that are components of or incidental to a primary procedure. These intra-operative services, incidental surgeries, or components of more major surgeries are not separately billable. See Chapter 23 for a description of mandatory edits to prevent separate payment for those procedures. Major surgical procedures are determined based on the MFSDB approved amount and not on the submitted amount from the providers. The major surgery, as based on the MFSDB, may or may not be the one with the larger submitted amount.

Also, see subsection D below for a description of the standard payment policy on multiple surgeries. However, these standard payment rules are not appropriate for certain procedures. Field 21 of the MFSDB indicates whether the standard payment policy rules apply to a multiple surgery, or whether special payment rules apply. Site of service payment adjustments (codes with an indicator of "1" in Field 27 of the MFSDB) should be applied before multiple surgery payment adjustments.

B. Billing Instructions

The following procedures apply when billing for multiple surgeries by the same physician on the same day.

Report the more major surgical procedure without the multiple procedures modifier "-51."

Report additional surgical procedures performed by the surgeon on the same day with modifier "-51."

There may be instances in which two or more physicians each perform distinctly different, unrelated surgeries on the same patient on the same day (e.g., in some multiple trauma cases). When this occurs, the payment adjustment rules for multiple surgeries may not be appropriate. In such cases, the physician does not use modifier "-51" unless one of the surgeons individually performs multiple surgeries. For information on carrier claims processing system requirements, please refer to Chapter 12, Physicians/Nonphysician Practitioners of the *Medicare Claims Processing Manual*.

Excerpt From the General Coding Policies Section of NCCI[2(p9)]

If the biopsy is performed on the same lesion on which the more extensive procedure is performed, it is separately reportable only if the biopsy is utilized for immediate pathologic diagnosis prior to the more extensive procedure, and the decision to proceed with the more extensive procedure is based on the result of the pathologic examination. Modifier -58 may be reported to indicate that the biopsy and the more extensive procedure were planned or staged procedures.

Interpretation

This guideline is very important in NCCI. Essentially, the NCCI policy states that if a biopsy is truly diagnostic and helps determine the need for a second procedure, both services should be coded. In this case, the second procedure should have a modifier 58 (staged procedure) appended to bypass the bundling edit. However, if a biopsy incidentally results from an excision and does not represent a separate and distinct diagnostic procedure, do not code the biopsy in addition to the excision.

Example

A patient presents with a lesion on his arm. The physician excises the lesion and sends the specimen to pathology.

If the physician initially excises the lesion and sends the excised lesion to pathology to determine the morphology, the biopsy is an *incidental* result of the excision and would not be separately coded. The decision to excise was not based on the result of the biopsy.

Example

A patient presents with a suspicious lesion on his arm. The physician takes a small portion of the lesion and sends that specimen for frozen section to determine the extent of disease and best treatment. The physician awaits the results of the frozen section. When the results of the frozen section are received, the physician makes the decision to proceed with a simple excision of the entire lesion and immediately excises the lesion.

In this case, the biopsy was truly diagnostic, and both the biopsy and excision may be coded because the decision for the excision was based on the biopsy results. Modifier 58 should be appended to the lesion excision.

Excerpt From the General Coding Policies Section of NCCI[2(p9-10)]

If a single lesion is biopsied multiple times, only one biopsy code may be reported with a single unit of service. If multiple lesions are non-endoscopically biopsied, a biopsy code may be reported for each lesion appending a modifier indicating that each biopsy was performed on a separate lesion. For endoscopic biopsies, multiple biopsies of a single or multiple lesions are reported with one unit of service of the biopsy code.

Interpretation

Code only one biopsy per lesion. Valid diagnostic results should be obtained from a single biopsy. Conversely, if different lesions are biopsied, each separate lesion biopsied may be coded. Skin lesion biopsies have add-on CPT codes to indicate separate lesions.

11100   Biopsy of skin, subcutaneous tissue and/or mucous membrane (including simple closure), unless otherwise listed; single lesion

+ 11101   each separate/additional lesion (List separately in addition to code for primary procedure)

Understand that the CPT code indicates single *lesion* as opposed to single *biopsy*.

If biopsies are performed endoscopically, the CPT code descriptions include multiple biopsies during a single endoscopic procedure:

45380   Colonoscopy, flexible, proximal to splenic flexure; with biopsy, single or multiple

As this code description includes one or more biopsies within a single endoscopy, only one code is used for endoscopic biopsies regardless of how many different polyps are biopsied during a single endoscopy. If different endoscopies of distinct anatomic sites are performed (eg, upper gastrointestinal endoscopy with biopsy and lower gastrointestinal endoscopy with biopsy), both may be coded.

Excerpt From the General Coding Policies Section of NCCI[2(p10)]

Exposure and exploration of the surgical field is integral to an operative procedure and is not separately reportable. For example, an exploratory laparotomy (CPT code 49000) is not separately reportable with an intra-abdominal procedure.

Interpretation

Again, the surgeon's work for a primary procedure includes accessing the body site as well as assessing landmarks and doing other integral procedures. Therefore, the surgical access should not be separately coded.

CPT Coding Tip: *NCCI edits do not include all codes for surgical access. Regardless, this is a guideline that should be followed. Do not code the surgical approach in addition to the primary procedure unless CPT guidelines specifically indicate to do so (eg, surgeries for skull-based tumors).*

> **Excerpt From the General Coding Policies Section of NCCI[2(p10)]**
>
> If removal, destruction, or other form of elimination of a lesion requires coincidental elimination of other pathology, only the primary procedure may be reported. For example, if an area of pilonidal disease contains an abscess, incision and drainage of the abscess during the procedure to excise the area of pilonidal disease is not separately reportable.

Interpretation

This guideline falls into the category of *not separately distinguishable*, as the primary procedure incidentally results in other disease being removed, and the incidental removal does not require additional effort on the part of the physician.

Example

If an open abdominal procedure is performed, and, in order to access the site of the procedure, the surgeon must lyse adhesions, the lysis of adhesions is a coincidental result of the access and should not be separately coded unless the adhesions were extensive, requiring unusual effort by the surgeon.

CPT Coding Tip: *Because extensive adhesions require work above and beyond what is usual, the surgeon may add a modifier 22 to the primary surgery CPT code to accurately represent the procedure performed. The documentation must clearly support the extensiveness of the adhesions and lysis.*

> **Excerpt From the General Coding Policies Section of NCCI[2(p10)]**
>
> An excision and removal (-ectomy) includes the incision and opening (-otomy) of the organ. A HCPCS/CPT code for an -otomy procedure should not be reported with an -ectomy code for the same organ.

Interpretation

The incision is a part of the approach for the procedure and, therefore, is not separately coded. (See earlier examples of laparotomy.)

> **Excerpt From the General Coding Policies Section of NCCI[2(p10-11)]**
>
> Multiple approaches to the same procedure are mutually exclusive of one another and should not be reported separately. For example, both a vaginal hysterectomy and abdominal hysterectomy should not be reported separately.

Interpretation

As mentioned earlier in this chapter, surgical approaches are incidental to the primary procedure and not separately reportable; therefore, never add a code for an approach. There are certain surgeries that may be performed through a variety of approaches (remember the hysterectomy examples). Because approaches are incidental to the procedure, additional CPT codes based solely on multiple approaches would be overcoding the surgery. Therefore, if two approaches are used to accomplish a single procedure, both approaches are still incidental to the primary procedure. If the CPT code is specific to the type of approach as in the example NCCI offers for hysterectomies, use the code for the most complex approach and do not add a code for the second approach.

CPT Coding Tip: *There are some CPT codes that separate the approach from the primary procedure (eg, skull-based tumor removal). For these codes, even though the approach is billed in addition to the root operation, only one approach may be coded. Two approaches should not be billed.*

Excerpt From the General Coding Policies Section of NCCI[2(p11)]

If a procedure utilizing one approach fails and is converted to a procedure utilizing a different approach, only the successful procedure may be reported. For example, if a laparoscopic hysterectomy is converted to an open hysterectomy, only the open hysterectomy procedure code may be reported.

Interpretation

When planning surgical procedures, physicians want to use the least invasive and/or most effective approach. On occasion, the planned approach is insufficient to the overall success of the procedure, and the surgeon must convert to a different approach during the procedure. Failed approaches, or approaches that are converted to different approaches, are incidental to successful approaches, and only the successfully approached procedure should be coded.

Example

For a shoulder arthroscopy with rotator cuff repair that must be converted to an open procedure due to poor visibility through the arthroscopy, only the open approach would be coded.

Excerpt From the General Coding Policies Section of NCCI[2(p11)]

If a laparoscopic procedure fails and is converted to an open procedure, the physician should not report a diagnostic laparoscopy in lieu of the failed laparoscopic procedure. For example, if a laparoscopic cholecystectomy is converted to an open cholecystectomy, the physician should not report the failed laparoscopic cholecystectomy nor a diagnostic laparoscopy.

Interpretation

If a failed therapeutic endoscopic procedure is converted to an open procedure, do not code a diagnostic endoscopy in lieu of the failed scope procedure. If the failed procedure was therapeutic, coding it as diagnostic would be misrepresenting the services performed.

Excerpt From the General Coding Policies Section of NCCI[2(p11)]

If a diagnostic endoscopy is the basis for and precedes an open procedure, the diagnostic endoscopy is separately reportable with modifier -58. However, the medical record must document the medical reasonableness and necessity for the diagnostic endoscopy. A scout endoscopy to assess anatomic landmarks and extent of disease is not separately reportable with an open procedure. When an endoscopic procedure fails and is converted to another surgical procedure, only the successful surgical procedure may be reported. The endoscopic procedure is not separately reportable with the successful procedure.

Interpretation

If an endoscopic procedure that precedes an open procedure is truly diagnostic, the diagnostic endoscopy may be coded in addition to the open procedure. The documentation within the record is critical here because it must clearly support that the endoscopy was diagnostic and not merely for land-marking the surgical site.

Learning Break Tip:
- *When coding, see if the preoperative diagnosis differs from the postoperative diagnosis, as this could be an indication of whether the endoscopy is truly diagnostic. If there is a symptom, or a rule-out diagnosis preoperatively, then that helps support the endoscopy as being diagnostic.*
- *There should be a procedure-indications section at the beginning of the operative note. This too can help clarify whether the endoscopy was diagnostic or not.*
- *Physicians should clearly document whether the endoscopy was diagnostic or not.*

NCCI edits state that when the diagnostic scope is performed prior to an open procedure, it may be coded by adding modifier 58 (staged procedure) to the diagnostic scope code. CPT guidelines for modifier 58 indicate that this modifier should be appended to the second (or later) procedure performed, rather than to the first procedure. This would indicate that modifier 58 should be appended to the open procedure. As discussed earlier in this chapter, modifier 58 should be appended to the second (or staged) procedure unless the payer denies the diagnostic scope code as bundled.

Excerpt From the General Coding Policies Section of NCCI[2(p11-12)]

Treatment of complications of primary surgical procedures are separately reportable with some limitations. The global surgical package for an operative procedure includes all intra-operative services that are normally a usual and necessary part of the procedure. Additionally the global surgical package includes all medical and surgical services required of the surgeon during the postoperative period of the surgery to treat complications that do not require return to the operating room. Thus, treatment of a complication of a primary surgical procedure is not separately reportable (1) if it represents usual and necessary care in the operating room during the procedure or (2) if it occurs postoperatively and does not require return to the operating room. For example, control of hemorrhage is a usual and necessary component of a surgical procedure in the operating room and is not separately reportable. Control of postoperative hemorrhage is also not separately reportable unless the patient must be returned to the operating room for treatment. In the latter case, the control of hemorrhage may be separately reportable with modifier -78.

Interpretation

Medicare guidelines indicate that postoperative complications are included in the surgery reimbursement and should not be separately coded unless they specifically require a return trip to the operating room. Modifier 78 should be appended to those procedures treating a postoperative complication that requires a return to the operating room. This modifier would allow bypassing of the bundling edit.

Example

If a patient has a postoperative wound infection at the site of the surgical incision, and the physician is able to treat the infection at bedside, that care should not be separately coded from the original surgery. If, however, the infection requires the surgeon to take the patient back to the operating room to re-open the site, perform debridement, apply vacuum-assisted closure, and redress the site, that could be coded with a modifier 78.

Evaluation and Management Services

NCCI edits incorporate Medicare Global Surgery Rules, and because reporting evaluation and management (E/M) services with procedures is covered by these rules, this section reviews those rules.

Excerpt From the General Coding Policies Section of NCCI[2(p9)]

Since NCCI edits are applied to same day services by the same provider to the same beneficiary, certain Global Surgery Rules are applicable to NCCI. An E&M service is separately reportable on the same date of service as a procedure with a global period of 000, 010, or 090 under limited circumstances.

Interpretation

NCCI edits apply only for services provided on a single date of service. NCCI screens for E/M CPT codes when the E/M service is billed on the same day as the procedure or surgery.

Examples

If a lesion excision and E/M service are billed for a patient on one calendar date, an NCCI edit potential would exist.

If an E/M service is billed with a date of service as yesterday, and a lesion is excised today, even if these services were billed on one claim, there would be no NCCI edit because of the different dates of service.

Excerpt From the General Coding Policies Section of NCCI[2(p12)]

If a procedure has a global period of 090 days, it is defined as a major surgical procedure. If an E&M is performed on the same date of service as a major surgical procedure for the purpose of deciding whether to perform this surgical procedure, the E&M service is separately reportable with modifier -57. Other E&M services on the same date of service as a major surgical procedure are included in the global payment for the procedure and are not separately reportable. NCCI does not contain edits based on this rule because Medicare Carriers have separate edits.

Interpretation

NCCI edits do not bundle E/M services into major surgeries. Chapter 12, Physicians/Nonphysician Practitioners (Section 40) of the *Medicare Claims Processing Manual*,[4] includes the guidelines for billing E/M services with major surgeries. Regardless of whether an edit exists or not, for Medicare claims, the guidelines should be followed.

Example

Hysterectomies are major surgeries with a 90 day global period. NCCI does not bundle E/M codes into the hysterectomy. Medicare guidelines for E/M services provided within global surgery care should be followed, regardless of whether an edit exists. If an E/M service was provided on the same day as the hysterectomy, and the E/M documentation met the definition for using modifier 57, the modifier should be appended and both services coded. If the E/M service performed did not meet modifier 57 criteria, only the hysterectomy should be coded as the E/M service is included in the global payment for the surgery.

Excerpt From the General Coding Policies Section of NCCI[2(p12-13)]

If a procedure has a global period of 000 or 010 days, it is defined as a minor surgical procedure. The decision to perform a minor surgical procedure is included in the payment for the minor surgical procedure and should not be reported separately as an E&M service. However, a significant and separately identifiable E&M service unrelated to the decision to perform the minor surgical procedure is separately reportable with modifier -25. The E&M service and minor procedure do not require different diagnoses.

Interpretation

NCCI contains some of the E/M edits for minor procedures, but not all. The guidelines for billing E/M services with minor procedures can be found in the Medicare manual, section 40, and should be followed, regardless of whether an edit exists.

Excerpt From the General Coding Policies Section of NCCI[2(p13)]

Procedures with a global surgery indicator of "XXX" are not covered by these rules. Many of these "XXX" procedures are performed by physicians and have inherent pre-procedure, intra-procedure, and post-procedure work usually performed each time the procedure is completed. This work should never be reported as a separate E&M code. Other "XXX" procedures are not usually performed by a physician and have no physician work relative value units associated with them. A physician should never report a separate E&M code with these procedures for the supervision of others performing the procedure or for the interpretation of the procedure. With most "XXX" procedures, the physician may, however, perform a significant and separately identifiable E&M service on the same day of service which may be reported by appending modifier -25 to the E&M code. This E&M service may be related to the same diagnosis necessitating performance of the "XXX" procedure but cannot include any work inherent in the "XXX" procedure, supervision of others performing the "XXX" procedure, or time for interpreting the result of the "XXX" procedure. Appending modifier -25 to a significant, separately identifiable E&M service when performed on the same date of service as an "XXX" procedure is correct coding.

Interpretation

If the physician performs an E/M service above and beyond the usual care for a procedure that is designated as an XXX procedure, modifier 25 may be appended to the E/M and both services allowed. Regardless, the documentation for the encounter must support a separate and distinct E/M service to be supported in addition to the XXX procedure.

Example

Chest radiographs (CPT code 71020) are designated as "XXX" procedures. Unless the provider performs a separately identifiable E/M service, only the chest radiograph should be coded. If a patient presents with chest pain, the provider assessing the patient will most likely perform a substantial work-up to determine the need for the radiograph. In this case, both the visit and radiograph should be billed. If, however, that patient returns on a second day for the radiograph, it would be unlikely that a separate E/M service would be required the day of the radiograph. In this case, only the radiograph would be billed.

Modifiers and Modifier Indicators

Modifiers are two-digit alphanumeric HCPCS/CPT suffix codes that help clarify a code and provide additional information for the HCPCS/CPT code. This section discusses the appropriate use of modifiers for NCCI edits.

Rule 1: Medical record documentation must support the modifier.

Rule 2: Modifiers should never be used solely to bypass an NCCI edit if Rule 1 is not met.

Rule 3: The most appropriate modifier should be used in all circumstances requiring a modifier.

The CMS-identified modifiers that could potentially bypass NCCI edits (when appropriate) include:

Anatomic modifiers: E1-E4, FA, F1-F9, TA, T1-T9, LT, RT, LC, LD, RC

Global surgery modifiers: -25, -58, -78, -79

Other modifiers: -27, -59, -91

Excerpt From the General Coding Policies Section of NCCI[2(p15)]

Although modifier -22 is not a modifier that bypasses an NCCI edit, its use is occasionally relevant to an NCCI edit and is discussed below.

Modifier -22: Modifier -22 is defined by the *CPT Manual* as an "unusual procedural service." This modifier should not be reported routinely but only when the service performed is significantly more extensive than that defined by the HCPCS/CPT code reported. Occasionally a provider may perform two procedures that should not be reported together based on an NCCI edit. If the edit allows use of NCCI-associated modifiers to bypass it and the clinical circumstances justify use of one of these modifiers, both services may be reported with the NCCI-associated modifier. However, if the NCCI edit does not allow use of NCCI-associated modifiers to bypass it and the procedure qualifies as an unusual procedural service, the physician may report the column one HCPCS/CPT code of the NCCI edit with modifier -22. The Carrier may then evaluate the unusual procedural service to determine whether additional payment is justified.

Interpretation

The CPT codebook updated the description of modifier 22 to read, "increased procedural service" in 2008. The previously mentioned guideline from NCCI indicates that, rather than billing both the Column 1 and Column 2 codes together, the documentation should be analyzed, and if there is substantial support that the overall procedure met the definition of increased procedural service for the Column 1 CPT code, modifier 22 may be appended to that code, rather than both codes being billed. This allows appropriate reflection of the complex nature of the procedure without violation of NCCI guidelines.

Example

A physician is performing a colectomy through an open abdominal incision. If the surgeon encounters extensive adhesions preventing access to the colon, and it is necessary to lyse the adhesions, the lysis is incidental to the colectomy. It would be inappropriate to code both services separately. However, if the adhesions were extremely dense and required substantial additional work and time to lyse, a modifier 22 may be appended to the colectomy code to indicate that the service was increased over the usual level of complexity for the colectomy.

Modifier 22 and Documentation Tip: *The documentation must be substantial to warrant appending a modifier 22. Use caution here and make sure the medical record supports extensive additional effort.*

Excerpt From the General Coding Policies Section of NCCI[2(p15-16)]

Modifier -25: The *CPT Manual* defines modifier -25 as a "significant, separately identifiable evaluation and management service by the same physician on the same day of the procedure or other service." Modifier -25 may be appended to an evaluation and management (E&M) CPT code to indicate that the E&M service is significant and separately identifiable from other services reported on the same date of service. The E&M service may be related to the same or different diagnosis as the other procedure(s).

Modifier -25 may be appended to E&M services reported with minor surgical procedures (global period of 000 or 010 days) or procedures not covered by global surgery rules (global indicator of XXX). Because minor surgical procedures and XXX procedures include pre-procedure, intra-procedure, and post-procedure work inherent in the procedure, the provider should not report an E&M service for this work. Furthermore, Medicare Global Surgery rules prevent the reporting of a separate E&M service for the work associated with the decision to perform a minor surgical procedure whether the patient is a new or established patient.

Interpretation

As discussed in the prior section (Evaluation and Management NCCI Policies), modifier 25 should be appended to the E/M code (and only E/M codes) when the documentation supports that the work performed for the E/M service was above and beyond the usual work for the separately billed service. Additional instruction on separately reportable E/M services are discussed in Chapter 3 of this book.

This is a challenging guideline because usual preprocedure and postprocedure care is very subjective, and it is often unclear whether the physician's documentation adequately supports modifier 25. The documentation should clearly support the E/M service as above and beyond the other service being coded. It is helpful if the documentation is separated within the record. Although not a requirement, separate documentation helps to clarify the physician's work dedicated to the E/M portion of the encounter and the physician's work on the procedural portion of the encounter.

Tip: The OIG performed a focused review of the use of modifier 25 and found that 35% of the services coded with modifier 25 did not have the documentation to support the modifier.[5] Figure 2-2 provides general rules for appending modifiers to bypass NCCI edits. Figure 2-3 shows the report cover page.

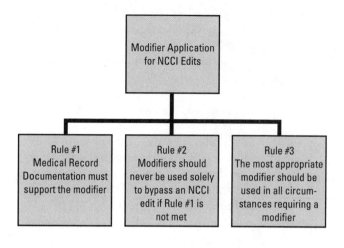

FIGURE 2-2 *Rules of Modifier Coding Within NCCI Edit Guidelines*

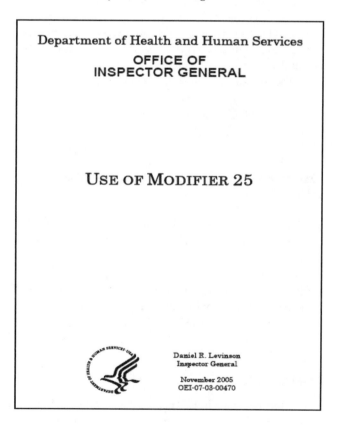

FIGURE 2-3 *Office of Inspector General Study on Modifier 25, Cover Page*[5]

Excerpt From Medicare Manual

Chapter 12, Physicians/Nonphysician Practitioners (Section 40.1) of the *Medicare Claims Processing Manual*[4]

Minor Surgeries and Endoscopies—Visits by the same physician on the same day as a minor surgery or endoscopy are included in the payment for the procedure, unless a significant, separately identifiable service is also performed. For example, a visit on the same day could be properly billed in addition to suturing a scalp wound if a full neurological examination is made for a patient with head trauma. Billing for a visit would not be appropriate if the physician only identified the need for sutures and confirmed allergy and immunization status.

Modifier 27—Multiple outpatient hospital E/M encounters on the same date

Modifier 27 is also listed as an NCCI modifier; however, its use is limited to hospital outpatient billing under the Ambulatory Payment Classification system. If a patient presented for outpatient medical care twice on one day, the hospital could bill each service (as long as medically necessary and appropriately documented) and append a modifier 27 on the second encounter. This modifier would allow both services to be considered for payment. Modifier 27 is not to be used for billing professional fee services.

Excerpt From the General Coding Policies Section of NCCI[2(p17)]

Modifier -59: Modifier -59 is an important NCCI-associated modifier that is often used incorrectly. For the NCCI its primary purpose is to indicate that two or more procedures are performed at different anatomic sites or different patient encounters. It should only be used if no other modifier more appropriately describes the relationships of the two or more procedure codes.

Interpretation

Two points are made in this part of the NCCI guidelines:
1. Modifier 59 is commonly misused, creating potential compliance risks if this modifier is used to bypass a bundling edit inappropriately (see the OIG study mentioned in the prior section).

2. Modifier 59 should be used when it is appropriate to bypass a bundling edit (based on the medical record documentation) and no other, more specific modifier exists. If another modifier is more specific and will also bypass the edit, the more specific modifier should be used.

Modifier 59 is not appropriate for E&M services.

Example

A patient presents with two lesions, one on the arm and another on the face. If the physician excises the lesion on the arm and takes a biopsy from the lesion on the face, both services may be coded. They are different services on different anatomic sites.

Remember, biopsies are incidental to excisions and will bundle into the excision code unless a modifier 59 is appended to the biopsy code to indicate a different anatomic site.

Excerpt From the General Coding Policies Section of NCCI[2(p18)]

An exception to this general principle about misuse of modifier -59 applies to some code pair edits consisting of a surgical procedure and a diagnostic procedure. If the diagnostic procedure precedes the surgical procedure and is the basis on which the decision to perform the surgical procedure is made, the two procedures may be reported with modifier -59 under appropriate circumstances. However, if the diagnostic procedure is an inherent component of the surgical procedure, it cannot be reported separately. If the diagnostic procedure follows the surgical procedure at the same patient encounter, modifier -59 may be utilized if appropriate.

Excerpt From the General Coding Policies Section of NCCI[2(p18)]

Use of modifier -59 to indicate different procedures/surgeries does not require a different diagnosis for each HCPCS/CPT coded procedure/surgery. Additionally, different diagnoses are not adequate criteria for use of modifier -59. The HCPCS/CPT codes remain bundled unless the procedures/surgeries are performed at different anatomic sites or separate patient encounters. From an NCCI perspective, the definition of different anatomic sites includes different organs or different lesions in the same organ. However, it does not include treatment of contiguous structures of the same organ. For example, treatment of the nail, nail bed, and adjacent soft tissue constitutes a single anatomic site.

Example: The column one/column two code edit with column one CPT code 38221 (bone marrow biopsy) and column two CPT code 38220 (bone marrow, aspiration only) includes two distinct procedures when performed at separate anatomic sites or separate patient encounters. In these circumstances, it would be acceptable to use modifier -59. However, if both 38221 and 38220 are performed through the same skin incision at the same patient encounter which is the usual practice, modifier -59 should NOT be used.

Interpretation

The requirement for appending modifier 59 to bypass the bundling edit is clearly distinct sites or encounters.

Example

A patient presents with nasal and throat symptoms, and a nasopharyngoscopy and a laryngoscopy are performed, based on symptoms in each site. Given that the nasopharynx and larynx are contiguous sites, only the laryngoscopy (Column 1 code) would be billed unless a different approach (one scope was inserted through the mouth for the laryngoscopy and the other through the nose for the nasopharyngoscopy) was clearly documented.

If different approaches or different encounters were documented for each procedure, then both could be coded and modifier 59 appended to the nasopharyngoscopy (Column 2 code).

In Chapter 1 of this book, we explained the correct coding modifier (CCM) indicator. This indicator (as seen in the third column of Table 2-1) provides information on whether a modifier will bypass the bundling edit.

CCM 1 indicates that when appropriate, the edit may be bypassed with a modifier, and both services will be allowed if no other reasons for denial (eg, medical necessity) exist.

CCM 0 indicates that even when a modifier is appended, no payment will be made for the Column 2 service (ie, the edit cannot be bypassed with a modifier).

CCM 9 indicates that the bundling edit is not applicable and can be ignored. If a code pair has a deletion date that is the same as the effective date, there will be a 9 indicator.

Standard Preparation/Monitoring Services for Anesthesia

Excerpt From the General Coding Policies Section of NCCI [2(p19)]

With few exceptions anesthesia HCPCS/CPT codes do not specify the mode of anesthesia for a particular procedure. Regardless of the mode of anesthesia, preparation and monitoring services are not separately reportable with anesthesia service HCPCS/CPT codes when performed in association with the anesthesia service. However, if the provider of the anesthesia service performs one or more of these services prior to and unrelated to the anticipated anesthesia service or after the patient is released from the anesthesia practitioner's postoperative care, the service may be separately reportable with modifier -59.

Interpretation

When a provider codes for anesthesia, all aspects of the anesthesia are included in the anesthesia CPT code. Services inherent in performing anesthesia are not separately billable unless clearly unrelated to the anesthesia service.

Example

An anesthesiologist billing for general anesthesia for a patient most often uses intravenous access, inserts an endotracheal tube, and performs other integral services to induce anesthesia. None of these services, nor any others necessary to induce anesthesia, would be coded separately from the anesthesia service.

Anesthesia Service Included in the Surgical Procedure

Excerpt From the General Coding Policies Section of NCCI[2(p20)]

Under the CMS Anesthesia Rules, with limited exceptions, Medicare does not allow separate payment for anesthesia services performed by the physician who also furnishes the medical or surgical service. In this case, payment for the anesthesia service is included in the payment for the medical or surgical service. For example, separate payment is not allowed for the physician's performance of local, regional, or most other anesthesia including nerve blocks if the physician also performs the medical or surgical procedure. However, Medicare may allow separate payment for moderate conscious sedation services (CPT codes 99143-99145) when provided by same physician performing the medical or surgical procedure except for those procedures listed in Appendix G of the *CPT Manual*.

Interpretation

If the physician who is performing a surgery also provides the anesthesia services for the surgery, separate CPT codes for the anesthesia may not be used. The anesthesia is included in the surgery when both services are performed by the same physician. An exception is for physicians using moderate sedation, and the CPT codebook identifies that the procedure is not one that includes moderate sedation.

CPT codebook's Appendix G

Appendix G of the CPT codebook includes those CPT codes that include moderate sedation. Additionally, the CPT codebook identifies those procedures that include moderate sedation with this symbol ⊙ preceding the code. For example:

31622 Bronchoscopy, rigid or flexible, with or without fluoroscopic guidance; diagnostic, with or without cell washing (separate procedure)

For the above code (or any with the ⊙ designation), the provider performing the procedure may not bill for moderate sedation additionally, as the code includes that service.

HCPCS/CPT Procedure Code Definition

This section discusses the NCCI principles based on the HCPCS/CPT code description. The code description is often the basis of an NCCI edit.

Excerpt From the General Coding Policies Section of NCCI[2(p20-21)]

Several general principles follow:

A family of CPT codes may include a CPT code followed by one or more indented CPT codes. The first CPT code descriptor includes a semicolon. The portion of the descriptor of the first code in the family preceding the semicolon is a common part of the descriptor for each subsequent code of the family.

For example, CPT code 70120, Radiologic examination, mastoids; less than 3 views per side; CPT code 70130 complete, minimum of 3 views per side.

The portion of the descriptor preceding the semicolon ("Radiologic examination, mastoids") is common to both CPT codes 70120 and 70130. The difference between the two codes is the portion of the descriptors following the semicolon. Often as in this case, two codes from a family may not be reported separately. A physician cannot report CPT codes 70120 and 70130 for a procedure performed on ipsilateral mastoids at the same patient encounter. It is important to recognize, however, that there are numerous circumstances when it may be appropriate to report more than one code from a family of codes. For example, CPT codes 70120 and 70130 may be reported separately if the two procedures are performed on contralateral mastoids or at two separate patient encounters on the same date of service.

Interpretation

When coding is done from a family of CPT codes, the description preceding the semicolon in the parent (or first-listed code) is shared with all the indented codes within that same family. There would be no need to add the parent code to capture the portion of the description that precedes the semicolon.

Example of Semicolon Interpretation

97010 Application of a modality to 1 or more areas; hot or cold packs

97012   traction, mechanical

97014   electrical stimulation (unattended)

97016   vasopneumatic devices

97018   paraffin bath

The above should be read as follows:

97010 Application of a modality to 1 or more areas; hot or cold packs

97012 Application of a modality to 1 or more areas; traction, mechanical

97014 Application of a modality to 1 or more areas; electrical stimulation (unattended)

97016 Application of a modality to 1 or more areas; vasopneumatic devices

97018 Application of a modality to 1 or more areas; paraffin bath

If the provider performed an application of a paraffin bath modality, CPT code 97018 includes the entire work, because the description before the semicolon in the parent code (CPT 97010) applies to all the indented codes within that same family. If hot or cold packs *and* paraffin were provided, it would be appropriate to use both codes.

Excerpt From the General Coding Policies Section of NCCI[2(p21)]

If a HCPCS/CPT code is reported, it includes all components of the procedure defined by the descriptor. For example, CPT code 58291 includes a vaginal hysterectomy with "removal of tube(s) and/or ovary(s)." A physician cannot report a salpingo-oophorectomy (CPT code 58720) separately with CPT code 58291.

Interpretation

This policy is self-explanatory, so just a word of caution: be sure to carefully read the CPT code description to make sure codes that duplicate one another are not added.

Excerpt From the General Coding Policies Section of NCCI[2(p21-22)]

CPT code descriptors often define correct coding relationships where two codes may not be reported separately with one another at the same anatomic site and/or same patient encounter. A few examples follow:

(a) A "partial" procedure is not separately reportable with a "complete" procedure.

(b) A "partial" procedure is not separately reportable with a "total" procedure.

(c) A "unilateral" procedure is not separately reportable with a "bilateral" procedure.

(d) A "single" procedure is not separately reportable with a "multiple" procedure.

(e) A "with" procedure is not separately reportable with a "without" procedure.

(f) An "initial" procedure is not separately reportable with a "subsequent" procedure.

Examples

Partial and Total CPT Codes

27125 Hemiarthroplasty, hip, partial (eg, femoral stem prosthesis, bipolar arthroplasty)

27130 Arthroplasty, acetabular and proximal femoral prosthetic replacement (total hip arthroplasty), with or without autograft or allograft

If these procedures were performed on the same hip during the same surgical session, do not bill both a partial (CPT code 27125) and total (CPT code 27130) procedure.

Unilateral and Bilateral CPT Codes

77055 Mammography; unilateral

77056   bilateral

When there is a bilateral code, do not bill the unilateral code instead of or in addition to the bilateral code when both procedures are performed at the same encounter.

Single and Multiple CPT Codes

10060 Incision and drainage of abscess (eg, carbuncle, suppurative hidradenitis, cutaneous or subcutaneous abscess, cyst, furuncle, or paronychia); simple or single

10061   complicated or multiple

When both procedures are performed during the same encounter, do not bill both the single and multiple CPT codes.

CPT Codebook and CMS Coding Manual Instructions

NCCI guidelines require that we follow any specific instructions within the CMS manuals or the CPT codebook. This section discusses this requirement.

One element of coding that even seasoned coding professionals sometimes fail to follow is reviewing the guidelines available through the CPT codebook. Additional instructions can be found in all sections of the CPT codebook. When coding services, especially when applying multiple CPT codes to a single encounter, one should review all the instructions provided. Additionally, as the CPT codebook is updated each year, it is an absolute must that all the changed guidelines be reviewed in detail.

> **Excerpt From the General Coding Policies Section of NCCI[2(p22)]**
>
> The American Medical Association publishes *CPT Assistant*, which contains coding guidelines. CMS does not review nor approve the information in this publication. In the development of NCCI edits, CMS occasionally disagrees with the information in this publication. If a physician utilizes information from *CPT Assistant* to report services rendered to Medicare patients, it is possible that Medicare Carriers and Fiscal Intermediaries may utilize different criteria to process claims.

Interpretation

Here, CMS is acknowledging the *CPT Assistant* information while indicating they do not necessarily subscribe to its contents. This is important to note when addressing NCCI edits. If *CPT Assistant* gives advice on bundling issues, CMS may or may not agree with the instruction. For appeals to denials, submitting information from *CPT Assistant* can prove beneficial. Use this resource when appropriate. *CPT Assistant* is a monthly publication by the American Medical Association (AMA) that provides additional instruction, information, and explanation of coding complex areas within medical records. The *CPT Assistant* may be purchased from the AMA through the Web site (www.amabookstore.com).

The Definition of a Separate Procedure

NCCI policies subscribe to the CPT codebook definition of *separate procedure*.

> **Excerpt From the General Coding Policies Section of NCCI[2(p22-23)]**
>
> If a HCPCS/CPT code descriptor includes the term "separate procedure," the HCPCS/CPT code may not be reported separately with a related procedure. CMS interprets this designation to prohibit the separate reporting of a "separate procedure" when performed with another procedure in an anatomically related region often through the same skin incision, orifice, or surgical approach.
>
> A HCPCS/CPT code with the "separate procedure" designation may be reported with another procedure if it is performed at a separate patient encounter on the same date of service or at the same patient encounter in an anatomically unrelated area often through a separate skin incision, orifice, or surgical approach. Modifier -59 may be appended to the "separate procedure" HCPCS/CPT code to indicate that it qualifies as a separately reportable service.

Interpretation

Whenever a CPT code description includes the term *separate procedure*, that service is usually incidental to other services provided during the same encounter on the same anatomic site. Do not code the separate procedure service in addition to another CPT code when both procedures are performed in the same anatomic region. However, if the separate procedure code service is performed in a different anatomic site or during a separate encounter than any other service also being coded, both services may be coded.

Example

A patient presents with a severe earache and headache that, after examining the patient, the physician believes could be due to sinus problems. The physician decides to perform a nasal endoscopy as well as a direct laryngoscopy. These were performed through different orifices (nose for nasal endoscopy and mouth for laryngoscopy) with different scopes.

31231 Nasal endoscopy, diagnostic, unilateral or bilateral (separate procedure)

31525 Laryngoscopy direct, with or without tracheoscopy; diagnostic, except newborn

The nasal endoscopy is designated as a separate procedure and would normally be bundled into the laryngoscopy, but because different scopes and approaches were used, both may be coded, with modifier 59 appended to the nasal endoscopy.

Example

A patient has bilateral wrist pain, and the physician performs a diagnostic arthroscopy of the right wrist and a therapeutic endoscopic carpal tunnel release of the left wrist.

29840 Arthroscopy, wrist, diagnostic, with or without synovial biopsy (separate procedure)

29848 Endoscopy, wrist, surgical, with release of transverse carpal ligament

The diagnostic arthroscopy is designated as a separate procedure and would normally be bundled into the therapeutic carpal tunnel release, but because they are on different wrists, both may be coded and the lateral modifiers (RT for right, LT for left) appended. Even though the guidelines indicate that modifier 59 is used to bypass separate procedure bundling edits, if a more appropriate modifier exists (in this case, the lateral modifiers), NCCI instructs that the more specific modifier be used.

 CMS Coding Tip: NCCI advises that modifier 59 may be appended to the separate procedure code; however, modifier 59 should be necessary only if the separate procedure code would otherwise be denied as bundled. Often, the codes themselves are clearly in separate anatomic sites. A good rule of thumb here is to check the edits to see if the codes bundle together, and, if they do, but the documentation supports billing both, then append the modifier 59 to the otherwise denied code.

Example

Upper and lower gastrointestinal endoscopies (CPT codes 43235 and 45378) are clearly in distinct anatomic locations and are accessed through different orifices (mouth and rectum, respectively). Even though these codes are designated as separate procedures, there should be no need to use a modifier 59 because the codes themselves represent the distinct sites. However, the NCCI edits should be checked to make sure both codes would be payable without appending the modifier. If necessary for appropriate payment, append the modifier 59.

More Extensive Procedures

Excerpt From the General Coding Policies Section of NCCI[2(p23)]

The *CPT Manual* often describes groups of similar codes differing in the complexity of the service. Unless services are performed at separate patient encounters or at separate anatomic sites, the less complex service is included in the more complex service and is not separately reportable.

Interpretation

Only the most complex procedure performed during a single encounter on a single anatomic site may be coded. The lesser services are incidental to the more complex procedure. This guideline is consistent with the other guidelines within NCCI. For example, failed procedures are incidental to successful procedures when performed during the same surgical session.

CMS provides several examples for the more complex guideline, including:

- *Simple* or *limited* procedures are included in *complex* or *complicated* procedures when performed at the same encounter on the same anatomic site.
- *Intermediate* procedures are included in *comprehensive* procedures when performed at the same encounter at the same anatomic site.

77261 Therapeutic radiology treatment planning; simple

77262   intermediate

77263   complex

If these services were performed on the same anatomic site, only the most complex service documented should be coded. Table 2-2 is an excerpt of the earlier referenced treatment planning NCCI edits.

Because CPT codes 77761 and 77762 are both bundled into CPT code 77763, if the services are performed on the same anatomic location, only the most complex service (CPT code 77763) should be coded.

- *Superficial* procedures are included in *deep* procedures when the procedures are performed at the same encounter at the same anatomic site.

20000 Incision of soft tissue abscess (eg, secondary to osteomyelitis); superficial

20005   deep or complicated

TABLE 2-2 *Excerpt From NCCI Edit Table for Treatment Planning Services*

Column 1	Column 2	Modifier 0 = not allowed 1 = allowed 9 = not applicable
77763	16030	0
77763	36000	1
77763	36410	1
77763	36425	0
77763	51701	0
77763	51702	0
77763	51703	0
77763	76873	0
77763	77761	1
77763	77762	1
77763	77785	1
77763	77786	1
77763	77787	1
77763	90760	1
77763	90765	1
77763	90772	1
77763	90774	1
77763	90775	1

If these services were performed at a single anatomic site during the same encounter, only the deep procedure should be coded. If, however, different abscesses at different sites are incised, each may be coded.

- *Incomplete* procedures are included in *complete* procedures when both procedures are performed at the same encounter at the same anatomic site.

  56620 Vulvectomy simple; partial

  56625 complete

If the above services were performed at a single anatomic site during the same encounter, only the complete procedure should be coded.

Misuse of Column 2 Codes With Column 1 Codes

As mentioned throughout this book, the NCCI edits are divided into two categories: Column 1/Column 2 codes and mutually exclusive codes. The NCCI guidelines warn about coding multiple CPT codes erroneously. The NCCI edits help to prevent erroneous billing of services. Additionally, the NCCI indicates edit code pairs that, when appropriate and supported by the documentation, may both be coded with a modifier appended to bypass the edit.

Excerpt From the General Coding Policies Section of NCCI[2(p26)]

… there are limited circumstances when the column two code may be reported on the same date of service as the column one code. Two examples follow:

(1) Three or more HCPCS/CPT codes may be reported on the same date of service. Although the column two code is misused if reported as a service associated with the column one code, the column two code may be appropriately reported with a third HCPCS/CPT code reported on the same date of service. For example, CMS limits separate payment for use of the operating microscope for microsurgical techniques (CPT code 69990) to a group of procedures listed in the online *Claims Processing Manual* (Chapter 12, Section 20.4.5 (Allowable Adjustments)). The NCCI has edits with column one codes of surgical procedures not listed in this section of the manual and column two CPT code of 69990. Some of these edits allow use of NCCI-associated modifiers because the two services listed in the edit may be performed at the same patient encounter as a third procedure for which CPT code 69990 is separately reportable.

(2) There may be limited circumstances when the column two code is separately reportable with the column one code. For example, the NCCI has an edit with column one CPT code of 80061 (lipid profile) and column two CPT code of 83721 (LDL cholesterol by direct measurement). If the triglyceride level is less than 400 mg/dl, the LDL is a calculated value utilizing the results from the lipid profile for the calculation, and CPT code 83721 is not separately reportable. However, if the triglyceride level is greater than 400 mg/dl, the LDL may be measured directly and may be separately reportable with CPT code 83721 utilizing an NCCI-associated modifier to bypass the edit.

Mutually Exclusive Procedures

A second category of NCCI edits is for procedures deemed mutually exclusive. The two codes should not be reported together because both services cannot be reasonably performed at the same anatomic site or during the same patient encounter.

Excerpt From the General Coding Policies Section of NCCI[2(p27)]

An example of a mutually exclusive situation is the repair of an organ that can be performed by two different methods. Only one method can be chosen to repair the organ. A second example is a service that can be reported as an "initial" service or a "subsequent" service. With the exception of drug administration services, the initial service and subsequent service cannot be reported at the same patient encounter.

Example

In normal anatomy, males have one prostate gland; therefore, if the prostate gland is resected, only one methodology could be used, and if two different prostate gland resections were billed for a single patient encounter, this would create a mutually exclusive code edit.

The following codes would create a mutually exclusive edit because they both represent prostate gland resections.

CPT Code Example

52601 Transurethral electrosurgical resection of prostate, including control of postoperative bleeding, complete (vasectomy, meatotomy, cystourethroscopy, urethral calibration and/or dilation, and internal urethrotomy are included)

55801 Prostatectomy, perineal, subtotal (including control of postoperative bleeding, vasectomy, meatotomy, urethral calibration and/or dilation, and internal urethrotomy)

Example

A single lesion might be destroyed or excised, and if both excision and destruction were coded for a single lesion, a mutually exclusive edit would be generated. However, because it is possible for a patient to have multiple lesions at the same time, this edit can be bypassed using a modifier 59 to indicate different anatomic sites.

CPT Code Example

17000 Destruction (eg, laser surgery, electrosurgery, cryosurgery, chemosurgery, surgical curettement), premalignant lesions (eg, actinic keratoses); first lesion

11400 Excision, benign lesion including margins, except skin tag (unless listed elsewhere), trunk, arms or legs; excised diameter 0.5 cm or less

The final coding should be:

11400

17000-59

Example

There is a code for both a right and left heart catheterization when the two procedures are performed together (**93526** Combined right heart catheterization and retrograde left heart catheterization). Therefore, the separate codes for right heart catheterization (CPT code 93501) and left heart catheterization (CPT code 93510) are mutually exclusive. The mutually exclusive edit for the heart catheterization codes may not be bypassed with a modifier.

CPT Code Example

93526 Combined right heart catheterization and retrograde left heart catheterization

93501 Right heart catheterization

93510 Left heart catheterization, retrograde, from the brachial artery, axillary artery or femoral artery; percutaneous

Gender-Specific Procedures

There are HCPCS/CPT codes that are gender specific, meaning the procedure would be performed only on either a male or female patient, but not both. NCCI created edits making conflicting gender-specific codes mutually exclusive, because it would be clinically impossible for both male and female gender-specific codes to be performed on a single patient.

There are codes for procedures performed on the female urethra (CPT code 53230), and the same procedure exists for the male urethra (CPT code 53235). These codes are listed as mutually exclusive and cannot be bypassed.

53230 Excision of urethral diverticulum (separate procedure); female

53235   male

Add-On Codes

In general, NCCI does not include edits for most add-on codes because edits related to the primary procedure(s) should be adequate to prevent inappropriate payment.

> **Excerpt From the General Coding Policies Section of NCCI[2(p28)]**
>
> (If an edit prevents payment of the primary procedure code, the add-on code will also not be paid.) However, NCCI does include edits for some add-on codes when coding edits related to the primary procedures must be supplemented. Examples include edits with add-on codes 69990 (microsurgical techniques requiring use of operating microscope) and 95920 (intraoperative neurophysiology testing).

Interpretation

Add-on CPT codes are those that cannot be billed alone. Add-on codes may be used only when the primary procedure counterpart is also coded. NCCI builds edits based on the primary codes; however, there are add-on codes that have multiple primary codes across different organ systems. For those, NCCI edits are created.

Example

The add-on code for skin biopsy (CPT code 11101) may be coded only in conjunction with the primary skin biopsy CPT code (11100) per CPT instructions. There is no NCCI edit for the add-on code, but NCCI edits do exist for the primary code.

11100   Biopsy of skin, subcutaneous tissue and/or mucous membrane (including simple closure), unless otherwise listed; single lesion

+ 11101   each separate/additional lesion (List separately in addition to code for primary procedure)

Per the CPT codebook:

(Use 11101 in conjunction with 11100)

Example

Per the CPT codebook: Do not report 69990 in addition to procedures where use of the operating microscope is an inclusive component (15756-15758, 15842, 19364, 19368, 20955-20962, 20969-20973, 22856-22861, 26551-26554, 26556, 31526, 31531, 31536, 31541, 31545, 31546, 31561, 31571, 43116, 43496, 49906, 61548, 63075-63078, 64727, 64820-64823, 65091-68850, 0184T).

The add-on code for operating microscope (CPT code 69990) may be coded in conjunction with many different primary codes per CPT instructions. The NCCI edits for this code expand the CPT codebook list of service, with which CPT code 69990 should not be billed.

+ 69990   Microsurgical techniques, requiring use of operating microscope (List separately in addition to code for primary procedure)

Medically Unlikely Edits

> **Excerpt From the General Coding Policies Section of NCCI[2(p30)]**
>
> CMS has established units of service edits referred to as Medically Unlikely Edit(s) (MUEs).
>
> An MUE for a HCPCS/CPT code is the maximum number of units of service (UOS) allowable by the same provider for the same beneficiary on the same date of service. The ideal MUE value for a HCPCS/CPT code is the unit of service that allows the vast majority of appropriately coded claims to pass the MUE.

Interpretation

Unlike the other NCCI edits in which two codes are compared to each other, the medically unlikely edits (MUEs) are line item edits on units of service. The units of service for an individual line item are compared to the CPT code, and if the unit of service on that line exceeds the CPT code established MUE value, the entire line is denied at the carrier, or the claim is returned to the provider at the fiscal intermediary.

Table 2-3 illustrates the MUE for certain inpatient E&M services. Note that the unit of service is limited to one. Chapter 12, section 30.6.9, of the *Medicare Claims Processing Manual*[4] states that all inpatient E/M services provided by a single physician on one day should be combined for a single E/M code; the unit of service is limited to one.

TABLE 2-3 *Example from Medically Unlikely Edits (MUE) Table*

HCPCS/CPT Code	Practitioner DME Supplier MUE
99217	1
99218	1
99219	1
99220	1
99221	1
99222	1
99223	1
99231	1
99232	1
99233	1
99234	1
99235	1
99236	1
99238	1
99239	1
99241	1

Chapter 12, Physicians/Nonphysician Practitioners (Section 30.6.9) of the *Medicare Claims Processing Manual*[4]

30.6.9—Payment for Inpatient Hospital Visits: General (Codes 99221 - 99239)

B. Two Hospital Visits, Same Day
Contractors pay a physician for only one hospital visit per day for the same patient, whether the problems seen during the encounters are related or not. The inpatient hospital visit descriptors contain the phrase *per day*, which means that the code and the payment established for the code represent all services provided on that date. The physician should select a code that reflects all services provided during the date of the service.

Excerpt From the General Coding Policies Section of NCCI[2(p31)]

If appropriate use of CPT modifiers (e.g., -59, -76, -77, -91, anatomic) causes the same HCPCS/CPT code to appear on separate lines of a claim, each line is separately adjudicated against the MUE value for that HCPCS/CPT code.

Interpretation

There may be clinical circumstances in which the same CPT code should be billed multiple times on separate line items. If documentation supports bypassing the MUE units of service value, separate the services on separate line items, and append the most appropriate modifier on the second line. This will bypass the edit.

Example

73560   Radiologic examination, knee; 1 or 2 views

The CPT code 73560 has an MUE value of two because there are two knees in normal anatomy. Limiting this service to two units of service is reasonable, but if bilateral, single-view knee radiographs were performed, with a fracture found on the right knee, and a postreduction single-view film of that knee was also performed, CPT code 73560 with two units of service should be billed on one line, and CPT 73560-76 (repeat procedure) with one unit of service should be billed on a separate line item.

SUMMARY

- The entire General Coding Policies section of NCCI should be read.

- Service components that are inherent and integral to the comprehensive CPT code should not be separately coded.

- Medical record documentation must support appending a modifier to bypass the edit.

- The NCCI guidelines and edits apply to all providers billing HCPCS/CPT codes.

- Three general principles are applied to the edits (standard of care, usually necessary, not separately distinguishable).

- The NCCI policies reinforce this guideline by including direction that anesthesia services provided by the surgeon should not be coded separately from the surgery.

- NCCI edits incorporate CMS reimbursement guidelines and CPT codebook instructions. Each of these resources should be thoroughly reviewed, evaluated, and incorporated in coding all Medicare services.

Definitions and Acronyms

Centers for Medicare and Medicaid Services (CMS): This is a branch of the Department of Health and Human Services (DHHS) responsible for overseeing the Medicare and Medicaid federal health care programs.

HCPCS: Healthcare Common Procedure Coding System: The code sets used for filing Medicare bills consisting of Level I CPT codes and Level II HCPCS codes.

Current Procedural Terminology® (CPT®): CPT codes are maintained by the American Medical Association (AMA) and distributed through the annual update of the AMA's CPT® 2009 *Professional Edition.*[1]

Level II HCPCS: CMS maintains Level II HCPCS codes. Updates to Level II codes are available through the CMS Web site (www.cms.hhs.gov) as well as through various vendor products, including hard copy books and software.

Chapter 2 begins to delve into the guidelines, policies, and issues relevant to all National Correct Coding Initiative (NCCI) edits. Within the General Correct Coding Policies section of the NCCI manual, CMS explains the general principles, issues, and policies for all edits. Chapter 2 briefly explains the specifics of the policies and offers examples. Analyzing the general principles is the best beginning step to understanding NCCI. Although the General Correct Coding Policies provide an overview of all the NCCI principles, the service-specific (Evaluation and Management [E/M], anesthesia, surgery, etc) issues, policies, and guidelines must also be reviewed and understood to make the right decision on each claim. The remaining chapters of this book review those service-specific guidelines.

CHAPTER EXERCISES

Determine, based on the provided information, which services can be coded separately and which cannot. There is no need to code the services, just indicate which may be coded or not and why.

1. Cystourethroscopy with fragmentation of ureteral calculus

   a. Separate codes for the two endoscopies   Y   N
   Why?

   b. Separate codes for the endoscopy and the fragmentation   Y   N
   Why?

   c. Separate code for nerve block for anesthesia   Y   N
   Why?

2. Heart transplant

   a. Thoracotomy   Y   N
   Why?

   b. Closure of surgical wound in layers with internal staples   Y   N
   Why?

3. Five skin lesions excised from various areas of the body

   a. Each lesion can be coded separately   Y   N
   Why?

ANSWERS TO CHAPTER EXERCISES

1a. Separate codes for the two endoscopies   Y   (N)

Why: Both endoscopies are included in a single CPT code and therefore not separately coded. There was only one endoscope used (no documentation that multiple encounters or scopes were used).

1b. Separate codes for the endoscopy and the fragmentation   Y   (N)

Why: Procedure approaches are an integral part of the primary procedure.

1c. Separate code for nerve block for anesthesia   Y   (N)

Why: This procedure is coded separately only when performed by someone other than the operating physician, as long as it is medically necessary for someone other than the surgeon to induce anesthesia.

2a. Thoracotomy Y

Why: Surgical approaches integral to performing the primary procedure (to gain access to the anatomic site) are included in the code for the primary procedure.

2b. Closure of surgical wound in layers with internal staples Y

Why: Usual closure for surgically created wounds is included in the global payment for the surgery and not coded separately.

3a. Each lesion can be coded separately Ⓨ N

Why: As long as the lesions are of distinct anatomical sites that are not adjacent, and separate incisions are made for the excision, each may be coded separately. This is not the case with endoscopic procedures or other surgeries in which the CPT code description includes multiple sites.

REFERENCES

1. American Medical Association. *Current Procedural Terminology CPT® 2009 Professional Edition.* Chicago, IL: American Medical Association; 2008.

2. Centers for Medicare and Medicaid Services. "Chapter I General Correct Coding Policies," In: NCCI Policy Manual for Medicare Services. www.cms.hhs.gov/NationalCorrectCodInitEd/01_overview.asp#TopOfPage. Accessed June 11, 2009.

3. Department of Health and Human Services, Office of Inspector General. *Use of Modifier 59 to Bypass Medicare's National Correct Coding Initiative Edits.* http://oig.hhs.gov/oei/reports/oei-03-02-00771.pdf. Accessed June 11, 2009.

4. Centers for Medicare and Medicaid Services. Physicians/Nonphysician Practitioners. In: *Medicare Claims Processing Manual.* www.cms.hhs.gov/manuals/downloads/clm104c12.pdf. Accessed June 11, 2009.

5. Department of Health and Human Services, Office of Inspector General. *Use of Modifier 25.* www.oig.hhs.gov/oei/reports/oei-07-03-00470.pdf. Accessed June 11, 2009.

NCCI Evaluation and Management Policies

Chapter 3 analyzes the National Correct Coding Initiative (NCCI) policies for evaluation and management services. The official Centers for Medicare and Medicaid Services (CMS) NCCI evaluation and management services (E/M) guidelines are incorporated in the guideline section, including medicine CPT codes (essentially, all CPT codes that begin with a first character of 9. Therefore, those services found in the Medicine section of the CPT codebook[1] (CPT codes 90281 through 99607) as well as services found in the E/M section of the CPT codebook (CPT codes 99201 through 99499) are located in the same section of the NCCI policies document. This book, however, divides the two categories of codes (ie, E/M and medicine services) to stay consistent with the CPT codebook format. This chapter delves into the guidelines, policies, and issues relevant to E/M NCCI edits.

Medicare coding and billing information for E/M services as well as documentation guidelines and manuals relative to E/M coding may be found on the CMS web site.

Introduction to NCCI Evaluation and Management Policies

Excerpt From the E/M Introduction Section of NCCI[1(p2)]

A. Introduction
The principles of correct coding discussed in Chapter I apply to the CPT codes in the range 90000-99999. Several general guidelines are repeated in this Chapter. However, those general guidelines from Chapter I not discussed in this chapter are nonetheless applicable.

Interpretation

This instruction means that the overall NCCI guidelines apply to each section of the CPT codebook and, even if they are not repeated within a service-specific chapter, they are nonetheless still a guideline to be followed. Refer back to Chapter 2 for a complete discussion of the general NCCI guidelines.

E/M Services and NCCI Edits

CPT codes for E/M services are principally included in the CPT code range of 99201 through 99499. There are also E/M-related services in the Medicine section of the CPT codebook, specifically, within the psychiatry and ophthalmology codes. The E/M CPT codes include such descriptions as the place of service (eg, office, hospital, nursing facility, emergency department) and the type of service (eg, new patient or initial encounter, established patient, follow-up or subsequent encounter, consultation), and they include various miscellaneous services (eg, prolonged physician service, care plan oversight service). E/M services are further classified by the complexity of the relevant clinical history, physical examination, and medical decision making. Time, in certain circumstances, is also included in the delineation between E/M CPT codes.

The purpose of this book is not to teach how to code services but rather how to properly address NCCI bundling edits. Please see the other excellent AMA products for coding instructions. This book provides applicable coding instructions that relate to NCCI edits.

Excerpt From the E&M Coding Policies Section of NCCI[1(p25)]

Rules governing the reporting of more than one E&M code for a patient on the same date of service are very complex and are not described herein.

Interpretation

Here the NCCI edit policy is simply reminding coders that CMS has extensive instructions for proper coding and billing of E/M services, most of which can be found on the CMS Web site. To repeat in the NCCI policies all of the instructions provided elsewhere is unnecessary and would prove too lengthy. It is important that the NCCI guidelines not be looked at in isolation of all the other regulations available. Use all available resources when coding and billing.

CMS manual guidelines with explanation and examples applicable to the individual NCCI guidelines will be incorporated within this chapter. Providers should refer to CMS manuals when coding services for federal payers.

The following is an example from the CMS manual[2] on Medicare guidance on coding and billing E/M services:

Excerpt from CMS Manual Section on E/M Coding

Chapter 12, Physicians/Nonphysician Practitioners (Section 30.6.5) of the *Medicare Claims Processing Manual*[2]

30.6.5 - Physicians in Group Practice

B. Office/Outpatient E&M Visits Provided on Same Day for Unrelated Problems

As for all other E&M services except where specifically noted, carriers may not pay two E&M office visits billed by a physician (or physician of the same specialty from the same group practice) for the same beneficiary on the same day unless the physician documents that the visits were for unrelated problems in the office or outpatient setting which could not be provided during the same encounter (eg, office visit for blood pressure medication evaluation, followed five hours later by a visit for evaluation of leg pain following an accident).

This CMS manual guideline instructs that only one office visit would be paid "per physician/per patient" on a single day, unless there were extenuating circumstances (ie, unforeseen and unrelated issues). As an example, a patient presents for a medical visit to manage chronic conditions, including diabetes, hypertension, and chronic obstructive pulmonary disease. If the physician managed only the diabetes during a morning visit and then evaluated the

other chronic conditions during a later visit on that same date, this should be billed as a single E/M service. If, on the other hand, a patient presents for management of chronic conditions, and then, later that day, the same patient falls down a flight of stairs and presents for treatment, the second visit could be separately billed. Clear documentation in these cases is critically important. There are many guidelines relative to coding multiple E/M services on a single date of service. These guidelines should be carefully assessed in coding.

Excerpt From the E/M Coding Policies Section of NCCI[1(p25)]

… the NCCI contains numerous edits based on several principles including, but not limited to:

1. A physician may report only one "new patient" code on a single date of service.

Interpretation

For E/M coding, *new patient* is defined by the CPT codebook and the Medicare manual as an encounter in which the physician has not provided a professional service with that patient within the past three years. Therefore, a second encounter on one day would be impossible to code as a new patient, because three years would not have elapsed between the visits. Do not bill for two new patient visits on a single date of service.

CPT Codebook E/M Introductory Guidelines Defining New Patient[3(p1-2)]

New and Established Patient
Solely for the purposes of distinguishing between new and established patients, **professional services** are those face-to-face services rendered by a physician and reported by a specific CPT code(s). A new patient is one who has not received any professional services from the physician or another physician of the same specialty who belongs to the same group practice, within the past three years.

Excerpt From CMS Manual Section on E/M Coding[3]

Chapter 12, Physicians/Nonphysician Practitioners (Section 30.6.5) of the *Medicare Claims Processing Manual*[2]

30.6.7 - Payment for Office or Other Outpatient Evaluation and Management (E&M) Visits (Codes 99201 - 99215)

Definition of New Patient for Selection of E&M Visit Code

Interpret the phrase "new patient" to mean a patient who has not received any professional services, i.e., E&M service or other face-to-face service (e.g., surgical procedure) from the physician or physician group practice (same physician specialty) within the previous 3 years. For example, if a professional component of a previous procedure is billed in a 3 year time period, e.g., a lab interpretation is billed and no E&M service or other face-to-face service with the patient is performed, then this patient remains a new patient for the initial visit. An interpretation of a diagnostic test, reading an x-ray or EKG, etc., in the absence of an E&M service or other face-to-face service with the patient does not affect the designation of a new patient.

Again, do not code two initial medical visits by a single physician or single, same specialty practice on the same date of service.

Example

Table 3-1 is an excerpt from the NCCI edits table for new patient E/M services.

TABLE 3-1 *Excerpt From NCCI Edits for New Patient E/M Services*

Column 1/Column 2 Edits		
Column 1	Column 2	Modifier 0 = not allowed 1 = allowed 9 = not applicable
99205	92002	0
99205	92004	0
99205	99201	0
99205	99202	0
99205	99203	0
99205	99204	0

Table 3-1 shows that the E/M CPT code 99205 (Level 5 new patient office visit) would include the following new patient E/M CPT codes:

92002-92004   New patient eye examinations

99201-99204   New patient Levels 1-4 outpatient E/M services

If multiple new patient E/M services are billed by the same provider for the same patient on a single date of service, the lesser E/M service would be denied per NCCI. Also, notice that these bundling edits cannot be bypassed with a modifier (modifier indicator is 0—see Chapter 1 of this book for additional information).

Example

The Medically Unlikely Edits (MUEs) limit initial (or new) patient visits to one unit of service per patient, per day. Table 3-2 shows the units of service edits for initial patient visits.

MUEs are based on units of service on a single line item and do not compare different line items. Therefore, this MUE edit would be generated only if a new patient E/M service were billed with a unit of service of two or more.

Excerpt From the E/M Coding Policies Section of NCCI[1(p25)]

… the NCCI contains numerous edits based on several principles including, but not limited to:
2. A physician may report only one code from a range of codes describing an initial E&M service on a single date of service.

TABLE 3-2 *Example of NCCI MUEs for New Patient E/M Services*

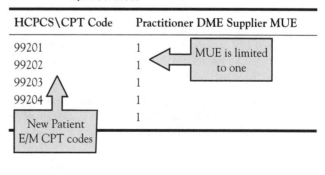

HCPCS\CPT Code	Practitioner DME Supplier MUE
99201	1
99202	1
99203	1
99204	1
	1

Interpretation

Within the E/M section of the CPT codebook, there are categories of initial services. Only one initial E/M service from a category may be billed per patient on a single day. As *initial* indicates the first, or primary, then there should be only one initial service per day.

Example

99221 **Initial hospital care,** per day, for the evaluation and management of a patient, which requires these three key components:
- **A detailed or comprehensive history;**
- **A detailed or comprehensive examination; and**
- **Medical decision making that is straightforward or of low complexity.**

Counseling and/or coordination of care with other providers or agencies are provided consistent with the nature of the problem(s) and the patient's and/or family's needs.

Usually, the problems requiring admission are of low severity. Physicians typically spend 30 minutes at the bedside and on the patient's hospital floor or unit.

99222 **Initial hospital care,** per day, for the evaluation and management of a patient, which requires these three key components:
- A comprehensive history;
- A comprehensive examination; and
- Medical decision making of moderate complexity.

Counseling and/or coordination of care with other providers or agencies are provided consistent with the nature of the problem(s) and the patient's and/or family's needs.

Usually, the problem(s) requiring admission are of moderate severity. Physicians typically spend 50 minutes at the bedside and on the patient's hospital floor or unit.

99223 **Initial hospital care,** per day, for the evaluation and management of a patient, which requires these three key components:
- A comprehensive history;
- A comprehensive examination; and
- Medical decision making of high complexity.

Counseling and/or coordination of care with other providers or agencies are provided consistent with the nature of the problem(s) and the patient's and/or family's needs.

Usually, the problem(s) requiring admission are of high severity. Physicians typically spend 70 minutes at the bedside and on the patient's hospital floor or unit.

Two or more of the above CPT codes could not be billed for a single patient because they represent initial visits and are "per day" codes per their CPT code description. To bill two initial services on a single date of service is counter to CMS and CPT codebook guidelines.

CPT Coding Tip: *A CPT code that designates a service as* initial *is not the same as a* new patient *code. New patient represents those patients who have not had professional services by the provider (or another provider in the same group with the same specialty) within the prior three years. Initial services are those that are the first for that patient for that episode or care or date of service. In our initial hospital care example, the physician billing these services could have a relationship with the patient or not;* initial *in this case simply means the first hospital service for the current hospital stay. The admitting physician would bill this care regardless of the prior relationship and knowledge of the patient.*

The following are the instructions found in the CPT codebook[1(p12)] regarding initial hospital care (emphasis added):

Initial Hospital Care (99221-99223)
New or Established Patient (99221-99223)

The following codes are used to report the ***first*** hospital inpatient encounter with the patient by the admitting physician.

99221 **Initial hospital care,** per day, for the evaluation and management of a patient which requires these three key components:
- **A detailed or comprehensive history;**
- **A detailed or comprehensive examination; and**
- **Medical decision making that is straightforward or of low complexity.**

Counseling and/or coordination of care with other providers or agencies are provided consistent with the nature of the problem(s) and the patient's and/or family's needs.

Usually, the problem(s) requiring admission are of low severity. Physicians typically spend 30 minutes at the bedside and on the patient's hospital floor or unit.

99222 **Initial hospital care,** per day, for the evaluation and management of a patient, which requires these three key components:
- **A comprehensive history;**
- **A comprehensive examination; and**
- **Medical decision making of moderate complexity.**

Counseling and/or coordination of care with other providers or agencies are provided consistent with the nature of the problem(s) and the patient's and/or family's needs.

Usually, the problem(s) requiring admission are of moderate severity. Physicians typically spend 50 minutes at the bedside and on the patient's hospital floor or unit.

99223 **Initial hospital care,** per day, for the evaluation and management of a patient, which requires these three key components:
- **A comprehensive history;**
- **A comprehensive examination; and**
- **Medical decision making of high complexity.**

Counseling and/or coordination of care with other providers or agencies are provided consistent with the nature of the problem(s) and the patient's and/or family's needs.

Usually, the problem(s) requiring admission are of high severity. Physicians typically spend 70 minutes at the bedside and on the patient's hospital floor or unit.

Example

Initial observation care codes are also per day services (boldface type is ours).

99218 Initial observation care, per day, for the evaluation and management of a patient, which requires these three key components:
- **A detailed or comprehensive history;**
- **A detailed or comprehensive examination; and**
- **Medical decision making that is straightforward or of low complexity.**

Counseling and/or coordination of care with other providers or agencies are provided consistent with the nature of the problem(s) and the patient's and/or family's needs.

Usually, the problem(s) requiring admission to "observation status" are of low severity.

99219 Initial observation care, per day, for the evaluation and management of a patient, which requires these three key components:
- **A comprehensive history;**
- **A comprehensive examination; and**
- **Medical decision making of moderate complexity.**

Counseling and/or coordination of care with other providers or agencies are provided consistent with the nature of the problem(s) and the patient's and/or family's needs.

Usually, the problem(s) requiring admission to "observation status" are of moderate severity.

99220 Initial observation care, per day, for the evaluation and management of a patient, which requires these three key components:
- **A comprehensive history;**
- **A comprehensive examination; and**
- **Medical decision making of high complexity.**

Counseling and/or coordination of care with other providers or agencies are provided consistent with the nature of the problem(s) and the patient's and/or family's needs.

Usually, the problem(s) requiring admission to "observation status" are of high severity.

Two or more of the above CPT codes could not be billed for a single patient because they represent initial visits and (and "per day" codes at that) per their CPT code description.

Excerpt From the E/M Coding Policies Section of NCCI[1(p26)]

… the NCCI contains numerous edits based on several principles including, but not limited to:
3. A physician may report only one "per diem" E&M service from a range of per diem codes on a single date of service.

Interpretation

If a CPT code description states *per diem*, that means *per day*, and all E/M services by the same provider on a single day should be combined for a single per diem CPT code. This NCCI instruction is also consistent with the instructions within the CMS manuals.

Excerpt from CMS Manual Section on E/M Coding

Chapter 12, Physicians/Nonphysician Practitioners (Section 30.6.9) of the *Medicare Claims Processing Manual*[2]

30.6.9 - Payment for Inpatient Hospital Visits - General (Codes 99221 - 99239)

Two Hospital Visits Same Day
Contractors pay a physician for only one hospital visit per day for the same patient, whether the problems seen during the encounters are related or not. The inpatient hospital visit descriptors contain the phrase "per day" which means that the code and the payment established for the code represent all services provided on that date. The physician should select a code that reflects all services provided during the date of the service.

B. Hospital Visits Same Day But by Different Physicians
In a hospital inpatient situation involving one physician covering for another, if physician A sees the patient in the morning and physician B, who is covering for A, sees the same patient in the evening, carriers do not pay physician B for the second visit. The hospital visit descriptors include the phrase "per day" meaning care for the day.

If the physicians are each responsible for a different aspect of the patient's care, pay both visits if the physicians are in different specialties and the visits are billed with different diagnoses. There are circumstances where concurrent care may be billed by physicians of the same specialty.

For example, two or more of the initial hospital care CPT codes (CPT 99221-99223) could not be billed for a single patient because they represent initial visits and are "per day" codes per their CPT code description.

Excerpt From the E/M Coding Policies Section of NCCI[1(p26)]

... the NCCI contains numerous edits based on several principles including, but not limited to:
4. A physician should not report an "initial" per diem E&M service with the same type of "subsequent" per diem service on the same date of service.

Interpretation

Codes that are per diem include all the same category services performed on a single date and combined for one comprehensive code. Therefore, *initial* and *subsequent* CPT codes within the same category that are designated as per diem should be combined for a single code. All the documentation for that date can be used to determine the level of service for that one code. However, if there are *initial* and *subsequent* CPT codes within the same category that are not designated as per diem, then there is an opportunity for billing both services, if services are supported by the documentation and patient need.

For example, if a provider admits a patient, performing an initial hospital care service (CPT code 99221-99223) and later that day, re-visits the patient to continue treatment, all the documentation on that date should be combined for a single initial hospital care CPT code. The subsequent hospital care codes (CPT code 99231-99233) should not be used for the second visit on the same date.

Excerpt From the E/M Coding Policies Section of NCCI[1(p26)]

... the NCCI contains numerous edits based on several principles including, but not limited to:
5. E&M codes describing observation/inpatient care services with admission and discharge on same date (CPT codes 99234-99236) should not be reported on the same date of service as initial hospital care per diem codes (99221-99223), subsequent hospital care per diem codes (99231-99233), or hospital discharge day management codes (99238-99239).

Interpretation

This is expanding the guideline for per diem services by stating that when there is a specific comprehensive code that includes all the services provided on that date, the comprehensive code should be used, rather than also coding the component services. In NCCI, as referenced earlier, the example of CPT codes that include admission and discharge care on the same date of service are used. To also code any of the component services would be incorrect. For a patient who is admitted and discharged on the same day, the comprehensive code should be used over the component parts.

This is a common guideline within NCCI—when there is a single comprehensive code, opt for that rather than applying multiple codes.

Excerpt from CMS Manual Section on E/M Coding

Chapter 12, Physicians/Nonphysician Practitioners (Section 30.6.9) of the *Medicare Claims Processing Manual*[2]

30.6.9.1 - Payment for Initial Hospital Care Services (Codes 99221 - 99223) and Observation or Inpatient Care Services (Including Admission and Discharge Services) (Codes 99234 - 99236)

C. Initial Hospital Care and Discharge on Same Day
When a patient has been admitted to inpatient hospital care for a minimum of 8 hours but less than 24 hours and discharged on the same calendar date, Observation or Inpatient Hospital Care Services (Including Admission and Discharge Services), from CPT code range 99234 - 99236, shall be reported.

CPT Codebook Evaluation and Management (E/M) Guidelines Surrounding Observation Care CPT Codes[3(p13-14)]

Observation or Inpatient Care Services (Including Admission and Discharge Services) (99234-99236)
The following codes are used to report observation or inpatient hospital care services provided to patients admitted and discharged on the same date of service. When a patient is admitted to the hospital from observation status on the same date, the physician should report only the initial hospital care code. The initial hospital care code reported by the admitting physician

(continued)

(continued)

should include the services related to the observation status services he/she provided on the same date of inpatient admission.

99234 **Observation or inpatient hospital care,** for the evaluation and management of a patient including admission and discharge on the same date, which requires these three key components:
- **A detailed or comprehensive history;**
- **A detailed or comprehensive examination; and**
- **Medical decision making that is straightforward or of low complexity.**

Counseling and/or coordination of care with other providers or agencies are provided consistent with the nature of the problem(s) and the patient's and/or family's needs.

Usually the presenting problem(s) requiring admission are of low severity.

99235 **Observation or inpatient hospital care,** for the evaluation and management of a patient including admission and discharge on the same date, which requires these three key components:
- **A comprehensive history;**
- **A comprehensive examination; and**
- **Medical decision making of moderate complexity.**

Counseling and/or coordination of care with other providers or agencies are provided consistent with the nature of the problem(s) and the patient's and/or family's needs.

Usually the presenting problem(s) requiring admission are of moderate severity.

99236 **Observation or inpatient hospital care,** for the evaluation and management of a patient including admission and discharge on the same date, which requires these three key components:
- **A comprehensive history;**
- **A comprehensive examination; and**
- **Medical decision making of high complexity.**

Counseling and/or coordination of care with other providers or agencies are provided consistent with the nature of the problem(s) and the patient's and/or family's needs.

Usually the presenting problem(s) requiring admission are of high severity.

Example

If the patient is admitted and discharged from an inpatient status on a single date of service, there is a specific and comprehensive code (see previous) for these services. To bill the component elements (admission and discharge) separately

is incorrect. Special note: CMS has time elements (8 hours) surrounding the use of these codes. Read these guidelines for observation services to make sure coding is compliant. (Hospitals have different guidelines for observation coding.)

Excerpt From the E/M Coding Policies Section of NCCI[1(p26)]

Evaluation and management services, in general, are cognitive services and significant procedural services are not included in the evaluation and management services. Certain procedural services that arise directly from the evaluation and management service are included as part of the evaluation and management service. For example, cleansing of traumatic lesions, closure of lacerations with adhesive strips, dressings, counseling and educational services are included in evaluation and management services.

Interpretation

This guideline is a reminder that only *significant* procedures are to be coded in addition to the E/M CPT code. Other procedures are incidental to the E/M services and are not to be coded separately. The following sections go into these details more specifically. Basically, any service that does not add significantly to the physician's work during the encounter is included in the allowance for that E/M service, and to bill separately for a service that does not add significantly to the work would be noncompliant with guidelines.

Excerpt From the E/M Coding Policies Section of NCCI[1(p26)]

Digital rectal examination for prostate screening (HCPCS code G0102) is not separately reportable with an evaluation and management code. CMS published this policy in the *Federal Register*, November 2, 1999, page 59414 as follows:

"As stated in the July 1999 proposed rule, a digital rectal exam (DRE) is a very quick and simple examination taking only a few seconds. We believe it is rarely the sole reason for a physician encounter and is usually part of an E&M encounter. In those instances when it is the only service furnished or it is furnished as part of an otherwise non-covered service, we will pay separately for code G0102. In those instances when it is furnished on the same day as a covered E&M service, we believe it is appropriate to bundle it into the payment for the covered E&M encounter."

Interpretation

CMS is stating that the digital rectal examination (DRE) should never be separately reported from an E/M service when both services are performed on a single date of service. Tip: Make a note in your CPT codebook to make certain these services are not erroneously unbundled.

HCPCS code G0102 (DRE) bundles into the E/M CPT codes, and you cannot bypass the edit with a modifier. See Table 3-3 for example edits for DRE services with E/M codes. CMS does have a correct coding modifier of 0, which means the DRE services should never be coded in addition to the E/M CPT code.

TABLE 3-3 *Digital Rectal Examination Edit Examples With E/M Services*

	Column 1/Column 2 Edits	
Column 1	Column 2	Modifier 0 = not allowed 1 = allowed 9 = not applicable
99195	99344	9
99201	G0101	9
99201	G0102	0
99201	G0104	9
99202	G0101	9
99202	G0102	0
99202	G0104	9
99203	G0101	9
99203	G0102	0
99203	G0104	9
99203	G0105	9
99204	G0101	9
99204	G0102	0
99204	G0104	9
99205	G0101	9
99205	G0102	0
99205	G0104	9
99205	G0105	9
99205	G0106	9
99205	G0107	9

Excerpt From the E/M Coding Policies Section of NCCI[1(p27)]

Because of the intensive nature of caring for critically ill patients, certain services beyond patient history, examination and medical decision making are included in the overall evaluation and management associated with critical care. Per CPT instructions, services including, but not limited to, the interpretation of cardiac output measurements (CPT codes 93561 and 93562), chest X-rays (CPT codes 71010 and 71020), blood gases, and data stored in computers (EKGs, blood pressures, hematologic data), gastric intubation (CPT code 91105), temporary transcutaneous monitoring (CPT code 92953), ventilator management (CPT codes 94002-94004, 94660, 94662), and vascular access procedures (HCPCS/CPT codes 36000, 36410, 36600) are included in critical and intensive care services and should not be reported separately.

Interpretation

Here CMS is supporting the CPT codebook guidelines on services that are included in the critical care CPT codes. The CPT codebook provides extensive guidance on what is included in the critical care CPT codes.

Excerpt From the E/M Coding Policies Section of NCCI[1(p27)]

Certain sections of CPT codes have incorporated codes describing specialty-specific services which primarily involve evaluation and management services. When codes for these services are reported, a separate evaluation and management service described by the range of CPT codes 99201-99499 is not to be reported on the same date of service. Examples of these codes include general and special ophthalmologic services and general and special diagnostic and therapeutic psychiatric services.

Interpretation

Several categories of CPT codes outside of the E/M section (CPT codes 99201-99499) include E/M services. It would be incorrect to add codes from the E/M section when specific CPT codes include E/M services.

Examples

Ophthalmological services:

92002 Ophthalmological services: medical examination and evaluation with initiation of diagnostic and treatment program; intermediate, new patient

92004 comprehensive, new patient, 1 or more visits

92012 Ophthalmological services: medical examination and evaluation, with initiation or continuation of diagnostic and treatment program; intermediate, established patient

92014 comprehensive, established patient, 1 or more visits

CPT Coding Tip: Codes 92002–92014 are for eye examinations and include all E/M services related to the examination. Other E/M CPT codes should not be billed in addition to these CPT codes.

Psychotherapy services:

90804 Individual psychotherapy, insight oriented, behavior modifying and/or supportive, in an office or outpatient facility, approximately 20 to 30 minutes face-to-face with the patient;

90805 with medical evaluation and management services

CPT Coding Tip: CPT code 90805 would be used when the clinician is providing outpatient psychotherapy and medical evaluation and management services on a single day for one patient. Other outpatient E/M CPT codes should not be billed in addition to these CPT codes. When one physician provides both the psychotherapy and medical evaluation and management care, it would be incorrect coding to bill CPT code 90804 and an E/M CPT code from 99201-99215. Likewise, it would be errant to code CPT code 90804 and CPT code 90805, as CPT code 90805 includes all the elements of CPT code 90804 (note the complete description for CPT code 90804 is before the semi-colon).

90816 Individual psychotherapy, insight oriented, behavior modifying and/or supportive, in an inpatient hospital, partial hospital or residential care setting, approximately 20 to 30 minutes face-to-face with the patient;

90817 with medical evaluation and management services

Excerpt From the E/M Coding Policies Section of NCCI[1(p27)]

> Procedural services involve some degree of physician involvement or supervision which is integral to the service. Separate evaluation and management services are not reported unless a significant, separately identifiable service is provided.

Interpretation

This reiterates that certain non-E/M CPT codes have an element of physician involvement. For those services, it would be incorrect to bill a separate E/M CPT code for the services that are integral to the procedural service CPT code. For example, Physical therapy (CPT code 97001) includes all evaluative services, and distinct procedures directly related to the physical therapy should be included in this evaluation and not separately billed.

Pertaining to the Physical Medicine and Rehabilitation codes 97001, Physical therapy evaluation, and 97003, Occupational therapy evaluation, the August 2006 issue of *CPT Assistant*[4] stated that "Codes 97001 and 97003 include the assessment of the patient, the documentation of the entire evaluation process, as well as the direct contact time spent performing the test or evaluation."

In an article on "Coding Communication: Physical Medicine and Rehabilitation Services," in the December 2003 issue of *CPT Assistant*,[5] the following guidelines were provided:

> … Since some of the physical medicine services include an assessment component as part of preservice work, use of these codes is dependent on whether the service being provided is a significant, separate service, or if it is simply a component of the more involved procedure. Since patient circumstances vary, choice of codes will depend on the specific patient encounter and the intent of the provider.

Physical Medicine Codes

The physical medicine codes 97001, *Physical therapy evaluation*, and 97002, *Physical therapy reevaluation*, are different from the evaluation and management (E/M) codes. They do not include management services and are strictly for the purposes of a comprehensive evaluation and reevaluation needed to support medical necessity for further care. These codes may only be used in addition to other services, if significant enough to report, and require separate effort from the provider in addition to other procedure(s). Codes 97001-97002 should not be used with modifier '25,' as this modifier is intended to be used for codes 99201-99499 included in the E/M section of CPT codebook. Codes 97001-97002 should be used when the physical therapy evaluation and reevaluation are not an inclusive component of the other procedure(s) being provided....

Clinical Example for CPT Code 97001

This is the initial visit with a 56-year-old female who has a medical diagnosis of right shoulder adhesive capsulitis. She is right handed. The patient presents with pain in the right shoulder at rest and during attempted motion. There are limitations in range of motion causing the inability to use the arm for the majority of her activities at work and home. Her medical history is significant for hypertension. She has had shoulder complaints for less than one month. The examination includes but is not limited to range of motion examination; joint integrity and mobility examination; muscle performance examination (including strength, power, and endurance) left as compared to right; respiration, heart rate, blood pressure assessment; consideration of environmental barriers at home and work.

Pre-service work includes coordination or discussion with other team members and review of any medical records including, but not limited to, pertinent imaging or operative reports.

Intra-service work includes examining the patient, obtaining a patient history, performing relevant systems reviews, and using data collection methods to elicit additional objective information; evaluation of the patient based on data gathered from the examination; organizing and interpreting the data to establish a diagnosis and/or obtaining such additional information as may be necessary; development of a plan of care including prognosis for functional improvement and selection of interventions to produce improvement in the patient's condition; education and instruction regarding the cause, prognosis, and plan of care for the patient's condition, which may include prevention and health promotion information.

Post-service work includes documenting the evaluation process (see intra-service work) and the results of the evaluation, as well as communicating with the family and/or caregiver relative to the patient's care and home program.

CPT Assistant is a monthly publication by the AMA that provides additional instruction, information, and explanation of coding complex areas within medical records.

The earlier referenced *CPT Assistant* helps explain what evaluative services are included in the physical therapy evaluation CPT code. In order to bill an additional E/M service for a patient visit with the physical therapy evaluation CPT code, the documentation would have to support

significant E/M services distinct from the CPT code 97001. In this case, it would need to be very substantial or completely separate from the physical therapy evaluation. These tips from the referenced *CPT Assistants* and CMS are useful, as is asking clinicians to clarify what evaluative services are usually performed as an incidental part of the non-E/M CPT code. Remember, for those services that are usual and incidental, payment is included in the CPT code, and only when additional and substantial E/M services are also provided—distinct from the non-E/M service—may an E/M CPT code be billed (often it will be necessary to append a modifier 25 to the E/M CPT code).

Another example would be for Osteopathic Manipulative Treatment (OMT) (98925-98929).

The CPT codebook instructs that E/M services may be reported separate from the OMT, using modifier 25, when the patient's condition requires a significant separately identifiable E/M service, above and beyond the usual preservice and postservice work associated with the procedure. The E/M service may be caused or prompted by the same symptoms or condition for which the OMT service was provided. As such, different diagnoses are not required for the reporting of the OMT and E/M service on the same date.

The August 2000 issue of *CPT Assistant*[6] addressed the issue of whether or not it was to report both an osteopathic manipulative treatment procedure with an evaluation and management (E/M) service when they printed this statement:

> Osteopathic manipulative treatment is a form of manual treatment applied by a physician to eliminate or alleviate somatic dysfunction and related disorders. As stated in the osteopathic manipulative treatment guidelines in CPT, the physician performing the osteopathic procedure may additionally report an E/M service, if the patient's condition requires a significant separately identifiable service, above and beyond the usual preservice and postservice work associated with the procedure. When performing a separate E/M service, the physician must perform the key components for a given level of service. Modifier '-25', Significant, separately identifiable evaluation and management service by the same physician on the same day of the procedure or other service, should be appended to the appropriate level of E/M service code.

Excerpt From the E/M Coding Policies Section of NCCI[1(p28)]

Medicare Global Surgery Rules define the rules for reporting evaluation and management (E&M) services with procedures covered by these rules. This section summarizes some of the rules.

Interpretation

NCCI edits incorporate the CMS guidelines surrounding global surgeries. The following is an excerpt from the CMS manual on global surgeries, and the following sections of this chapter will review them in detail and provide examples. This entire section of the manual should be reviewed prior to billing for global surgery care.

Excerpt From the CMS Manual Section 30.6.6

Chapter 12, Physicians/Nonphysician Practitioners (Section 30.6.6) of the *Medicare Claims Processing Manual*[2]

30.6.6 - Payment for Evaluation and Management Services Provided During Global Period of Surgery

A. CPT Modifier "-24" - Unrelated Evaluation and Management Service by Same Physician During Postoperative Period

Carriers pay for an evaluation and management service other than inpatient hospital care before discharge from the hospital following surgery (CPT codes 99221-99238) if it was provided during the postoperative period of a surgical procedure, furnished by the same physician who performed the procedure, billed with CPT modifier "-24," and accompanied by documentation that supports that the service is not related to the postoperative care of the procedure. They do not pay for inpatient hospital care that is furnished during the hospital stay in which the surgery occurred unless the doctor is also treating another medical condition that is unrelated to the surgery. All care provided during the inpatient stay in which the surgery occurred is compensated through the global surgical payment.

B. CPT Modifier "-25" - Significant Evaluation and Management Service by Same Physician on Date of Global Procedure

Medicare requires that Current Procedural Terminology (CPT) modifier -25 should only be used on claims for evaluation and management (E&M) services, and only when these services are provided by the same physician (or same qualified nonphysician practitioner) to the same patient on the same day as another procedure or other service. Carriers pay for an E&M service provided on the day of a procedure with a global fee period if the physician indicates that the service is for a significant, separately identifiable E&M service that is above and beyond the usual pre- and post-operative work of the procedure.

(continued)

(continued)

Different diagnoses are not required for reporting the E&M service on the same date as the procedure or other service. Modifier -25 is added to the E&M code on the claim.

Both the medically necessary E&M service and the procedure must be appropriately and sufficiently documented by the physician or qualified nonphysician practitioner in the patient's medical record to support the claim for these services, even though the documentation is not required to be submitted with the claim.

If the physician bills the service with the CPT modifier "-25," carriers pay for the service in addition to the global fee without any other requirement for documentation unless one of the following conditions is met:

- When inpatient dialysis services are billed (CPT codes 90935, 90945, 90947, and 93937), the physician must document that the service was unrelated to the dialysis and could not be performed during the dialysis procedure;
- When preoperative critical care codes are being billed on the date of the procedure, the diagnosis must support that the service is unrelated to the performance of the procedure; or
- When a carrier has conducted a specific medical review process and determined, after reviewing the data, that an individual or a group has high use of modifier "-25" compared to other physicians, has done a case-by-case review of the records to verify that the use of modifier was inappropriate, and has educated the individual or group, the carrier may impose prepayment screens or documentation requirements for that provider or group. When a carrier has completed a review and determined that a high usage rate of modifier "-57," the carrier must complete a case-by-case review of the records. Based upon this review, the carrier will educate providers regarding the appropriate use of modifier "-57." If high usage rates continue, the carrier may impose prepayment screens or documentation requirements for that provider or group.

Carriers may not permit the use of CPT modifier "-25" to generate payment for multiple evaluation and management services on the same day by the same physician, notwithstanding the CPT definition of the modifier.

C. CPT Modifier "-57" - Decision for Surgery Made Within Global Surgical Period

Carriers pay for an evaluation and management service on the day of or on the day before a procedure with a 90-day global surgical period if the physician uses CPT modifier "-57" to indicate that the service resulted in the decision to perform the procedure. Carriers may not pay for an evaluation and management service billed with the CPT modifier "-57" if it was provided on the day of or the day before a procedure with a 0 or 10-day global surgical period.

Interpretation

Three modifiers are applicable to E/M coding within a surgery's global period. Modifiers 24, 25, and 57 are modifiers applied only to E/M codes and only to request payment outside a surgery or procedure's reimbursement. Only modifiers 25 and 57 can bypass NCCI edits (when appropriately documented). However, modifier 24 allows bypassing of global surgery bundling.

Excerpt From the E/M Coding Policies Section of NCCI[1(p28)]

All procedures on the Medicare Physician Fee Schedule are assigned a Global period of 000, 010, 090, XXX, YYY, or ZZZ. The global concept does not apply to XXX procedures. The global period for YYY procedures is defined by the Carrier. All procedures with a global period of ZZZ are related to another procedure, and the applicable global period for the ZZZ code is determined by the related procedure.

Interpretation

A 0-day global period means that procedure's reimbursement includes all care directly related to the performance of that procedure and normal follow-up on the date of the procedure only. If the patient presented the next day for additional, related services, the global period is over, and the care the next day is not considered a part of the procedure—it would be separately reimbursed.

A 10-day global period means that procedure's reimbursement includes all care directly related to the performance of that procedure and normal follow-up care on the date of the procedure and during the following 10 days.

A 90-day global period means that procedure's reimbursement includes all care directly related to the performance of that procedure and normal follow-up care on the date immediately preceding the date of the surgery, the actual date of the surgery, and the following 90 days. Medicare also tells us that surgeries with a 90-day global period are major surgeries.

An MMM-day global period is reserved CPT codes for maternity and means that procedure does not follow the usual global period. The global period would be driven by the payer.

A ZZZ-day global period means that procedure is considered an add-on to another procedure, and the global care is included in the main procedure's reimbursement. Because these codes are never billed alone, there is no need to assign a global period to them.

A YYY-day global period means that the individual carrier will determine the number of global days for that code (it will be 0-90).

Example

CPT code 59400 has an MMM global period.

59400 Routine obstetric care including antepartum care, vaginal delivery (with or without episiotomy, and/or forceps) and post-partum care

This code includes, as is shown by the CPT code description, the usual antepartum and postpartum (before and after birth) care in the maternity care reimbursement. Those prepartum and postpartum visits that are usual to the maternity care should not be billed separately from the maternity codes. Note that this guideline is in effect even though these services are not going to be performed on the same date as the delivery.

Example

CPT 11100 has a global period of 0.
CPT 11101 has a ZZZ global period.

11100 Biopsy of skin, subcutaneous tissue and/or mucous membrane (including simple closure), unless otherwise listed; single lesion

+ 11101 each separate/additional lesion (List separately in addition to code for primary procedure)

CPT 11100 has a global period of 0; therefore, related and not separately distinct E/M services provided on the same date would be included in this code and not billed in addition to the biopsy. However, CPT 11101 is an add-on code, and for add-on codes, the global period is tied to the primary code. The primary CPT code global period applies to the add-on code as well.

Excerpt From the E/M Coding Policies Section of NCCI[1(p28)]

Since NCCI edits are applied to same day services by the same provider to the same beneficiary, certain Global Surgery Rules are applicable to NCCI. An E&M service is separately reportable on the same date of service as a procedure with a global period of 000, 010, or 090 under limited circumstances.

If a procedure has a global period of 090 days, it is defined as a major surgical procedure. If an E&M is performed on the same date of service as a major surgical procedure for the purpose of deciding whether to perform this surgical procedure, the E&M service is separately reportable with modifier -57. Other E&M services on the same date of service as a major surgical procedure are included in the global payment for the procedure and are not separately reportable. NCCI does not contain edits based on this rule because Medicare Carriers have separate edits.

Interpretation

Figure 3-1 illustrates how surgery care extends beyond what happens during the procedure itself. Services in each phase are either included in the surgery reimbursement or are paid separately. Our job when coding is to determine which is billable separately and make sure we capture it.

A global surgical fee includes all necessary services performed by the physician before, during, and after a surgical procedure. Medicare payment for a given surgical procedure includes applicable preoperative and intraoperative services, complications, and postoperative care.

Reimbursement for the surgery also includes payment for any preoperative care, the surgery itself, and appropriate and normal follow-up care. Determining which services are acceptable to report in addition to the main procedure is a challenge. The global surgical package is essential to access and understand in order to appropriately code and bill. Global periods are assigned to almost every surgical procedure. That period can range from 0 to 90 days. Regardless of whether or not a procedure has a global period assigned, each and every code will have a designation as to the global aspect of the reimbursement for that procedure. Codes with a 0 or 10-day global period are minor procedures and endoscopies. Codes with a 90-day global period are considered major surgeries.

Carriers apply the national definition of a global surgical package to all procedures with the appropriate entry in Field 16 of the Medicare Fee Schedule Database (MFSDB) or Physician Fee Schedule (PFS). The current MFSDB/PFS can be downloaded from the CMS Web site at www.cms.hhs.gov. Table 3-4 is an excerpt from the PFS, illustrating global days.

The Medicare-approved amount for these procedures includes payment for the following services related to the surgery when they are furnished by the physician who performs the surgery.

- **Preoperative visits** after the decision is made to operate beginning with the day before the day of surgery for major procedures and the day of surgery for minor procedures
- **Intraoperative services** that are normally a usual and necessary part of a surgical procedure
- **Complications following surgery** that do not require additional trips to the operating room
- **Postoperative visits** that are related to recovery from the surgery
- **Postsurgical pain management** by the surgeon
- **Supplies**
- **Miscellaneous services:** Items such as dressing changes; local incisional care; removal of operative pack; removal of cutaneous sutures and staples, lines, wires, tubes, drains, casts, and splints; insertion, irrigation, and removal of urinary catheters, routine peripheral intravenous lines, nasogastric and rectal tubes; and changes and removal of tracheostomy tubes.

The services included in the global surgical package may be furnished in any setting, for example, in hospitals, Ambulatory Surgery Centers (ASCs), physicians' offices. Visits to a patient in an intensive care or critical care unit are also included if made by the surgeon. However, critical care services (99291 and 99292) are payable separately in some situations.

FIGURE 3-1 *Illustration Inclusive Components of a Surgical Code*

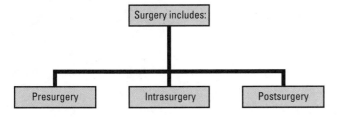

TABLE 3-4 *Excerpt From Medicare Fee Schedule for Global Day Periods*

HCPCS	Description	Global Days
15321	Apply sknallogrft f/n/hfg add	ZZZ
15330	Apply acell alogrft t/arm/leg	090
15331	Apply acell grft t/a/l add-on	ZZZ
15335	Apply acell graft, f/n/hf/g	090
15336	Apply acell grft f/n/hf/g add	ZZZ
15340	Apply cult skin substitute	010
15341	Apply cult skin sub add-on	ZZZ
15360	Apply cult derm sub, t/a/l	090
15361	Apply cult derm sub t/a/l add	ZZZ
15365	Apply cult derm sub f/n/hf/g	090
15366	Apply cult derm f/hf/g add	ZZZ

See the earlier explanation of global days found within this chapter. This will help to determine how many days are applicable to the code.

The Medicare-approved amount for procedures does not include payment for the following services. These services may be paid separately.

- **The initial consultation or evaluation** of the problem by the surgeon to determine the need for surgery. Please note that this policy applies only to major surgical procedures. The initial evaluation is always included in the allowance for a minor surgical procedure
- **Services of other physicians** except where the surgeon and the other physician(s) agree on the transfer of care
- **Visits unrelated to the diagnosis** for which the surgical procedure is performed, unless the visits occur due to complications of the surgery
- **Treatment for the underlying condition** or an added course of treatment that is not part of normal recovery from surgery
- **Diagnostic tests and procedures**
- **Clearly distinct surgical procedures** during the postoperative period that are not re-operations or treatment for complications
- **Treatment for postoperative complications that require a return trip to the operating room**
- If a less extensive procedure fails, and a **more extensive procedure** is required, the second procedure is payable separately if on a different date than the original procedure
- **Splints and casting supplies** are payable separately under the reasonable charge payment methodology
- **Immunosuppressive therapy for organ transplants**
- **Critical care services (codes 99291 and 99292) unrelated to the surgery**

CMS Tip: *Medicare screens for high use of modifiers 25 and 57. This should not discourage their use when appropriate documentation supports them. Other payers use modifiers 25 and 57 differently from Medicare. Understanding their requirements is a must. Accounts receivable management personnel must do a good job of evaluating payments, denials, and reductions.*

Payers should be asked the following questions:

1. *Do you follow CPT guidelines of surgical packaging and modifier application? If they do, use the CPT book definition of surgical packages. If they do not, request their guidelines.*
2. *Do you follow Medicare's global surgery guidelines, including the global surgery days? If they do, ask for a copy of the Medicare guidelines they follow and review for variations from Medicare. If they do not, ask for their guidelines.*

We have seen some payers who use modifier 25 instead of modifier 57 or vice versa and some payers who do not acknowledge either. Challenge them to make sure both parties are in agreement contractually.

Bottom Line for Modifiers 25 and 57

Modifier 57 indicates that the E/M service resulted in the decision to perform major surgery. Medicare carriers pay for an E/M service on the day of, or the day before, a procedure with a 90-day global period, if the service resulted in the decision to perform the procedure. It would not be appropriate to bill E/M services with modifier 57 if the services were provided on the day before, or the day of, a procedure with a 0 or 10-day global surgical period. Also, modifier 57 would not be appropriate for preoperative visits. With preoperative visits, the decision for surgery has already been made. Scheduled preoperative visits the day before or day of surgery are included in the global package and should not be billed with a modifier 57. This also applies to minor procedures, those with 0 to 10 global days, and modifier 25. Preoperative care is part of the global package for major and minor procedures.

For NCCI edits, this is an issue only for those E/M services performed on the same date as the minor procedure (modifier 25) or major surgery (modifier 57).

Excerpt From the E/M Coding Policies Section of NCCI[1(p28)]

If a procedure has a global period of 000 or 010 days, it is defined as a minor surgical procedure. The decision to perform a minor surgical procedure is included in the payment for the minor surgical procedure and should not be reported separately as an E&M service. However, a significant and separately identifiable E&M service unrelated to the decision to perform the minor surgical procedure is separately reportable with modifier -25. NCCI does contain some edits based on these principles, but the Medicare Carriers have separate edits. Neither the NCCI nor Carriers have all possible edits based on these principles.

Interpretation

Modifier 25 is a difficult modifier to interpret correctly because there is no specific guideline for the level of documentation required for the E/M service to be considered significantly separate from the procedure performed on the same date of service. Modifier 25 use will be more closely reviewed in the next section of this chapter.

A medical visit encounter is paid separate from a minor procedure when the visit is where the decision for the procedure is made if:

1. the medical visit portion of the encounter exceeds what is usual preoperative preparation or evaluation for the procedure *and*
2. the medical visit portion supports an E/M level "on its own" separate from the procedure note.

When these criteria are met, modifier 25 is used on the E/M to designate a separately identifiable medical visit in addition to a minor procedure when performed on the same date. Again, if the procedures are performed on a separate date, no modifier is necessary to support the distinct E/M care. The medical visit portion of the encounter may be for a related, same, or different diagnosis than the procedure.

Some quick examples:
1. A physician sees a patient in the office on Monday and determines that the patient needs major surgery, which is performed on Tuesday. Modifier 57 is appended to the E/M code for the office visit on Monday to indicate that it represents the decision for surgery and should not be included in the surgical package.
2. A physician is requested to perform a consultation on a patient with abdominal pain. The physician meets the consultation criteria (ie, documents findings, communicates with the requesting physician). The requesting physician agrees with the consultant's findings and transfers care to the consultant. The patient consents to the surgery for repair of a perforated ulcer, which is performed later that day. The surgeon reports the consultation E/M with modifier 57 and reports the surgery CPT code.

CPT Coding Tip: *The medical visit portion of the encounter for a minor procedure must be above and beyond what is usual work-up. That means if a patient presents with a laceration, and a minimal work-up is performed to determine the need for the surgery (ie, examination of that immediate site only), then the E/M with modifier 25 is not supported. However, if the medical visit extends to include a neurological work-up, or medical decision making supports an unclear picture as to the problem and solution, those visits should be justifiably coded with modifier 25.*

Medicare states that the initial evaluation is always included in the payment for a minor procedure. An example would be if a patient presents for a planned epidural steroid injection (ESI) for pain management. The provider takes the patient's vital signs, makes sure there have been no clinically significant changes since the last visit, obtains consent for the procedure, and proceeds with the ESI. In this example, there is nothing to support an E/M service separate from the ESI service. It is a planned procedure, and minimal history and examination are performed, which are usual for the procedure.

Another example would be for a patient who presents with leg spasms. The provider takes a detailed history from the patient to determine the location, duration, severity, any associated signs and symptoms of the current problem as well as inquiring about pertinent other systems and the patient's personal, family, and social history. Additionally, the physician performs an expanded, problem-focused examination and finally determines that an ESI will be given to the patient to see if that alleviates the pain and schedules the patient to return in four weeks after some radiographs are obtained. In this example, clearly there should be enough documentation for both the E/M and ESI to be billed. A modifier 25 would be appended to the E/M service.

Excerpt From the E/M Coding Policies Section of NCCI[1(p29)]

Procedures with a global surgery indicator of "XXX" are not covered by these rules. Many of these "XXX" procedures are performed by physicians and have inherent pre-procedure, intra-procedure, and post-procedure work usually performed each time the procedure is completed. This work should never be reported as a separate E&M code. Other "XXX" procedures are not usually performed by a physician and have no physician work relative value units associated with them. A physician should never report a separate E&M code with these procedures for the supervision of others performing the procedure or for the interpretation of the procedure. With most "XXX" procedures, the physician may, however, perform a significant and separately identifiable E&M service on the same day of service which may be reported by appending modifier –25 to the E&M code. This E&M service may be related to the same diagnosis necessitating performance of the "XXX" procedure but cannot include any work inherent in the "XXX" procedure, supervision of others performing the "XXX" procedure, or time for interpreting the result of the "XXX" procedure. Appending modifier –25 to a significant, separately identifiable E&M service when performed on the same date of service as an "XXX" procedure is correct coding.

Interpretation

An XXX-day global period means that the code has no global concept affiliated with it—the global period does not apply. However, many codes include a certain level of oversight that should not be coded separately with an E/M code. An example would be for chest x-rays (CPT code 71020, which has an XXX global period). Plain films have no global period. The NCCI guidelines for radiology services and E/M (to be covered in the radiology chapter of this book) instruct that when physicians must interact with a patient in order to accomplish the radiograph, that interaction is usually limited to pertinent history, obtaining informed consent, discussion of follow-up, and reviewing the medical record. In that case, the E/M portion of the plain film would not be separately reported. However, if the physician who is performing the plain film is also assessing the patient's presenting complaints, determining the need for a radiograph, and performing the elements necessary to support a separate E/M CPT code, then the E/M could be billed.

SUMMARY

- NCCI edits incorporate CMS reimbursement guidelines and CPT codebook instructions. Each of these resources should be thoroughly reviewed, evaluated, and incorporated in coding all Medicare services.

- For the most part, E/M coding is based on the total care provided to a patient on a single day; therefore, all documentation for a single patient for a day should be reviewed prior to coding.

- E/M coding is primarily found in the 99201-99499 range of CPT codes; however, there are codes in other sections of HCPCS codes (ophthalmology medicine, psychotherapy medicine, HCPCS Level II) that include E/M-type services. Guidelines applicable to E/M would also apply to these other codes unless otherwise instructed.

Definitions and Acronyms

Centers for Medicare and Medicaid Services (CMS): This is a branch of the Department of Health and Human Services (DHHS) responsible for overseeing the Medicare and Medicaid federal health care programs.

Documentation guideline: Medicare (as well as many payers) follows documentation guidelines to determine how levels of E/M services are documented to support the differing levels of E/M CPT codes. Two versions of the official guidelines are used: 1995 and 1997. These documentation guidelines can be downloaded from the CMS web site, www.cms.hhs.gov.

Healthcare Common Procedure Coding System (HCPCS): These are the code sets used for filing Medicare bills consisting of Level I CPT codes and Level II HCPCS codes.

CHAPTER EXERCISES

1. A new patient presents for evaluation of arthritis, hypertension, and diabetes. The history, examination, and medical decision making support code 99202. During the examination, the patient's shoulder is hurting badly, and the physician decides to do a joint injection, which is done. Is modifier 25 supported?

2. A physician examines an established patient exhibiting pain in the elbow and performs a joint injection. Documentation supports a code 99214. The above-mentioned symptoms prompted the patient's visit to his physician; however, the patient did not visit his physician with the intention of having a joint injection procedure performed, and on examination by the physician, it was determined that a joint injection would be performed. Is modifier 25 supported?

3. A patient presents with severe abdominal pain. During the history and physical examination, the need for a cholecystectomy is determined, and the procedure is scheduled for the next day. Is modifier 57 supported?

4. The same patient has a personal emergency and reschedules the surgery for one week later, and the physician performs a preoperative assessment the day of surgery. Is modifier 57 supported for the preoperative assessment?

ANSWERS TO CHAPTER EXERCISES

1. Yes. A modifier 25 is supported because the joint injection has no direct relationship to evaluating and managing the chronic conditions.

2. We do not know with this example. Although the level of service (99214) seems to indicate there is extensive documentation, the documentation would need to be carefully reviewed to see if a Level 4 E/M is supported in addition to the joint injection. It is very likely that an E/M is supported as medically necessary, but it would seem odd that a Level 4 would be warranted in addition to billing the joint injection. Remember, portions of the visit are related to and incorporated in the joint injection's reimbursement and should not be separately coded. Most likely, a lower level E/M service with a modifier 25 would be billed in addition to the joint injection, depending on the documentation.

3. Yes, as long as the E/M service is well documented, the E/M should be billed with a modifier 57.

4. No. The decision for surgery has been made, and the preoperative assessment is included in the surgery's reimbursement and should not be separately coded.

REFERENCES

1. Centers for Medicare and Medicaid Services. "Chapter XI Medicine, Evaluation and Management Services," In: NCCI Policy Manual for Medicare Services. www.cms.hhs.gov/ NationalCorrectCodInitEd/01_overview.asp#TopOfPage. Accessed June 11, 2009.

2. Centers for Medicare and Medicaid Services. Physicians/ Nonphysician Practitioners. In: *Medicare Claims Processing Manual.* www.cms.hhs.gov/manuals/downloads/clm104c12.pdf. Accessed June 11, 2009.

3. American Medical Association. *Current Procedural Terminology CPT® 2009 Professional Edition.* Chicago, IL: American Medical Association; 2008.

4. American Medical Association. "Medicine: Physical medicine and rehabilitation, 97001, 97003 (Q&A)," *CPT® Assistant.* 2006; 16(8):11.

5. American Medical Association. "Coding communication, physical medicine and rehabilitation services, Part I," *CPT® Assistant.* 2003;13(12):4.

6. American Medical Association. "Coding consultation, evaluation and management, 98925-98929, 00025 (Q&A)," *CPT® Assistant.* 2000;10(8):11.

Chapter 4

Anesthesia Services

For anesthesiologists and other providers who provide anesthesia care, these guidelines are important. The National Correct Coding Initiative (NCCI) policies applicable to anesthesia services are found within the second section of the NCCI guidelines. The related *Current Procedural Terminology CPT® 2009 Professional Edition*[1] codes are found in the anesthesia section of CPT code range 00100-01999. This chapter analyzes the NCCI policies for anesthesia services and provides interpretations as well as examples of the guidelines. As with all chapters of NCCI edits, the policies in the General NCCI Policies chapter (Chapter 2 of this book) apply to the anesthesia services as well.

 CMS Tip: *NCCI edits are updated quarterly, and the institutional version is one calendar quarter behind the physician version. As of January 1, 2009, anesthesia edits are applicable to institutional claims. Prior to this date, these edits were not applied to institutional services.*

Background About Anesthesia

Anesthesia is the administration of a drug or gas to induce partial or complete loss of consciousness. As mentioned earlier, services involving the administration of anesthesia are billed using the CPT anesthesia codes (00100-01999) and an appropriate modifier. Surgery codes are not appropriate for billing anesthesia services, although there are times when the anesthesiologist or certified registered nurse anesthetist (CRNA) may perform a procedure outside of what is included in the anesthesia service, and a nonanesthesia code would be needed.

Introduction to NCCI Policies Regarding Anesthesia Services

Excerpt From the Anesthesia Section of NCCI[1(p2)]

A. Introduction
The principles of correct coding discussed in Chapter I apply to the CPT codes in the range 00100-01999. Several general guidelines are repeated in this Chapter. However, those general guidelines from Chapter I not discussed in this chapter are nonetheless applicable.

Interpretation

The instruction indicates that the overall NCCI guidelines apply to each section of the CPT codebook, and, even if they are not repeated within a chapter, they are nonetheless a guideline to be followed. The introductory guidelines were reviewed comprehensively in Chapter 2 of this book. Review Chapter 2 completely before proceeding to this chapter.

CPT codes for anesthesia capture those services provided by an anesthesia provider. The Centers for Medicare and Medicaid Services (CMS) indicates that the providers for anesthesia include physicians, CRNAs, or anesthesia assistants (AAs) with appropriate medical direction. CMS recognizes both CRNAs and AAs as nonphysician anesthesia providers; however, CRNAs may provide anesthesia with or without medical direction, whereas AAs must provide services only under medical direction by an anesthesiologist. In cases of medical direction, both the anesthesiologist and the CRNA would bill Medicare for their component of the procedure. Each provider should use the appropriate anesthesia modifier. See Table 4-1 for anesthesia modifiers used by providers.

TABLE 4-1 *Anesthesia Modifiers*

Anesthesiologist Modifier	Description
AA	Anesthesia services personally performed by the anesthesiologist
QY	Medical direction of one CRNA by an anesthesiologist
QK	Medical direction of two, three, or four concurrent anesthesia procedures
AD	Supervision, more than four procedures

These modifiers are separate from the potential modifiers related to NCCI edits discussed in this chapter.

Excerpt From the Anesthesia Coding Policies Section of NCCI[1(2-3)]

The anesthesia care package consists of preoperative evaluation, standard preparation and monitoring services, administration of anesthesia, and post-anesthesia recovery care. Preoperative evaluation includes a sufficient history and physical examination so that the risk of adverse reactions can be minimized, alternative approaches to anesthesia planned, and all questions regarding the anesthesia procedure by the patient answered. Types of anesthesia include local, regional, epidural, general, moderate conscious sedation, or monitored anesthesia care (MAC). The anesthesia practitioner assumes responsibility for the post-anesthesia recovery period which includes all care until the patient is released to the surgeon or another physician. Anesthesia services include, but are not limited to, preoperative evaluation of the patient, administration of anesthetic, other medications, blood, and fluids, monitoring of physiological parameters, and other supportive services.

Interpretation

The anesthesiologist is a perioperative physician who provides care to each patient throughout the surgical experience as it relates to the anesthesia the patient will receive. This includes medically evaluating the patient before surgery (preoperative), consulting with the surgical team, providing pain control, supporting life functions during surgery (intraoperative), supervising care after surgery (postoperative), and often medically discharging the patient from the recovery unit. All of these are incidental to the payment for the anesthesia service and should not be billed separately. To do so would violate the NCCI and CPT codebook guidelines.

CPT Codebook Anesthesia Introductory Guidelines[2(p37)]

These services include the usual preoperative and post-operative visits, the anesthesia care during the procedure, the administration of fluids and/or blood, and the usual monitoring services (eg, ECG, temperature, blood pressure, oximetry, capnography, and mass spectrometry).

For example, if a patient presents for a scheduled colectomy surgery to be performed under general anesthesia and the anesthesiologist evaluates the patient in the preoperative suite to ensure that he is able to safely undergo general anesthesia. This includes a review of the patient's intake chart, a meeting with the patient to include a brief history and examination—all of which are oriented toward the patient's readiness for general anesthesia. Once the patient is in the operating room, the anesthesiologist induces the anesthesia and monitors the patient during the procedure. When the procedure is complete, the anesthesiologist would evaluate the patient in the post-anesthesia care unit (PACU) to make sure he has recovered (adequacy of breathing, circulation, level of consciousness, oxygen saturation) and that his pain is under control.

Excerpt From the Anesthesia Coding Policies Section of NCCI[1(p3)]

Anesthesiologists may personally perform anesthesia services or may supervise anesthesia services performed by a CRNA or AA. CRNAs may perform anesthesia services independently or under the supervision of an anesthesiologist. An AA always performs anesthesia services under the direction of an anesthesiologist. Anesthesiologists personally performing anesthesia services and non-medically directed CRNAs bill in a standard fashion in accordance with CMS regulations as outlined in the *Internet-Only Manuals (IOM)*, *Medicare Claims Processing Manual*, Publication 100-04, Chapter 12, Sections 50 and 140.2 CRNAs and AAs practicing under the medical direction of anesthesiologists follow instructions and regulations regarding this arrangement as outlined in the above sections of the *Medicare Claims Processing Manual*.[3]

Interpretation

Under Medicare regulations, an anesthesia procedure is considered "personally performed" by the anesthesiologist if the physician is continuously involved in a single case. When the anesthesiologist or CRNA personally performs the anesthesia service for a patient, the provider may not leave the operating room to perform other medical procedures. He or she must remain physically present in the operating room during the entire procedure. Medically directed anesthesia is defined as a single anesthesia case that involves oversight by a provider other than the provider who remains in the room with the patient, with both providers having clinical responsibility for the patient's anesthesia.

The NCCI guideline highlights the importance of correctly representing whether the case is personally performed or medically directed, because there are different coding guidelines and payment methodologies for these. Also, the licensure of the performing provider determines whether medical direction is optional (CRNA) or mandatory (AA).

When coding for anesthesia, one should review the appropriate anesthesia resources on the CMS Web site.[2] There are many references available—a few of which are shown in Table 4-2.

Example

Two separate claims must be filed for medically directed anesthesia procedures when a physician and CRNA are the providers. One of the claims is for the anesthesiologist, and one is for the CRNA. The payment is limited to 50% for each provider so that the reimbursement mimics what a single provider would receive. Here are some of the coding guidelines important to know:

- When an anesthesiologist is medically directing one CRNA, the anesthesiologist would bill with the QY modifier, and the CRNA would bill with the QX modifier. Medicare reimbursement is divided between the two providers, with each receiving 50% of the allowed amount.
- When an anesthesiologist is medically directing two, three, or four CRNAs, the anesthesiologist would bill with the QK modifier, and the CRNAs would bill with the QX modifier. The Medicare payment would be divided between the two providers, with each provider receiving 50% of the allowable amount.

Anesthesia Policies and NCCI

> **Excerpt From the Anesthesia Coding Policies Section of NCCI**[1(p3-4)]
>
> Anesthesia codes describe a general anatomic area or service which usually relates to a number of surgical procedures, often from multiple sections of the *CPT Manual*. For Medicare purposes, only one anesthesia code is reported unless the anesthesia code is an add-on code. In this case, both the code for the primary anesthesia service and the anesthesia add-on code are reported according to *CPT Manual* instructions.

Interpretation

According to this guideline, only one anesthesia CPT code may be used per anesthetic (surgery) session. If there are

TABLE 4-2 *Screen Shot of CMS Web Site for Anesthesia Resources*

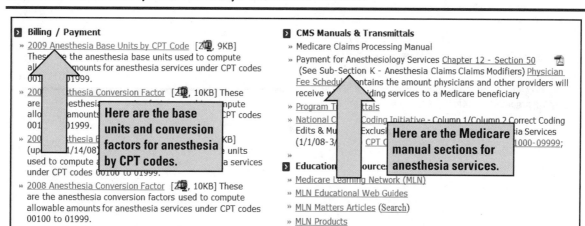

multiple codes that apply to the surgical session, only the most complex anesthesia code should be billed. However, the time for the entire anesthesia service should be used for the units of service. This guideline is applicable only to single surgery sessions. If a patient returns to the operating room for another procedure on the same date of service as the original surgery, and if the second procedure required anesthesia, the second anesthetic encounter may be coded with an appropriate modifier (eg, repeat procedure would require modifier 76 or 77, staged procedure would require modifier 58, unrelated procedure, modifier 59). The NCCI modifiers would be in addition to the anesthesia modifiers (AA, QY, etc).

 CMS Tip: There are few edits within the NCCI to bundle multiple anesthesia procedures, so the provider must understand the guidelines and bill appropriately. Medicare instructs to report one anesthesia code per encounter (unless there is an appropriate add-on code); however, there are Medicare training manuals that instruct all codes to be billed, and Medicare will pay only one. Be careful to avoid overpayments and compliance risks. So, as an example, if a patient is having multiple procedures performed during a single operative session due to trauma (gunshot wound), and multiple anesthesia codes would apply, only the highest-based anesthesia CPT code should be used. See the following CPT codes for this example:

01480 Anesthesia for open procedures on bones of lower leg, ankle, and foot; not otherwise specified

Base unit - 3

00770 Anesthesia for all procedures on major abdominal blood vessels

Base unit - 15

01740 Anesthesia for open or surgical arthroscopic procedures of the elbow; not otherwise specified

Base unit - 4

For this scenario, the base unit of 15 would be used to calculate reimbursement, and the other procedures would be bundled into the 15. Remember, however, total time for the entire procedure would be used to calculate the units of service.

Example

01951 Anesthesia for second- and third-degree burn excision or debridement with or without skin grafting, any site, for total body surface area (TBSA) treated during anesthesia and surgery; less than 4% total body surface area

Base unit - 3

+ 01953 each additional 9% total body surface area or part thereof (List separately in addition to code for primary procedure)

Base unit - 1

Because 01953 is an add-on code (never billed alone), both the base units (3 + 1) would be used to calculate the reimbursement.

Example

A patient is returned to the operating room on the same day as the original surgery to repair a complication from the first procedure. The same anesthesiologists provided the anesthesia for each session. The second procedure should be billed with a modifier 78 (Unplanned Return to the Operating/Procedure Room by the Same Physician Following Initial Procedure for a Related Procedure During the Postoperative Period). Table 4-3 illustrates how the claim would be billed.

 CMS Tip: Base units can be obtained from the CMS web site.[3]

TABLE 4-3 *Billing Snapshot, Example 3*

Provider	Date of Service	Procedure	Modifier
Anesthesiologist	01/01/2009	00740	AA, First service
Anesthesiologist	01/01/2009	00810	AA, 78, Return to operating room

Excerpt From the Anesthesia Coding Policies Section of NCCI[1(p4)]

A unique characteristic of anesthesia coding is the reporting of time units. Payment for anesthesia services increases with time. In addition to reporting a basic unit value for an anesthesia service, the anesthesia practitioner reports anesthesia time. Anesthesia time is defined as the period during which an anesthesia practitioner is present with the patient. It starts when the anesthesia practitioner begins to prepare the patient for anesthesia services in the operating room or an equivalent area and ends when the anesthesia practitioner is no longer furnishing anesthesia services to the patient. Anesthesia time is a continuous time period from the start of anesthesia to the end of an anesthesia service. In counting anesthesia time, the anesthesia practitioner can add blocks of time around an interruption in anesthesia time as long as the anesthesia practitioner is furnishing continuous anesthesia care within the time periods around the interruption.

Interpretation

According to CMS guidelines, anesthesia time begins when the anesthesiologist starts to prepare the patient for the procedure. This preparation does not include the minimal history and physical examination portion of care, but rather the actual preparing the patient for the anesthesia. This preparation usually occurs in the operating room, but on occasion the preparation may begin in another location (ie, preoperative suite). Anesthesia time is a continuous time period from the start of anesthesia to the end of an anesthesia service (personal attendance of the anesthesiologist). However, if an interruption in the anesthesiologist's care for the patient occurs, the time where anesthesia care is not being provided should not count toward the total time for the anesthesia, and this should be clearly documented by the anesthesiologist to ensure appropriate billing.

Only the time spent actually administering anesthesia should be counted toward the units of service. Figure 4-1 illustrates what is counted in anesthesia time.

FIGURE 4-1 *Anesthesia Time*

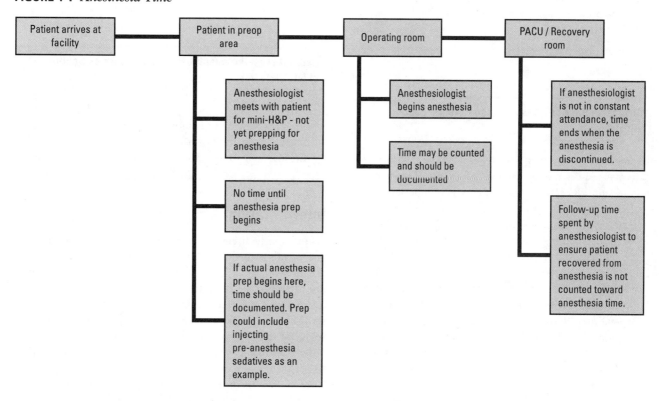

Calculating Anesthesia Services

CMS follows this calculation when processing claims for anesthesia services:

(time units + base units) × conversion factor
= allowance

One time unit is allowed for each 15-minute interval, or fraction thereof, starting from the time the physician begins to prepare the patient for induction and ending when the patient may safely be placed under postoperative supervision, and the physician is no longer in personal attendance. Steps:

1. The 15-minute time interval is divided into the total time indicated on the claim.
   Example:
   95 minutes ÷ 15 = 6.33 = 6.3
   79 minutes ÷ 15 = 5.26 = 5.3
2. The total units derived from Step 1 constitute the total units for time.
3. The time units are added to the relative value units (base units) assigned to the anesthesia procedure code.
4. Total units derived from Steps 1 through 3 are then multiplied by the conversion factor. The final step results in the calculation amount compared to the billed charge.

Excerpt From the Anesthesia Coding Policies Section of NCCI[1(p4)]

Example: A patient who undergoes a cataract extraction may require monitored anesthesia care. This may require administration of a sedative in conjunction with a peri/retrobulbar injection for regional block anesthesia. Subsequently, an interval of 30 minutes or more may transpire during which time the patient does not require monitoring by an anesthesia practitioner. After this period, monitoring will commence again for the cataract extraction and ultimately the patient will be released to the surgeon's care or to recovery. The time that may be reported would include the time for the monitoring during the block and during the procedure. The interval time and the recovery time are not to be included in the anesthesia time calculation. Also, if unusual services not bundled into the anesthesia service are required, the time spent delivering these services before anesthesia time begins or after it ends may not be included as reportable anesthesia time.

Interpretation

This is a great example for the time element of anesthesia coding and billing. For this procedure, the example CMS offers is an interruption of 30 minutes between the anesthesiologist beginning to prepare the patient (administering the sedative) and the intraoperative monitoring of the patient. Those 30 minutes would not be included in the total time for the cataract extraction anesthesia because it did not require the anesthesiologist's presence or monitoring of the patient. This example also includes an instruction that if there are other services the anesthesiologist provides that are not otherwise bundled into the anesthesia service, those services may be separately coded, but the time to perform the additional services may not be used in the anesthesia time calculation.

Another example would be an anesthesiologist who spends 15 minutes inserting a Swan-Ganz catheter to monitor the patient. The total intraoperative service by the anesthesiologist was 120 minutes (including the time of inserting the catheter). Because the Swan-Ganz catheter insertion (CPT code 93503) is separately reportable, the 15 minutes should be deducted from the 120 minutes for the anesthesia services. To include the 15 minutes would create double reimbursement for the Swan-Ganz catheter insertion service.

Excerpt From the Anesthesia Coding Policies Section of NCCI[1(p4)]

... if it is medically necessary for the anesthesia practitioner to continuously monitor the patient during the interval time and not perform any other service, the interval time may be included in the anesthesia time.

Interpretation

As previously discussed, only the time the anesthesiologist spends actively involved in the patient's anesthesia preparation, induction and monitoring, and discontinuing anesthesia to the point the patient may safely be turned over to postoperative care is billable. Any time necessary for the anesthesiologist to monitor the patient should be included in the total time billed. So, if the anesthesia provider administers a sedative to the patient 30 minutes prior to performing a nerve block, and during that 30-minute interval, it is medically necessary for the anesthesiologist to monitor the patient, the 30 minutes may be included in the billed time. So, for a patient who undergoes a cataract extraction with MAC, the anesthesiologist administers a sedative in conjunction with a peri/retrobulbar injection for regional block anesthesia and must monitor the patient for the 30 minutes between the sedative injection and the regional block. If the anesthesiologist spends 30 minutes monitoring the patient before surgery and 30 minutes during the procedure and through recovery, the total time for this anesthesia service is 60 minutes. Note that the anesthesiologist is constantly monitoring the patient during the 60 minutes.

Excerpt From the Anesthesia Coding Policies Section of NCCI[1(p5)]

It is standard medical practice for an anesthesia practitioner to perform a patient examination and evaluation prior to surgery. This is considered part of the anesthesia service and is included in the base unit of the anesthesia code. The evaluation and examination are not reported in the anesthesia time. If surgery is canceled, subsequent to the preoperative evaluation, payment may be allowed to the anesthesiologist for an evaluation and management service and the appropriate E&M code (usually a consultation code) may be reported. (A non-medically directed CRNA may also report an E&M code under these circumstances if permitted by state law.)

Interpretation

Remember from the earlier instructions in this chapter that time spent preoperatively evaluating the patient should not be counted toward the total time for the anesthesia. However, on occasion surgeries are canceled for the well being of the patient. If that occurs, the anesthesiologist would not bill for anesthesia, because there would be no anesthesia. Rather, the anesthesiologist would bill for the appropriate level E/M code, based on the documented preoperative evaluation. The E/M service billed must be supported by the documentation. Take a patient who is scheduled for a coronary artery bypass graft procedure, and, prior to the surgery, the anesthesiologist visits with the patient to make sure the patient is ready for the surgery and general anesthesia. On evaluating the patient, the anesthesiologist discovers that the patient is nauseated and that the patient ate breakfast against warnings otherwise. The anesthesiologist and surgeon decide that the surgery would be unsafe at that point and cancel the surgery, to reschedule several days later. In this example, there is no surgery and no anesthesia; however, the anesthesiologist may bill for the preoperative evaluation. The E/M level assigned would be based on the documentation by the anesthesiologist. Therefore, this encounter should be well documented, coded, and billed.

Excerpt From the Anesthesia Coding Policies Section of NCCI[1(p5)]

Similarly, routine postoperative evaluation is included in the basic unit for the anesthesia service. If this evaluation occurs after the anesthesia practitioner has safely placed the patient under postoperative care, neither additional anesthesia time units nor evaluation and management codes should be reported for this evaluation. Postoperative evaluation and management services related to the surgery are not separately reportable by the anesthesia practitioner except when an anesthesiologist provides significant, separately identifiable ongoing critical care services.

Interpretation

The time billed for anesthesia services stops once the anesthesiologist ceases active anesthesia care including monitoring the patient and ensuring that the patient safely wakes from anesthesia. Postoperative evaluation after that point is included in the base unit for the service and is not separately billable.

Excerpt From the Anesthesia Coding Policies Section of NCCI[1(p5)]

Anesthesia practitioners other than anesthesiologists cannot report evaluation and management codes except as described above when a surgical case is canceled.

Interpretation

Nonphysician anesthesia providers (CRNAs, AAs) may not bill for E/M services. Any evaluation of the patient is included in the anesthesia services being provided and billed. However, as noted in Medicare guidelines, CRNAs may bill an E/M, when performed, if the surgery is canceled.

Excerpt From the Anesthesia Coding Policies Section of NCCI[1(p5)]

Anesthesia practitioners if permitted by state law may separately report significant, separately identifiable postoperative management services after the anesthesia service time ends. These services include, but are not limited to, postoperative pain management and ventilator management unrelated to the anesthesia procedure.

Interpretation

Once the anesthesia time is completed, the anesthesia provider may bill for other services if those services are performed within their licensure and if medically necessary. As an example, consider a patient who has undergone a major surgery with general anesthesia is released from the recovery area. Once the patient is back in the hospital room, the anesthesia provider is called to provide postoperative pain management. The anesthesia provider performs a nerve block for the patient to relieve the pain. This service may be billed in addition to the anesthesia provided to the same patient on the same day.

 Documentation Tip: The documentation should be very clear that the time spent on the separately billable service is not included in the reported anesthesia time. It might be helpful to dictate a note separate from the anesthesia record.

Note: Postoperative pain management performed by the surgeon would not be separately paid, as it is included in the global surgery package. See Chapter 3 of this book for additional information.

> **Excerpt From the Anesthesia Coding Policies Section of NCCI**[1(p5-6)]
>
> Management of epidural or subarachnoid drug administration (CPT code 01996) is separately payable on dates of service subsequent to surgery but not on the date of surgery. If the only service provided is management of epidural/subarachnoid drug administration, then an evaluation and management service should not be reported in addition to CPT code 01996. Payment for management of epidural/subarachnoid drug administration is limited to one unit of service per postoperative day regardless of the number of visits necessary to manage the catheter per postoperative day (CPT definition). While an anesthesiologist or non-medically directed CRNA may be able to report this service, only one payment will be made per day.

Interpretation

01996 Daily hospital management of epidural or subarachnoid continuous drug administration

This code is bundled into the anesthesia code for the day of the surgery but is separately billable on subsequent days. If on subsequent days the service provided is solely for the management of the continuous drug administration, no separate E/M service should be billed in addition to the drug management. However, if there is a medically necessary E/M service performed and documented, it may be billed with a modifier 25.

Because the CPT code 01996 is a "per diem" or daily code, it should be coded only once per day regardless of how many encounters the provider has with the patient.

> **Excerpt From the Anesthesia Coding Policies Section of NCCI**[1(p6)]
>
> Postoperative pain management services are generally provided by the surgeon who is reimbursed under a global payment policy related to the procedure and shall not be reported by the anesthesia practitioner unless separate, medically necessary services are required that cannot be rendered by the surgeon. The surgeon is responsible to document in the medical record the reason care is being referred to the anesthesia practitioner.

Interpretation

As mentioned previously, postoperative pain management is bundled into the surgeon's global surgery payment but is reimbursed if provided by the anesthesiologist. In order to avoid patient dumping, the surgeon must document within the patient's chart why the anesthesiologist is performing the pain management. Actually, many surgeons discover that the anesthesiologists have refined techniques, and surgeons will consult with the anesthesiologists for difficult patients.

> Patient dumping is the intentional transfer of certain portions of a patient's care to another provider solely because those services would not be paid if performed by the transferring physician.

> **Excerpt From the Anesthesia Coding Policies Section of NCCI**[1(p6)]
>
> In certain circumstances critical care services are provided by the anesthesiologist. It is currently national CMS policy that CRNAs cannot be reimbursed for evaluation and management services in the critical care area. In the case of anesthesiologists, the routine immediate postoperative care is not separately reported except as described above.

Interpretation

This NCCI guideline notes that, when necessary, critical care may be billed by the anesthesiologist as long as the critical care is not a part of active surgical anesthetic management. The same guidelines for critical billing exist for anesthesiologists as with other physicians:

1. The patient must be critically ill or injured.
2. The care provided by the physician (anesthesiologist) must be needed to support vital system functions or vital organ failure or to prevent life-threatening deterioration.

CRNAs are not paid for critical care services.

As an example, consider a patient who is in critical condition following a motor vehicle accident, with acute respiratory arrest as well as multiple organ injuries creating cardiovascular and gastrointestinal problems. The critical care anesthesiologist-intensivist performs diagnostic, monitoring, and therapeutic activities, including bronchoscopy, invasive and noninvasive hemodynamic and respiratory monitoring, metabolic assessment, airway intubation; institution, management of, and weaning from mechanical ventilation; tube thoracostomy; cardiopulmonary resuscitation; cardioversion; electrical cardiac pacing; mechanical and pharmacologic support of the circulation; parenteral and enteral nutrition; fluid, electrolyte, and acid-base support; management of extracorporeal membrane oxygenation; oxygen therapy; intra-aortic balloon counterpulsation; and analgesia and sedation for both acute and chronic pain.

The critical care services could be billed by the anesthesiologist as well as any other procedures separately billable from the critical care.

Excerpt From the Anesthesia Coding Policies Section of NCCI[1(p6)]

Certain procedural services such as insertion of a Swan-Ganz catheter, insertion of a central venous pressure line, emergency intubation (outside of the operating suite), etc. are separately payable to anesthesiologists as well as non-medically directed CRNAs if these procedures are furnished within the parameters of state licensing laws.

Interpretation

Anesthesiologists and CRNAs (working within their licensure) may bill for procedures in addition to their anesthesia services as outlined by the NCCI edits (see earlier excerpt) and the CPT codebook. The remainder of this chapter summarizes the services incidental to anesthesia and not separately billable.

CPT Codebook Anesthesia Introductory Guidelines[2(p37)]

The reporting of anesthesia services is appropriate by or under the responsible supervision of a physician. These services may include but are not limited to general, regional, supplementation of local anesthesia, or other supportive services in order to afford the patient the anesthesia care deemed optimal by the anesthesiologist during any procedure. These services include the usual preoperative and postoperative visits, the anesthesia care during the procedure, the administration of fluids and/or blood, and the usual monitoring services (eg, ECG, temperature, blood pressure, oximetry, capnography, and mass spectrometry). Unusual forms of monitoring (eg, intra-arterial, central venous, and Swan-Ganz) are not included.

Excerpt From the Anesthesia Coding Policies Section of NCCI[1(6-7)]

Anesthesia HCPCS/CPT codes include all services integral to the anesthesia procedure such as preparation, monitoring, intra-operative care, and post-operative care until the patient is released by the anesthesiologist to the care of another physician.

Interpretation

NCCI gives a fairly complete listing of services that are included in reimbursement for the anesthesia CPT code. These services should not be coded separately from the anesthesia care when provided by the same provider for the same patient during a single surgical session. It would be useful to make a note in the billing system next to each CPT code for these services indicating that they are not separately billable. There are NCCI edits for most of these services; however, if these services are performed outside the active surgical anesthesiology, service there is a potential for coding in addition to the anesthesia by appending a modifier (58 Staged or Related Procedure or Service by the Same Physician During the Postoperative Period, 59 Distinct Procedural Service, etc.).

In a later section of this chapter, CMS provides specific CPT codes that are included in the anesthesia CPT code reimbursement. Therefore, an anesthesiologist providing general anesthesia services for a patient undergoing a hysterectomy would use anesthesia CPT code 00846:

00846 Anesthesia for intraperitoneal procedures in lower abdomen including laparoscopy; radical hysterectomy

Included in the reimbursement for this anesthesia would be the insertion of the endotracheal tube and intraoperative monitoring of the patient's blood pressure, heart rate, respirations, oximetry, capnography, temperature, etc. None of these services should be separately coded from the 00846 CPT code.

Excerpt From the Anesthesia Coding Policies Section of NCCI[1(p7)]

The NCCI contains many edits bundling standard preparation, monitoring, and procedural services into anesthesia CPT codes. Although some of these services may never be reported on the same date of service as an anesthesia service, many of these services could be provided at a separate patient encounter unrelated to the anesthesia service on the same date of service. Providers may utilize modifier -59 to bypass the edits under these circumstances.

Interpretation

Throughout NCCI it is noted that separate sessions of care are usually coded individually and not bundled together (there is an exception for E/M services and some global surgical care), and the same is true with anesthesia services. If there is a distinctly separate encounter with the patient—that means not related to the anesthesia care provided perioperative (immediately before, during, and after the operation)—the separate service may be coded with a modifier 59 (or other appropriate modifier, depending on the circumstances) for billing.

As in our prior example, a hysterectomy patient is taken to the PACU and is later released to a hospital room. Several hours after that, the patient spikes a fever, has additional complications, and is transferred to critical care. The anesthesiologist assumes care for the critically ill patient and can bill those services in addition to the perioperative anesthesia care from earlier in the day. A modifier 25 should be appended to the critical care service. Modifier 25 would be used, rather than modifier 59, in this example because modifier 59 is not applicable for E/M services.

However, if, rather than being taken to critical care, the hysterectomy patient is taken back to the operating room for a second procedure to repair an intestinal injury resulting from the earlier procedure, the second anesthesia service may be coded in addition to the original by appending a modifier 78 (Unplanned Return to the Operating/Procedure Room by the Same Physician Following Initial Procedure for a Related Procedure During the Postoperative Period).

Excerpt From the Anesthesia Coding Policies Section of NCCI[1(p7-9)]

CPT codes describing services that are integral to an anesthesia service include, but are not limited to, the following:

31505, 31515, 31527 (Laryngoscopy) (Laryngoscopy codes are for diagnostic or surgical services)

31622, 31645, 31646 (Bronchoscopy)

36000, 36010-36015 (Introduction of needle or catheter)

62310-62311, 62318-62319 (Injection of diagnostic or therapeutic substance): CPT codes 62310-62311 and 62318-62319 may be reported on the date of surgery if performed for postoperative pain relief rather than as the means for providing the regional block for the surgical procedure. If a narcotic or other analgesic is injected through the same catheter as the anesthetic, CPT codes 62310-62319 should not be billed. Modifier -59 will indicate that the injection was performed for postoperative pain relief but a procedure note should be included in the medical record.

90760-90776 (Injections, IV infusions, and drug administration)

93307-93308 (Transthoracic echocardiography when displayed for monitoring purposes.) However, when performed for diagnostic purposes with documentation of a formal report, this service will be considered a significant, separately identifiable, and separately payable service.

93312-93317 (Transesophageal echocardiography) However, when performed for diagnostic purposes with documentation of a formal report, this service will be considered a significant, separately identifiable, and separately payable service.

93922-93981 (Extremity arterial venous studies) When performed diagnostically with a formal report, this will be considered a significant, separately identifiable, and if medically necessary, a payable service.

94002-94004, 94660-94662 (Ventilation management/CPAP services) If performed as management for maintenance ventilation during a surgical procedure, this is part of the anesthesia service. This is separately payable if performed as an ongoing service after transfer out of the operating room or post-anesthesia recovery to a hospital unit/ICU. Modifier -59 would be necessary to signify that this was a separate service.

94760-94770 (Oximetry)

99201-99499 (Evaluation and management)

(Please note: This is not a comprehensive list of all services included in anesthesia services. Please refer to the NCCI manual for the more exhaustive list.)

Interpretation

Within the NCCI guidelines for the anesthesia edits, Medicare provides a listing of CPT codes believed to be included in the anesthesia CPT code reimbursement and not separately billable. This is not an exhaustive list of codes but gives a very good perspective of what CPT codes are deemed incidental to anesthesia. The following is an example provided in the NCCI guidelines.

Excerpt From the Anesthesia Coding Policies Section of NCCI[1(p8-9)]

Example: A patient has an epidural block with sedation and monitoring for arthroscopic knee surgery. The anesthesiologist reports CPT code 01382 (Anesthesia for diagnostic arthroscopic procedures of knee joint). The epidural catheter is left in place for postoperative pain management. The anesthesiologist should not also report CPT codes 62311 (injection of diagnostic or therapeutic substance) or 01996 (daily management of epidural) on the date of surgery. CPT code 01996 may be reported with one unit of service per day on subsequent days until the catheter is removed. On the other hand, if the anesthesiologist performs general anesthesia reported as CPT code 01382 and reasonably believes that postoperative pain is likely to be sufficient to warrant an epidural catheter, CPT code 62319-59 may be reported indicating that this is a separate service from the anesthesia service. In this instance, the service is separately payable whether the catheter is placed before, during, or after the surgery. If the epidural catheter was placed on a different date than the surgery, modifier -59 would not be necessary. Effective January 1, 2004, daily hospital management of continuous epidural or subarachnoid drug administration performed on the day(s) subsequent to the placement of an epidural or subarachnoid catheter (CPT codes 62318-62319) may be reported as CPT code 01996.

Interpretation

The NCCI permits the reporting of a pain procedure along with an anesthesia service when appropriate (ie, when the pain procedure is not used as regional anesthesia for surgery). The NCCI edits would be bypassed with a modifier 59 as long as the postoperative pain service is medically necessary, cannot be performed by the surgeon, and the surgeon requests, in writing, that the anesthesiologist provide this service.

Various *CPT Assistant* articles have offered further clarification of coding for pain management procedures performed in conjunction with anesthesia services. For instance, the February 1997 issue stated:

> An anesthesiologist could perform a therapeutic nerve block for pain management before or at the conclusion of the surgical procedure, or insert a catheter into the spinal column to induce continuous postoperative analgesia for therapeutic pain management. In the latter case, if an epidural catheter is inserted into the lumbar region, report code 62279. This code includes insertion of the catheter and initial injection of the analgesic medication or fluid mixture that may then be connected to and controlled by an external infusion pump. Subsequent daily monitoring of the patient may be reported separately using an appropriate E/M code or anesthesia code 01996 because code 62279 does not include daily monitoring. Payor coverage and reporting requirements for daily monitoring services may vary.[4]

The July 1998 issue of *CPT Assistant* addressed the issue of whether one can code a pain management service (64400-64530) in conjunction with an operative anesthesia service. In this case, the pain management injection (64400-64530) is not the operative anesthesia, but is administered pre-, inter- or post-operatively for the purpose of postoperative pain management. The *CPT Assistant* stated:

> It is appropriate to report a code from 64400-64530 in conjunction with an operative anesthesia service if an injection, as described by these codes, was also given. The February 1997 issue of *CPT Assistant* published an article on anesthesia and the coding of procedural services. Under 'Reporting Additional Procedural Services' it reads:
>
> Additional procedural services provided in conjunction with basic anesthesia administration are separately reportable and coded according to standard CPT coding guidelines applicable to the given code and the respective CPT section (eg, Surgery or Medicine sections) in which they are listed. Do not code procedural services with anesthesia coding guidelines.[5]

Also, the October 2001 *CPT Assistant* dealt with whether or not it is appropriate to report pain management procedures, including the insertion of an epidural catheter or the performance of a nerve block, for postoperative analgesia separately from the administration of a general anesthetic. The publication stated that,

> [i]f, on the other hand, the block procedure is used primarily for the anesthesia itself, the service should be reported using the anesthesia code alone.[6]

In May 2007, the *CPT Assistant* dealt with several issues surrounding the time spent placing nerve blocks for postoperative pain control, spinals, arterial lines, etc. Questions they addressed included: Can the time be deducted from main anesthesia start and stop times, or would the time spent placing these items need to be deducted from the anesthesia time for the operation? Is there a difference between the arterial line, etc, being placed prior to the patient "going to sleep" or after in regards to discounting this "placement" time? The guideline provided was this:

The Anesthesia guidelines in the CPT codebook indicate that placement of monitoring devices such as central venous lines, arterial lines, and Swan-Ganz catheters are separately reportable from an anesthesia service. Placement of these monitoring devices has no time associated with them. If a nerve block or epidural is performed for the purpose of postoperative pain management and not as part of the anesthesia for the surgical procedure, then it too is reported separately. When these procedures are performed before the start of anesthesia time, the time spent on them should not be added to the reported anesthesia time because they are separate and distinct from the anesthesia service. If the procedure is performed after induction of the primary anesthetic, it is not necessary to deduct the time spent on the procedure from reported anesthesia time.[7]

Excerpt From the Anesthesia Coding Policies Section of NCCI[1(p10-11)]

C. Radiologic Anesthesia Coding
In keeping with standard anesthesia billing guidelines for Medicare, only one anesthesia code may be reported for anesthesia services provided in conjunction with radiological procedures. Radiological Supervision and Interpretation (S & I) codes will usually be applicable to radiological procedures being performed.

The appropriate S & I code may be reported by the appropriate provider (radiologist, cardiologist, neurosurgeon, radiation oncologist, etc.). Accordingly, S & I codes are not included in anesthesia codes referable to these procedures; only the appropriate provider, however, may bill for S & I services.

Interpretation

When anesthesia is used in the performance of radiologic services, as with any other anesthesia coding, only a single anesthesia code should be used, but the total anesthesia

time may be billed. Medicare notes that anesthesia for radiology is usually for those services that have a supervision and interpretation (S&I) code in addition to an invasive service code (eg, stent placement). The S&I code is billed by the performing provider and is not considered incidental or integral to the anesthesia service. However, it is unlikely that the anesthesiologist would be performing that part of the care. Take the example of a patient presenting for intravascular stent placement in his or her renal artery under MAC. The interventional radiologist would bill CPT codes 37205 and 75960. The anesthesiologist would code 01924.

01924 Anesthesia for therapeutic interventional radiological procedures involving the arterial system; not otherwise specified

37205 Transcatheter placement of an intravascular stent(s), (except coronary, carotid, and vertebral vessel), percutaneous; initial vessel

75960 Transcatheter introduction of intravascular stent(s) (except coronary, carotid, and vertebral vessel), percutaneous and/or open, radiological supervision and interpretation, each vessel

---

Excerpt From the Anesthesia Coding Policies Section of NCCI[1(p11)]

CPT code 01920 (Anesthesia for cardiac catheterization including coronary angiography and ventriculography [not to include Swan-Ganz catheter]) can be reported for monitored anesthesia care (MAC) in patients who are critically ill or critically unstable. If the physician performing the radiologic service places a catheter as part of that service, and, through the same site, a catheter is left and used for monitoring purposes, it is inappropriate for either the anesthesiologist/certified registered nurse anesthetist or the physician performing the radiologic procedure to bill for placement of the monitoring catheter (eg, CPT codes 36500, 36555-36556, 36568-36569, 36580, 36584, 36597).

Interpretation

This guideline indicates that although anesthesia may be performed, coded, and billed for a cardiac catheterization, there are some NCCI policies that apply, namely:

1. The anesthesia must be performed by someone other than the physician performing the cardiac catheterization.
2. Catheter placement is a part of the cardiac catheterization and should not be billed separately by anyone involved in the case, as it is included in the

reimbursement for the cardiac catheterization CPT codes. However, should a separate catheter be placed by the anesthesia provider specifically for monitoring anesthesia, it may be separately coded if of a nature that is not incidental to the usual anesthesia service.

Excerpt From the Anesthesia Coding Policies Section of NCCI[1(p11)]

D. Monitored Anesthesia Care (MAC)
Monitored anesthesia care involves the intraoperative monitoring by a physician or qualified individual under the medical direction of a physician of the patient's vital physiological signs in anticipation of the need for administration of general anesthesia or of the development of adverse physiological patient reaction to the surgical procedure. It also includes the performance of a preanesthetic examination and evaluation, prescription of the anesthesia care required, administration of any necessary oral or parenteral medications and provision of indicated postoperative anesthesia care.

Interpretation

If the anesthesia used for a procedure is monitored anesthesia care, that anesthesia reimbursement still includes the perioperative anesthesia management (preoperative evaluation, intraoperative induction and monitoring, and postoperative recovery), just as other forms of anesthesia do. Do not code these services in addition to the monitored anesthesia care.

Excerpt From the Anesthesia Coding Policies Section of NCCI[1(p12)]

E. General Policy Statements
2. Physicians should not report drug administration CPT codes 90760-90776 for anesthetic agents or other drugs administered between the patient's arrival at the operative center and discharge from the post-anesthesia care unit.

Interpretation

The anesthesia CPT code reimbursement includes the administration of anesthetic drugs as an inherent part of the anesthesia care. This administration should not be billed separately. To illustrate through an example, if as a part of general anesthesia, the anesthesiologist intravenously injects etomidate to induce anesthesia, followed by desflurane via inhalation to maintain the anesthesia, both the intravenous injection and the inhalation procedure are incidental to the anesthesia care and should not be separately billed.

Excerpt From the Anesthesia Coding Policies Section of NCCI[1(p12)]

3. With limited exceptions Medicare Anesthesia Rules prevent separate payment for anesthesia for a medical or surgical service when provided by the physician performing the service. The physician should not report CPT codes 00100-01999. Additionally, the physician should not unbundle the anesthesia procedure and report component codes individually. For example, introduction of a needle or intracatheter into a vein (CPT code 36000), venipuncture (CPT code 36410), or drug administration (CPT codes 90760-90776) should not be reported when these services are related to the delivery of an anesthetic agent.

Interpretation

As explained in Chapter 1 of this book, the physician performing the procedure should not bill separately if he or she provided the anesthesia service. The reimbursement for the anesthesia is included in the procedure allowance. Any aspect of inducing or monitoring anesthesia by the physician performing the procedure should not be coded in addition to the procedure.

Example

A patient presents for outpatient excision of a lesion, and the surgeon injects a local anesthetic to deaden the area of excision. Because the surgeon is providing the anesthesia, the injection of the local anesthetic is not separately reported from the lesion excision.

Excerpt From the Anesthesia Coding Policies Section of NCCI[1(p12)]

Medicare may allow separate payment for moderate conscious sedation services (CPT codes 99143-99145) when provided by the same physician performing the medical or surgical procedure except for those procedures listed in Appendix G of the CPT Manual.

Interpretation

Moderate sedation is a drug-induced depression of consciousness during which patients respond purposeful to verbal commands and perhaps some tactile stimulation. There are no interventions required to maintain the patient's airway because spontaneous ventilation is adequate.

If the physician who is performing the procedure also provides the moderate sedation for the procedure, payment may be made for the conscious sedation services using CPT codes 99143-99145. However, please be sure to check appendix G of the CPT codebook for a listing of services for which conscious sedation may not be separately billed.

CPT Coding Tip: CPT provides information on what is included in the moderate sedation codes. This should be referenced when coding services for a physician who is performing moderate sedation.

CPT Codebook Moderate Sedation Guidelines[1(p447)]

When providing moderate sedation, the following services are included and NOT reported separately:
- Assessment of the patient (not included in intraservice time);
- Establishment of IV access and fluids to maintain patency, when performed;
- Administration of agent(s);
- Maintenance of sedation;
- Monitoring of oxygen saturation, heart rate, and blood pressure; and
- Recovery (not included in intraservice time).

99143   Moderate sedation services (other than those services described by codes 00100-01999) provided by the same physician performing the diagnostic or therapeutic service that the sedation supports, requiring the presence of an independent trained observer to assist in the monitoring of the patient's

level of consciousness and physiological status; younger than 5 years of age, first 30 minutes intra-service time

99144   age 5 years or older, first 30 minutes intra-service time

+ 99145   each additional 15 minutes intra-service time (List separately in addition to code for primary service)

SUMMARY

- The entire Anesthesia Coding Policies Section of NCCI should be read.

- Documentation for anesthesia care must carefully capture the actual attendance time by the billing provider as well as clearly separate those services that are billed in addition to the anesthesia CPT code.

- If services by the anesthesia provider are performed at different encounters on the same day, they should be billed and separately documented within the medical record.

- All usual anesthetic perioperative care is included in the base unit for the anesthesia service billed and should not be separately reported. Additionally, time for the preoperative and postoperative evaluations is not added to the actual anesthesia time, as these are included in the base unit for the anesthesia CPT code.

Definitions and Acronyms

moderate (conscious) sedation: This is drug-induced depression of consciousness during which patients respond purposefully to verbal commands, either alone or accompanied by light tactile stimulation. It does not include minimal sedation, deep sedation, or monitored anesthesia care.

monitored anesthesia care (MOC): Monitored anesthesia care involves intraoperative monitoring, by a physician or qualified individual under the medical direction of a physician, of a patient's vital signs in anticipation of the need for administration of general anesthesia or of the development of a patient's adverse physiological reaction to the surgical procedure.

patient dumping: The intentional transfer of certain portions of a patient's care to another provider solely because those services would not be paid if performed by the transferring physician.

perioperative: Activity immediately surrounding a surgery (before, during, and after).

post-anesthesia care unit (PACU): Patients are placed in the PACU for close monitoring as they recover from surgery and the effects of anesthesia outside the operating room.

CHAPTER EXERCISES

1. A patient is scheduled for emergency Broviac catheter placement under monitored anesthesia care. Preoperatively, the anesthesiologist speaks with the patient and performs an examination, at which point the anesthesiologist diagnoses congestive cardiac failure. The surgeon decides to proceed with the catheter placement. The anesthesiologist gives the patient furosemide 40 mg intravenously. The surgeon injects lidocaine at the incision site, and suddenly the patient's CO_2 level drops from 38 mmHg to 15 mmHg, and her oxygen saturation drops to 83%. The anesthesiologist provides mask ventilation with 100% oxygen, and the patient's O_2 saturation increases to 94%. It is discovered that the patient has a pneumothorax. The anesthesiologist treats the pneumothorax with tube thoracostomy, which takes about four minutes. More furosemide is given, and the patient's vital signs return almost to baseline levels over a period of 10 to 20 minutes. The procedure is concluded after a total of 48 minutes in the operating room suite.

   What services may the anesthesiologist bill and why?

2. A patient presents for a nephrectomy to be performed under general anesthesia. The anesthesiologist preoperatively evaluates the patient to determine the best method to proceed. Once the patient is in the operating room, a sedative is provided, and inhalation anesthesia begun for the anesthesia. The operation concludes 95 minutes later, and the anesthesiologist brings the patient out of anesthesia within 3 minutes thereafter and releases the patient to the recovery area. In recovery, the anesthesiologist revisits the patient as a final check to ensure no ill effects of the anesthesia.

   The surgeon requests that the anesthesiologist provide postoperative pain management for the patient on an as-needed basis, which the anesthesiologist provides by simple oral administration of opioids.

   What services may the anesthesiologist bill and why?

3. A patient presents for a nephrectomy to be performed under general anesthesia. The anesthesiologist preoperatively evaluates the patient to determine the best method to proceed. Once the patient is in the operating room, a sedative is given and inhalation anesthesia begun for the anesthesia. The operation is concluded 95 minutes later, and the anesthesiologist brings the patient out of anesthesia within 3 minutes thereafter and releases the patient to the recovery area. In recovery, the anesthesiologist revisits the patient as a final check to ensure no ill effects of the anesthesia.

   The surgeon requests that the anesthesiologist provide postoperative pain management for the patient, as he believes it will require more than routine pain management. The surgeon requests that the anesthesiologist evaluate the situation and advise regarding the best course of treatment. The anesthesiologist determines that continuous infusions will provide the appropriate level of pain control, and the anesthesiologist manages this drug administration for the day of the procedure and the day after, before discontinuing it.

   What services may the anesthesiologist bill and why?

ANSWERS TO CHAPTER EXERCISES

1. The anesthesiologist may bill for the anesthesia services for the Broviac catheter placement as well as the tube thoracostomy; however, the time spent inserting the thoracostomy tube must be subtracted from the total procedure time with only 44 minutes (48 minus 4) billed for the anesthesia service. The preoperative evaluation is included in the anesthesia CPT code.

   CPT codes:

   00532 Anesthesia for access to central venous circulation

   Bill for 44 minutes of anesthesia time on this code.

   32551 Tube thoracostomy, includes water seal (eg, for abscess, hemothorax, empyema), when performed (separate procedure)

2. The anesthesiologist may bill only the anesthesia care service for 98 minutes. There is no medical necessity supported for the anesthesiologist to provide the postoperative pain management that is included in the surgeon's global surgery allowance.

   00862 Anesthesia for extraperitoneal procedures in lower abdomen, including urinary tract; renal procedures, including upper one-third of ureter, or donor nephrectomy

3. The anesthesiologist may bill for the anesthesia service, the placement of the epidural catheter (because it is not part of the surgery anesthesia and is solely for the purpose of postoperative pain management) with a modifier 59, and the subsequent day's management. The management of the pain medications administered through the epidural would not be separately reported on the day of the procedure. The time for the epidural insertion is not included in the time for anesthesia.

   00862 Anesthesia for extraperitoneal procedures in lower abdomen, including urinary tract; renal procedures, including upper one-third of ureter, or donor nephrectomy

   The code for the epidural catheter placement would be determined by the procedure note details.

REFERENCES

1. Centers for Medicare and Medicaid Services. "Chapter II Anesthesia Services," In: NCCI Policy Manual for Medicare Services. www.cms.hhs.gov/NationalCorrectCodInitEd/01_overview.asp#TopOfPage. Accessed June 11, 2009.

2. American Medical Association. *Current Procedural Terminology CPT® 2009 Professional Edition.* Chicago, IL: American Medical Association; 2008.

3. Center for Medicare and Medicaid Services. *Anesthesiologists Center.* www.cms.hhs.gov/center/anesth.asp. Accessed June 11, 2009.

4. American Medical Association. "Anesthesia: coding for procedural services," *CPT Assistant.* 1997;7(2):4.

5. American Medical Association. "Coding consultation, nervous system, 64400-64530 (Q&A)," *CPT Assistant.* 1998;8(7):10.

6. American Medical Association. "Coding correction, coding clarification: anesthesia and postoperative pain management," *CPT Assistant.* 2001;11(10):9.

7. American Medical Association. "Coding communication: anesthesia," *CPT Assistant.* 2007;17(5):9.

The Integumentary System

Chapter 5 provides background about the integumentary system, reviews the National Correct Coding Initiative (NCCI) coding guidelines for procedures performed on the integumentary system, and provides examples to reflect the logic behind the edits. As with the other chapters, this chapter provides an NCCI guideline followed by our interpretation, an example, or both.

The first rule in correct coding is to understand the service or procedure being coded. Without the clinical knowledge or understanding of a service or procedure, it is difficult to correctly code the service or decide whether a bundling edit should be bypassed. Coders should remember to read all the instructions within that section (eg, Integumentary) of *Current Procedural Terminology (CPT®) 2009 Professional Edition*[1] and refer to it for additional instructions. The NCCI guidelines should also be reviewed to make sure information is being coded correctly, optimally, and compliantly.

For CPT coding, the integumentary system is divided by categories as outlined in Figure 5-1.

Figure 5-1 illustrates the main categories of CPT coding for the integumentary system.

Integumentary System and NCCI Guidelines

Excerpt From the NCCI Section on the Integumentary System[2(p2)]

A. Introduction
The principles of correct coding discussed in Chapter I apply to the CPT codes in the range 10000-19999. Several general guidelines are repeated in this chapter. However, those general guidelines from Chapter I not discussed in this chapter are nonetheless applicable.

Interpretation

The instruction indicates that the overall NCCI guidelines apply to each section of the CPT codebook, and even if they are not repeated within a chapter, they are nonetheless still a guideline to be followed. The introductory guidelines were covered comprehensively in Chapter 2 of this book, those introductory guidelines that have clear application within the integumentary system are reiterated in this chapter.

FIGURE 5-1 *CPT Codebook Breakdown for Integumentary System Format*

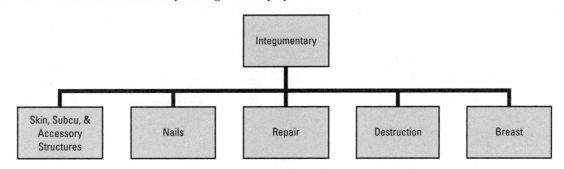

Remember from the General Correct Coding Policies that a biopsy performed at the time of another more extensive procedure (eg, excision, destruction, removal) is only separately reportable under specific circumstances. An example would be for a biopsy being performed on a separate lesion, then an excision would be separately reportable. So, if a patient presents with multiple benign lesions (one on the hand, one on the face, and one on the back), and the physician performs the following services:

Hand lesion—biopsy only

Face lesion—removal with requested biopsy

Back lesion—removal with requested biopsy

The appropriate coding would be: Hand lesion Code the biopsy, because that is all that was performed.

11100 Biopsy of skin, subcutaneous tissue and/or mucous membrane (including simple closure), unless otherwise listed; single lesion[2]

Face lesion
Code only the removal, because the biopsy was not separately supported.
From CPT code range: Excision—Benign Lesions (11440-11446) depending on the size of the lesion.

Back lesion
Code only the removal, because the biopsy was not separately supported.
From CPT code range: Excision—Benign Lesions (11400-11406) depending on the size of the lesion.
The hand lesion is coded because it is on a separate site.

Another policy from the General Guidelines states that if a biopsy is sent for pathologic evaluation, and the evaluation will be completed after the excision or more extensive procedure is performed, the biopsy may not be separately coded in addition to the more extensive procedure. Using the prior example, the face lesion biopsy and back lesion biopsy are not separately billable from the excisions of those lesions. The indication is that the biopsy is performed after the more extensive procedure (ie, the removal). Therefore, only the more extensive procedure (removal) should be coded. Modifier 59 would be necessary on the biopsy of the hand lesion because it was performed and is coded in addition to the other lesion excisions. Use modifier 59 only if the service would otherwise be denied.

Taking this guideline one step further, if a biopsy is performed on the same lesion on which the more extensive procedure is performed, the biopsy is appropriately coded only if the biopsy is for immediate pathologic diagnosis before performing the more extensive procedure. That means that the decision to proceed with the more extensive procedure is based on the result of the biopsy's evaluation. Modifier -58 may be reported to indicate that the biopsy and the more extensive procedure were planned or staged procedures. If the guidelines are closely reviewed, one can notice that the decision for the more major procedure is based, at least in part, on the results of the biopsy. In this scenario, the biopsy is clearly a diagnostic service driving the decision for the therapeutic service. Modifier 58 (staged or related procedure) is appended to the second, more extensive procedure rather than modifier 59.

As an example, take a patient who presents for a biopsy of a breast mass. During the biopsy procedure, the tissue sample is sent for frozen section, and the surgeon awaits the pathology results. The results come back indicating a diagnosis that results in the physician deciding to perform a mastectomy, which was performed during the same surgical setting.

Appropriate coding would be to code the breast biopsy and the mastectomy, with a modifier 58 appended to the mastectomy code.

Explanation

The biopsy was truly an independent diagnostic step in the procedure and drove the treatment decision. Therefore, both services may be coded. Remember to use modifier 58, not modifier 59; however, a lateral modifier to indicate which breast was involved would be appropriately applied to each code.

The physician must document clearly that either there were distinct anatomic sites for the biopsies versus the more extensive procedures or that the physician awaited the results of the pathology examination prior to performing the more extensive procedures. Without sufficient documentation, only the more extensive procedure should be coded.

Excerpt From the General Correct Coding Policies Section of NCCI[3(p10)]

If a definitive surgical procedure requires access through diseased tissue (eg, necrotic skin, abscess, hematoma, seroma), a separate service for this access (eg, debridement, incision and drainage) is not separately reportable. For example, debridement of skin to repair a fracture is not separately reportable.

Interpretation

Approaches and access for procedures are always bundled into the procedure and not separately coded. The thought here is that because the site had to be accessed for the primary surgery, that access (or approach) did not add to the physician's work sufficiently to warrant an additional code. This is true even if that access results in treating an independent condition. Take a patient who presents with a traumatic wound to the arm, which resulted in a fracture and, over the site of the fracture, there is an abscess (caused by the trauma). The physician's treatment involves creating an incision at the abscess site in order to reach and treat the fracture. The primary procedure is an open fracture repair. The approach for the open fracture repair is at the site of the abscess, and by incising the abscess, the abscess drains. In this scenario, only the fracture repair should be coded, because:

1. The abscess drainage was caused by the incision.
2. The incision was to reach and treat the fracture, so the incision was inherent in the open fracture repair.
3. The incision was not documented as adding significant work by the provider.

CPT Coding Tip: *It is sometimes difficult to determine when a service is inherent or incidental to another and when it can be separately coded. Remember, it is inherent if it must be performed in order to perform the deeper or more major procedure. It is incidental if it does not add significant work by the physician.*

Excerpt From the General Correct Coding Policies Section of NCCI[3(p22)]

CMS often publishes coding instructions in its rules, manuals, and notices. Physicians must utilize these instructions when reporting services rendered to Medicare patients.

The *CPT Manual* also includes coding instructions which may be found in the "Introduction", individual chapters, and appendices. In individual chapters the instructions may appear at the beginning of a chapter, at the beginning of a subsection of the chapter, or after specific CPT codes. Physicians should follow *CPT Manual* instructions unless CMS has provided different coding or reporting instructions.

Interpretation

NCCI guidelines instruct coders to follow the guidelines in the CPT codebook unless CMS provides different instructions. For example, the CPT codebook[1(p54)] instructs that lesion excisions include a simple closure of the excised site. The guideline precedes the lesion excision section (beginning with CPT code 11400) and is as follows:

> Excision (including simple closure) of benign lesions of skin (eg, neoplasm, cicatricial, fibrous, inflammatory, congenital, cystic lesions), includes local anesthesia.[1]

It would violate NCCI *and* CPT coding guidelines if a simple repair were coded in addition to a lesion excision (of the same site). Even though simple closure (simple suturing, strip closure, dressing changes) is included in the excision of lesions (whether malignant or benign) and not billed separately, remember that intermediate or complex repairs can be billed separately.

CPT Coding Tip: *According to NCCI guidelines, excision of benign lesions of 0.5 cm or less (CPT code 11400) includes all kinds of repairs (simple, intermediate, complex).*

Excerpt From the General Correct Coding Policies Section of NCCI[3(p23)]

The *CPT Manual* often describes groups of similar codes differing in the complexity of the service. Unless services are performed at separate patient encounters or at separate anatomic sites, the less complex service is included in the more complex service and is not separately reportable.

Interpretation

If the physician attempts treatment of a problem with a less complex procedure and discovers that a more extensive service is necessary for greater success, only the most complex procedure should be coded. CMS will not allow additional coding for failed treatment followed by successful treatment—only the more extensive treatment should be coded. The less extensive services are incidental to the more extensive one if of the same site, for the same problem, during the same session.

Example

The following CPT codes represent debridement services:

11040 Debridement; skin, partial thickness

11041   skin, full thickness

11042   skin, and subcutaneous tissue

11043   skin, subcutaneous tissue, and muscle

11044   skin, subcutaneous tissue, muscle, and bone

If a provider debrides the skin at a single site, then continues through to the subcutaneous tissue and continues further with the debridement to the muscle, at one anatomic site, only the most extensive code (skin, subcutaneous, muscle) (CPT code 11043) should be used, as it clearly includes all the other tissues. The lesser services are integral to the code. See further information on debridement procedures in the following.

CPT Coding Tip
Excision—Debridement (11000-11044): The documentation must support the intensity of the debridement. The codes are driven by site and intensity (or depth) of nonviable tissue being removed:
- *Partial thickness skin*
- *Full thickness skin*
- *Skin and subcutaneous tissue*
- *Skin, subcutaneous tissue, and muscle*
- *Skin, subcutaneous tissue, muscle, and bone*

If the physician doesn't document intensity, the lowest level must be selected, which, in this case, would be partial-thickness skin graft.

The February 1997 issue of *CPT Assistant*[4] provided this coding tip pertaining the debridement of multiple sites:

> To report debridement of multiple sites, CPT codes 11040-11044 may be used more than one time, for a single patient encounter. For each site, select the appropriate code based on the intensity of the wound.
>
> When reporting debridement of more than one site, the physician reports the secondary code (ie, the second code listed) with the -59 modifier appended, to indicate the different areas that were given attention.

Decontamination or debridement: Debridement is considered a separate procedure only when gross contamination requires prolonged cleansing, when appreciable amounts of devitalized or contaminated tissue are removed, or when debridement is carried out separately without immediate primary closure.

Introductory Section of NCCI Integumentary System Guidelines

Excerpt From the NCCI Section on the Integumentary System[2(p2)]

Physicians should report the HCPCS/CPT code that describes the procedure performed to the greatest specificity possible. A HCPCS/CPT code should be reported only if all services described by the code are performed. A physician should not report multiple HCPCS/CPT codes if a single HCPCS/CPT code exists that describes the services. This type of unbundling is incorrect coding.

Interpretation

If a single code encompasses the entire procedure, use that code, rather than separating parts of the procedure. This is true regardless of whether an edit exists in NCCI. If one CPT code includes the entire work performed, do not code separate components.

Example

11975 Insertion, implantable contraceptive capsules

11976 Removal, implantable contraceptive capsules

11977 Removal with reinsertion, implantable contraceptive capsules

If, during a single encounter, the physician removed and reinserted an implantable contraceptive capsule, CPT code 11977 should be coded, as it encompasses the entire procedure. It would be incorrect to code 11975 and 11976, and there is not an edit available for these two codes.

Evaluation and Management Services (99201-99499) and NCCI Guidelines

Evaluation and management (E/M) services represent the medical encounter between a clinician and patient. Often, there may be an E/M service provided at the same encounter as a procedure, and thus the NCCI guidelines instruct when both an E/M CPT code and a procedure CPT code maybe be billed.

Excerpt From NCCI Section on the Integumentary System[2(p3)]

Example: If a physician determines that a new patient with head trauma requires sutures, confirms the allergy and immunization status, obtains informed consent, and performs the repair, an E/M service is not separately reportable. However, if the physician also performs a medically reasonable and necessary full neurological examination, an E/M service may be separately reportable.

Interpretation

The physician must document sufficiently that a separate and distinct medical visit was needed (medical necessity) and was performed (work). If the visit exceeds what is considered normal preprocedure work, and that work is clearly documented, then a visit may be coded and a modifier 25 appended to the visit's E/M code.

Skin, Subcutaneous, and Accessory Structures Incision and Drainage (10040-10180) and NCCI Guidelines

The majority of the integumentary system procedures are found within this section of the CPT codebook. NCCI addresses several of the categories of procedures for skin, subcutaneous and accessory structures. The NCCI guidelines are explained by category within this section of this chapter.

Excerpt From the NCCI Section on the Integumentary System[2(p5)]

Incision and drainage services, as related to the integumentary system, generally involve cutaneous or subcutaneous drainage of cysts, pustules, infections, hematomas, seromas, or fluid collections. If it is necessary to incise and drain a lesion as a part of another procedure or in order to gain access to an area for another procedure, the incision and drainage is not separately reportable if performed at the same patient encounter.

HCPCS/CPT codes for incision and drainage should not be reported separately with other procedures such as excision, repair, destruction, and removal when performed at the same anatomic site at the same patient encounter.

Example

CMS offers the example of a case in which the physician's intent for a procedure is the excision of a pilonidal cyst (CPT code 11770). The physician may incise and drain the cyst as a part of the excision (the incision causes the drainage) or for access. In either case, the incision and drainage is an inherent part of the excision and should not be coded separately.

Excision of Lesions (11400-11646) and NCCI Guidelines

The CPT codebook defines lesion excisions as the full thickness (through the dermis) removal of a lesion, including margins, and includes simple (nonlayered) closure when performed.

Excerpt From the NCCI Section on the Integumentary System[2(p6)]

HCPCS/CPT codes define different types of removal codes such as destruction (eg, laser, freezing), debridement, paring/cutting, shaving, or excision. Only one HCPCS/CPT removal code may be reported for a lesion. If a removal is begun by one method but is converted to another method for completion of the procedure, only the HCPCS/CPT code describing the completed procedure may be reported.

Interpretation

It is clear that the NCCI guidelines are instructing that for a given lesion, only the successful service should be coded. So, in the case in which an initial attempt using a less invasive procedure was followed by a more invasive lesion removal, the more complex procedure used would be appropriately reported, but not both procedures. For example, if the physician begins the procedure by shaving a lesion (CPT codes 11300-11313) but discovers that the lesion is deeper than suspected and must perform a full-thickness excision (CPT codes 11400-11646), only the full-thickness excision should be coded, because one lesion is being treated and the most extensive or successful service should be coded. If multiple, distinct lesions are removed using different methods, an anatomic modifier or the -59 modifier would be used to indicate a different site, a different method, or a different lesion.

Excerpt From NCCI Section on the Integumentary System[2(p6)]

If multiple lesions are included in a single removal procedure (eg, single excision of skin containing three nevi) only one removal HCPCS/CPT code may be reported for the procedure. … If multiple lesions are removed separately, it may be appropriate depending upon the code descriptors for the procedures to report multiple HCPCS/CPT codes utilizing anatomic modifiers or modifier -59 to indicate different sites or lesions.

The medical record must document the appropriateness of reporting multiple HCPCS/CPT codes with these modifiers.

Interpretation

A CPT code should be assigned for each lesion excised, unless the lesions are excised through the same incision. Because the work involves only one actual excision, it is inappropriate to code as if separate procedures were performed. However, if separate excisions were performed, each may be coded. For example, if the physician documents that there are three adjacent lesions on the arm and through a single incision all three are excised, do not code each lesion separately. A single lesion excision would be coded by combining the sizes of all lesions.

Excerpt From NCCI Section on the Integumentary System[2(p7)]

Lesion removal may require closure (simple, intermediate, or complex), adjacent tissue transfer, or grafts. If the lesion removal requires dressings, strip closure, or simple closure, these services are not separately reportable. Thus, CPT codes 12001-12021 (simple repairs) are integral to the lesion removal codes. Intermediate or complex repairs, adjacent tissue transfer, and grafts may be separately reportable if medically reasonable and necessary. However, excision of benign lesions with excised diameter of 0.5 cm or less (CPT codes 11400, 11420, 11440) includes simple, intermediate, or complex repairs which should not be reported separately.

Interpretation

Both the CPT codebook and NCCI (see previous) instruct that a simple closure is included in the lesion excision codes. Therefore, when lesions are excised, and the site is then closed with simple suturing, it would be incorrect to add a code for the repair. However, NCCI takes this guideline one step further by adding that small lesion excisions (those lesions that are 0.5 cm or less) also include any level of repair other than flap or graft closures. To illustrate, a patient presents for an excision of multiple lesions. One is on the back and measures 1.2 cm, another is on the arm and measures 0.5 cm, and a third is on the cheek and measures 0.3 cm. The physician excises each lesion and closes the arm lesion by simple suturing. The back and cheek lesions require a layered closure.

The appropriate coding follows:

Arm

11400   Excision, benign lesion including margins, except skin tag (unless listed elsewhere), trunk, arms or legs; excised diameter 0.5 cm or less

Back

11402   excised diameter 1.1 to 2.0 cm

12031   Repair, intermediate, wounds of scalp, axillae, trunk and/or extremities (excluding hands and feet); 2.5 cm or less

Cheek

11440   Excision, other benign lesion including margins, except skin tag (unless listed elsewhere), face, ears, eyelids, nose, lips, mucous membrane; excised diameter 0.5 cm or less

Explanation

Based on CPT coding guidelines, adding the repair for the cheek would be appropriate, but because of the size of the lesions, NCCI instructs that the repair may not be coded.

Questions to Ask When Coding Lesion Excisions

- Is the lesion benign or malignant?
  Codes vary by lesion morphology.
- Was the lesion removed by excision? Destruction? Other method?
  If excised, use the 11400-11646 codes. If destroyed, see the 17000-17250 codes.
- Is the excision followed by simple closure? Intermediate? Complex? Adjacent tissue transfer? Graft? Other type of repair?
  Simple closure is included in the excision. Complex and intermediate closure may be added to the excision.
- Did the depth of the lesions extend beyond the integument?
  If so, search other systems for a more appropriate code.
- What is the size of the lesion?
  Use the lesion diameter plus the most narrow margin required, not the entire area removed.
- Where is the lesion located?
  Body site drives one part of code selection.
- Is this a re-excision on the same site? If so, was the original lesion malignant?
  If so, code as a malignant excision, even if the pathology report returns as benign.

Mohs Micrographic Surgery (17311-17315) and NCCI Guidelines

Excerpt From the NCCI Section on the Integumentary System[2(p7-8)]

Mohs micrographic surgery (CPT codes 17311-17315) is performed to remove complex or ill-defined cutaneous malignancy. A single physician performs both the surgery and pathologic examination of the specimen(s). The Mohs micrographic surgery CPT codes include skin biopsy and excision services (CPT codes 11000-11001, 11600-11646, and 17260-17286) and pathology services (88300-88309, 88329-88332). Reporting these latter codes in addition to the Mohs micrographic surgery CPT codes is inappropriate. However, if a suspected skin cancer is biopsied for pathologic diagnosis prior to proceeding to Mohs micrographic surgery, the biopsy (CPT codes 11000, 11001) and frozen section pathology (CPT code 88331) may be reported separately utilizing modifier -59 or -58 to distinguish the diagnostic biopsy from the definitive Mohs surgery. Although the *CPT Manual* indicates that modifier -59 should be utilized, it is also acceptable to utilize modifier -58 to indicate that the diagnostic skin biopsy and Mohs micrographic surgery were staged or planned procedures. Repairs, grafts, and flaps are separately reportable with the Mohs micrographic surgery CPT codes.

Interpretation

Because a single physician performs the removal and pathological interpretation, the CPT codes for Mohs micrographic surgery and CMS reimbursement inherently include both portions. Because the codes are all-inclusive, it would be incorrect coding to add the pathology examination to the Mohs codes. It would also be incorrect to code different CPT codes for true Mohs techniques—in other words, do not substitute lesion excision (CPT codes 11400-11646) in order to add the pathology service (CPT codes 88300-88309, 88329-88332) codes.

NCCI also instructs that if the biopsy and pathology service are performed prior to and distinct from the Mohs (usually as the true diagnostic tool), the biopsy and pathology service may be added. Then, it would be appropriate to add a modifier 58 to the Mohs procedure code to illustrate that the Mohs service was related to, but more extensive than, the biopsy service. A case in point would be a patient who has a suspected lesion on her face, and the physician biopsies the lesion. When the frozen section is returned, the physician determines that a Mohs procedure is the best treatment for the lesion and begins the Mohs service. In this case, the biopsy and Mohs may be coded, and the Mohs service should be appended with modifier 58.

Repair and Tissue Transfers (12001-14350) and NCCI Guidelines

Excerpt From the NCCI Section on the Integumentary System[2(p8-9)]

The CPT Manual classifies repairs (closure) (CPT codes 12001-13160) as simple, intermediate, or complex. If closure cannot be completed by one of these methods, adjacent tissue transfer or rearrangement (CPT codes 14000-14350) may be utilized.

Adjacent tissue transfer or rearrangement procedures include excision (CPT 11400-11646) and repair (CPT 12001-13160). Thus, CPT codes 11400-11646 and 12001-13160 should not be reported separately with CPT codes 14000-14350 for the same lesion or injury.

Additionally, debridement necessary to perform a tissue transfer procedure is included in the procedure.

Interpretation

When lesion excision is of such an extent that closure cannot be accomplished by simple, intermediate, or complex closure, other methodology must be employed. Frequently, ATT or tissue rearrangement is employed (Z-plasty, W-plasty, flaps, etc). This family of codes (CPT codes 14000-14350) includes excision of the lesion and repair by ATT. Because CPT codebook instructions within the ATT section of codes state that the ATT includes the excision,

it would be violating a CPT coding as well as an NCCI guideline if both the excision and ATT of a single site were coded separately.

Additionally, because only one repair of a single site may be coded, only the most extensive repair should be coded; therefore, the simple-complex repairs are incidental to the ATT repair services.

 Coding ATTs Tip: *Skin grafts necessary to close a secondary defect are an additional procedure. These codes do not apply when direct closure or rearrangement of traumatic wounds incidentally (unintentionally) results in these configurations. The goal of the physician must be to perform an ATT.*

Skin Replacement Surgery and Skin Substitutes (15002-15431) and NCCI Guidelines

Excerpt From the NCCI Section on the Integumentary System[2(p5)]

CPT codes describing skin grafts and skin substitutes are classified by size, location of recipient site, and type of graft or skin substitute. For most combinations of location and type of graft/skin substitutes, there are two or three CPT codes, including a primary code and one or two add-on codes. The primary code describes one size of graft/skin substitute and should not be reported with more than one unit of service. Larger size grafts or skin substitutes are reported with add-on codes.

The primary graft/skin substitute codes (eg, 15100, 15120, 15200, 15220) are mutually exclusive since only one type of graft/skin substitute can be utilized at a single anatomic site. If multiple sites require different types of grafts/skin substitutes, the different graft/skin substitute CPT codes should be reported with anatomic modifiers or modifier 59 to indicate the different sites.

Interpretation

NCCI explains that for a single anatomic site, only one primary code should be used, and if the size of the graft is larger, then the add-on codes should be coded until the complete size is accounted for; however, NCCI guidelines also indicate that separate sites repaired with different types of grafts should be coded separately. When that is the case, modifier 59 should be appended to the second primary code to ensure that a clear picture of the procedure is presented on the bill. Although NCCI instructs that anatomic modifiers, rather than modifier 59, may be used, it is recommended that modifier 59 be used, because these CPT codes include multiple anatomic sites, and the anatomic modifiers would not clearly indicate the specific location. For instance, a patient presents for skin grafting of wounds (resulting from prior injury) on both arms. The wounds are extensive and results in split-thickness grafting of 150 cm² on the left arm and 55 cm² full-thickness grafting on the right arm. The correct coding would be as follows:

Right arm

15220×1 + 15221×2

15220 Full thickness graft, free, including direct closure of donor site, scalp, arms, and/or legs; 20 sq cm or less

+ 15221 each additional 20 sq cm, or part thereof (List separately in addition to code for primary procedure)

Left arm

15100×1-59 + 15101×1

15100 Split-thickness autograft, trunk, arms, legs; first 100 sq cm or less, or 1% of body area of infants and children (except 15050)

+ 15101 each additional 100 sq cm, or each additional 1% of body area of infants and children, or part thereof (List separately in addition to code for primary procedure)

Because there are two primary sites repaired by different types of grafts, each of those may be billed separately by modifying one with -59.

For a specific location, a primary code is defined and followed by a supplemental code for additional coverage area. As a result of this coding structure, for a given area of involvement, the initial code is limited to one unit of service; the supplemental code may have multiple units of service depending on the area to be covered. Medicare currently has an MUE in place for these codes.

Additional Information on Flaps and Grafts

Flaps are attached to the donor site and are usually obtained from tissue adjacent to or near the recipient site. Grafts are not attached to the donor site and are most often obtained from tissue remote from the recipient site.

The donor site is where the wound is created by the surgeon—in other words, where the graft or flap material was obtained. The recipient site is where the wound was repaired by the surgeon—in other words, where the graft or flap material was applied.

Questions to ask when coding flaps and grafts:

Into which category does the repair fall (flap or graft)? *If the repair is a flap, it does not really matter from a coding perspective what type of flap was used (Z plasty, V-Y, other). If the repair is a graft, the type of graft (pinch, split-thickness or full-thickness, skin substitute) must be specified.*

What are the measurements of the original wound site (determined by multiplying the dimensions)?
Was a lesion excised?
If so for ATTs, do not code the excision, because it is included in the repair. If so for skin grafts, code lesion excision codes.

Was there site preparation other than for lesion excision?
Was the donor site repaired with a flap or graft? *If so, add that as well.*

Breast Procedures (19000-19499) and NCCI Guidelines

Excerpt From the NCCI Section on the Integumentary System[2(p10)]

Since a mastectomy (CPT codes 19300-19307) describes removal of breast tissue including all lesions within the breast tissue, breast excision codes (19110-19126) generally are not separately reportable unless performed at a site unrelated to the mastectomy. However, if the breast excision procedure precedes the mastectomy for the purpose of obtaining tissue for pathologic examination which determines the need for the mastectomy, the breast excision and mastectomy codes are separately reportable. (Modifier -58 may be utilized to indicate that the procedures were staged.) If a diagnosis was established preoperatively, an excision procedure for the purpose of obtaining additional pathologic material is not separately reportable.

Interpretation

The most extensive procedure (mastectomy) would be billed, rather than separately reporting the less extensive excision codes. The exception to this, which is quite common, is when the lesser procedure is the diagnostic determining factor to proceed with the more extensive procedure. Coders will often see cases in which a physician removes some tissue and, during the same surgical encounter, awaits the frozen section results prior to continuing to the mastectomy. In that case, as long as the documentation is clear, both the lesser and more extensive procedures may be billed, with a modifier 58 appended to the more extensive and later procedure (eg, mastectomy).

Excerpt From the NCCI Section on the Integumentary System[2(p10)]

Similarly, diagnostic biopsies (eg, fine needle aspiration, core, incisional) to procure tissue for diagnostic purposes to determine whether an excision or mastectomy is necessary at the same patient encounter are separately reportable with modifier -58. However, biopsies (eg, fine needle aspiration, core, incisional) are not separately reportable if a preoperative diagnosis exists.

Interpretation

Because an excision of lesions occurs in the course of performing a mastectomy, breast excisions are not separately reported from a mastectomy unless performed to establish the malignant diagnosis before proceeding to the mastectomy. If the excision is performed to obtain tissue to determine a pathologic diagnosis of malignancy prior to proceeding to a mastectomy, the excision is coded separately with modifier 58. This reiterates that the biopsy may be coded in addition to the more major procedure only if it serves a true diagnostic purpose. This, of course, must be clearly documented. The more extensive procedure would be coded in addition to the diagnostic biopsy with a modifier 58.

 CPT Coding Tip: *The preoperative diagnosis might differ from the postoperative diagnosis in this case.*

Excerpt From the NCCI Section on the Integumentary System[2(p10)]

Some codes describe mastectomies with lymphadenectomy and/or removal of muscle tissue. The latter procedures are not separately reportable.

Interpretation

This instruction from NCCI indicates that if an additional part of the operation is included in the CPT code description, it should not be separately billed when performed at the same session as the primary surgery.

Example

To better understand this instruction, review the following codes:

19300   Mastectomy for gynecomastia

19301   Mastectomy, partial (eg, lumpectomy, tylectomy, quadrantectomy, segmentectomy);

19302   with axillary lymphadenectomy

19303   Mastectomy, simple, complete

19304   Mastectomy, subcutaneous

19305   Mastectomy, radical, including pectoral muscles, axillary lymph nodes

19306   Mastectomy, radical, including pectoral muscles, axillary and internal mammary lymph nodes (Urban type operation)

19307   Mastectomy, modified radical, including axillary lymph nodes, with or without pectoralis minor muscle, but excluding pectoralis major muscle

38500   Biopsy or excision of lymph node(s); open, superficial

38505   by needle, superficial (eg, cervical, inguinal, axillary)

38510   open, deep cervical node(s)

38520   open, deep cervical node(s) with excision scalene fat pad

38525   open, deep axillary node(s)

38530   open, internal mammary node(s)

NCCI and CPT codebook guidelines indicate that if mastectomies with lymphadenectomies or removal of muscle tissue are performed during a single operative session, it would be incorrect to separate these services into two different codes (eg, 19300 and 38525), rather than using the comprehensive code (eg, 19305).

Excerpt From the NCCI Section on the Integumentary System[2(p10-11)]

Except for sentinel lymph node biopsies, ipsilateral lymph node excisions are not separately reportable. Contralateral lymph node excisions may be separately reportable with appropriate modifiers (e.g., -LT, -RT).

Interpretation

Ipsilateral means of the same side, whereas *contralateral* means of the opposite side. Therefore, if procedures are performed on the same side, do not code separately from the comprehensive procedure. If procedures are performed on the opposite side, both may be coded, and the lateral modifiers should be appended to each code to clarify that separate sites are involved.

Excerpt From the NCCI Section on the Integumentary System[2(p11)]

Sentinel lymph node biopsy is separately reportable when performed prior to a localized excision of breast or a mastectomy without lymphadenectomy. However, sentinel lymph node biopsy is not separately reportable with a mastectomy procedure that includes lymphadenectomy in the anatomic area of the sentinel lymph node biopsy.

Interpretation

This guideline is similar to those for the biopsy codes that are discussed in prior sections. If the sentinel lymph node biopsy is performed prior to and as the diagnostic component determining the need for the more extensive procedure, both services may be coded, and the mastectomy should be appended with modifier 58.

CPT Coding Tip: CPT codes 19000 and 19001 are for puncture aspirations of a cyst. Each aspiration is coded, and CPT 19001 is for each additional cyst aspirated on the same breast. If both breasts have puncture aspirations, use 19000 for each initial cyst per breast by using modifiers RT/LT or 50.

Code 19101 is for an open incisional biopsy, but if the entire lesion is removed, use code 19120 instead. Do not add codes 19101 to 19120 for the same lesion.

Code 19120 is for excision of one of more masses within a single incision. Assign CPT code 19120 for each lesion excised through separate incision sites. If an excision of a lesion coincidentally results in the excision of an adjacent lesion through the same incision, do not code it separately.

Phrases in the body of the operative report or on the pathology report that indicate that the lesion was removed and not just biopsied include:
- *The mass was excised.*
- *Excised margins are clear of abnormal tissue.*
- *Specimen is received in toto.*

Physicians will often use the terms incisional breast biopsy and excisional breast biopsy synonymously. Carefully review the operative report to determine

whether the lesion was biopsied (19101) or excised (19120).

CPT code 19125 may be reported once with modifier -50 appended if needle localization and excision are performed on the right and left breast.

If there is a skin lesion excision, do not code the procedure as an excision of a breast mass but rather a skin lesion excision.

Fine-needle aspiration biopsies, core biopsies, open incisional or excisional biopsies, and related procedures performed to procure tissue from a lesion for which an established diagnosis exists are not to be reported separately at the time of a lesion excision unless performed on a different lesion or on the contralateral breast. However, if a diagnosis is not established, and the decision to perform the excision or mastectomy is dependent on the results of the biopsy, then the biopsy is separately reported. Modifier 58 may be used appropriately to indicate that the biopsy and the excision or mastectomy are staged or planned procedures.

Because excisions of lesions occur in the course of performing a mastectomy, breast excisions are not separately reported from a mastectomy unless performed to establish the malignant diagnosis before proceeding to the mastectomy. Specifically, CPT codes 19110-19126 (breast excision) are in general included in all mastectomy CPT codes (19300-19307) of the same side. However, if the excision is performed to obtain tissue to determine a pathologic diagnosis of malignancy prior to proceeding to a mastectomy, the excision is separately reportable with the mastectomy. Modifier 58 should be used in this situation.

SUMMARY

- The entire integumentary system section from the NCCI manual should be read.

- Biopsies are bundled into excisions unless they are performed for diagnostic purposes.

- Less extensive services are bundled into more complex services when they are performed on a single anatomic location during a single surgical session.

- All of the instructions within the CPT codebook for integumentary system procedures should be reviewed. They are often consistent with the NCCI guidelines.

Definitions and Acronyms

adjacent tissue transfer/rearrangement (ATT): This is the transfer of tissue to repair a defect such as traumatic avulsion or an area where a large defect exists as the result of lesion excision. This procedure involves moving or lifting a normal, healthy section of skin (that remains connected at one or two of its borders) to an adjacent or nearby defect for the repair of the defect.

American Academy of Dermatology (AAD): The specialty society devoted to dermatologists. Excellent coding-related resources are provided on the society's Web site (www.aad.org). The AAD also provides a coding publication available by subscription.

carrier: Medicare payer for physician professional fee services

Centers for Medicare and Medicaid Services (CMS): This is a branch of the Department of Health and Human Services (DHHS) responsible for overseeing the Medicare and Medicaid federal health care programs.

contralateral: Referring to the opposite side of the body

dermis: Referring to the innermost layer of skin

epidermis: Referring to the outermost layer of skin

fiscal intermediary: The Medicare payer for hospital services (inpatient and outpatient)

hypodermis: Referring to the subcutaneous layer (layer beneath the dermis) of the skin

ipsilateral: Referring to the same side of the body

Medicare administrative contractor (MAC): Medicare is replacing its current fiscal intermediary and carrier contractors with MACs. MACs will process both Part A and Part B claims.

CHAPTER EXERCISE

Review the following case information:

Operative Report

Diagnosis: Basal cell carcinoma of the right nasal ala and multicentric basal cell carcinoma of the top of the left shoulder.

Operation: Excision of basal cell carcinoma from the right nasal ala and frozen section control for margins and reconstruction with a quadrilateral focal rotation flap and excision of basal cell carcinoma from the top of the left shoulder and frozen section for margins.

Procedure: With the patient in the supine position and draped in such a manner as to expose the nasal area, the

#15 scalpel is used to excise the lesion on the right nasal ala with an ellipse of skin measuring 2 × 1 cm. The specimen is sent for frozen section evaluation. Report is that the margin is free of tumor. Consideration is then given to closure of the wound with a full-thickness skin graft or a local rotation flap. The patient prefers a local rotation flap, and, therefore a quadrilateral flap is based laterally and rotated into the defect over the nasal ala. The skin flaps are sutured with interrupted 5-0 nylon suture.

The scalpel is then used to excise the lesion from the top of the left shoulder. An ellipse of skin measuring 4 × 2 cm is used for excision, and the specimen is tagged at the 12 o'clock position margin and sent for frozen section evaluation. Report is that the margin is free of tumor. The wound margins are undermined to allow for eversion and advancement and then approximated with interrupted 4-0 nylon suture. The patient tolerates the procedure well and is taken to the holding area in satisfactory condition.

The patient is given prescriptions for propoxyphene 100 mg and doxycycline 100 mg. He will be able to change the dressing daily and will be seen in the office in eight days for evaluation and suture removal.

What would be coded in this case and why?

Originally coded:

14060RT	Adjacent tissue transfer or rearrangement, eyelids, nose, ears and/or lips; defect 10 sq cm or less. Modifier RT represents right side.
11642RT	Excision, malignant lesion including margins, face, ears, eyelids, nose, lips; excised diameter 1.1 to 2.0 cm. Modifier RT represents right side.
14000LT59	Adjacent tissue transfer or rearrangement, trunk; defect 10 sq cm or less. Modifier LT represents left side. Modifier 59 represents distinct service.
11604LT59	Excision, malignant lesion including margins, trunk, arms, or legs; excised diameter 3.1 to 4.0 cm. Modifier LT represents left side. Modifier 59 represents distinct service.

ANSWERS TO CHAPTER EXERCISES

Originally coded:	Should be coded:
14060RT	**14060** (no modifier)
11642RT	not coded—incidental to 14060
14000LT59	not coded—not documented
11604LT59	**11604-59** (to indicate separate site from 14060)

Comments:

Physician report is unclear about size of ATT.

Modifier 59 is necessary on CPT code 11604 because there is an NCCI edit.

Lateral modifiers are unnecessary on these codes according to CMS. The codes inherently include multiple anatomic sites; therefore, lateral modifiers do not specify a site.

REFERENCES

1. American Medical Association. *Current Procedural Terminology CPT® 2009 Professional Edition*. Chicago, IL: American Medical Association; 2008.

2. Centers for Medicare and Medicaid Services. "Chapter III Surgery: Integumentary System," In: NCCI Policy Manual for Medicare Services. www.cms.hhs.gov/NationalCorrectCodInitEd/01_overview.asp#TopOfPage. Accessed June 12, 2009.

3. Centers for Medicare and Medicaid Services. "Chapter I General Correct Coding Policies," In: NCCI Policy Manual for Medicare Services. www.cms.hhs.gov/NationalCorrectCodInitEd/01_overview.asp#TopOfPage. Accessed June 12, 2009.

4. American Medical Association. "Coding tip, debridement of multiple sites," *CPT Assistant*. 1997;7(2):7.

The Musculoskeletal System

Chapter 6 provides background about the musculoskeletal system, reviews the National Correct Coding Initiative (NCCI) coding guidelines for procedures performed on the musculoskeletal system, and provides examples to reflect the logic behind the edits. As in the other chapters, an NCCI guideline is followed by our interpretation, an example, or both.

There are several categories of musculoskeletal procedures within *Current Procedural Terminology (CPT®) 2009 Professional Edition 2009*[1], and this section is the largest within the surgery CPT codes. See Figure 6-1 for the breakdown of CPT codebook musculoskeletal service categories.

CPT Coding Tip: *The first section of musculoskeletal surgery CPT codes is for general procedures, which means services that could belong to most anatomic sites. Become familiar with the CPT codes in this section, and if there is not a more appropriate code in the specific anatomical section of musculoskeletal system coding guidelines, then look here. Always use a more specific procedure, if available.*

The musculoskeletal system section of CPT is classified into a general section and grafts, and then moves through all the anatomical sites starting with the head and working through the spine, extremities, and so forth. Coding for each anatomical site addresses incision, excision, introduction or removal, repair, revision or reconstruction, fracture or dislocation, manipulation, arthrodesis, amputation, and miscellaneous procedures. The CPT codebook is arranged to guide the coder logically to the appropriate site and code.

CPT Coding Tip:

20000 Incision of soft tissue abscess (eg, secondary to osteomyelitis); superficial

20005 deep or complicated

What is the difference between superficial and deep?

One definition of superficial is "above the fascia" and deep means anything deeper than that. See the CPT 2010 codebook for the definitions. Work with the physicians to determine the difference. Perhaps, superficial is just below the integumentary system (hypodermis), and deep is anything beyond that.

FIGURE 6-1 *CPT Codebook Surgery Categories Regarding the Musculoskeletal System*

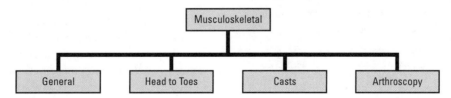

Musculoskeletal System and NCCI Guidelines

Excerpt From the Musculoskeletal System Section of NCCI Guidelines[2(p2)]

Introduction

The principles of correct coding discussed in Chapter I apply to the CPT codes in the range 20000-29999. Several general guidelines are repeated in this chapter. However, those general guidelines from Chapter I not discussed in this Chapter are nonetheless applicable.

Interpretation

This instruction indicates that the overall NCCI guidelines apply to each section of the CPT codebook, and, even if they are not repeated within a chapter, they are nonetheless a guideline to be followed. The introductory guidelines were reviewed comprehensively in Chapter 2 of this book; however, those introductory guidelines that have clear application within the musculoskeletal system are reiterated in this chapter.

Excerpt From the General Correct Coding Policies Section of NCCI Guidelines[3(p10)]

Exposure and exploration of the surgical field is integral to an operative procedure and is not separately reportable. If exploration of the surgical field results in additional procedures other than the primary procedure, the additional procedures may generally be reported separately. However, a procedure designated by the CPT code descriptor as a "separate procedure" is not separately reportable if performed in a region anatomically related to the other procedure(s) through the same skin incision, orifice, or surgical approach.

Interpretation

Approaches, access, and explorations for procedures are always bundled into the primary procedure and not separately coded. Because invasive procedures require reaching the body part, the access (or approach) does not add to the physician's work sufficiently to warrant an additional code. Also, during the procedure the surgeon should assess the entire surgical field to decide the best route for approach and determine the extent of the condition (disease, injury) and whether any other procedures are needed. All of these services are usual for an invasive procedure and not separately coded. However, if during that exploration, the surgeon determines that another procedure is needed, the additional procedure should be coded unless it is bundled into the primary procedure for other reasons (separate procedure, NCCI edits, etc). For example, in performing an open rotator cuff repair, the physician must cut into the shoulder joint to access the rotator cuff ligaments. This incision and any exploration of the joint is included in the rotator cuff surgery.

Another example would be when, during the open rotator cuff repair (see example 1), the surgeon determines that the patient also required a distal claviculectomy. Both the rotator cuff repair and the claviculectomy may be coded. These services do not bundle, based on NCCI edits.

Excerpt From the General Correct Coding Policies Section of NCCI Guidelines[3(p11)]

If a diagnostic endoscopy is the basis for, and precedes, an open procedure, the diagnostic endoscopy is separately reportable with modifier -58. However, the medical record must document the medical reasonableness and necessity for the diagnostic endoscopy. A scout endoscopy to assess anatomic landmarks and extent of disease is not separately reportable with an open procedure. When an endoscopic procedure fails and is converted to another surgical procedure, only the successful surgical procedure may be reported. The endoscopic procedure is separately reportable with the successful procedure.

Interpretation

This guideline indicates that if both a diagnostic endoscopy and an open procedure of the same body area are performed on a single date of service (regardless of whether they are within the same procedure session), both may be coded. Important here is that the endoscopy (arthroscopy for musculoskeletal joint procedures) must be diagnostic. A diagnostic endoscopic procedure will often help determine whether and which therapeutic procedure should be performed. The more major procedure (or open procedure) is based, at least in part, on the results of the diagnostic endoscopy.

The guideline also indicates that modifier 58 (staged or related procedure) is appended to the endoscopy. Lastly, obviously, if the endoscopy was performed at a different anatomic site than the open procedure, both may be coded.

For instance, a patient presents to an orthopaedic surgeon complaining of increased shoulder pain. Magnetic resonance imaging is completed, but no definitive diagnosis or treatment is determined. The surgeon decides to perform a diagnostic arthroscopy of the shoulder for diagnosis and treatment. During the diagnostic arthroscopy of the shoulder, the surgeon discovers a massive tear in the patient's rotator cuff and decides to repair the tear through an open procedure. The diagnostic arthroscopy is completed and an open repair performed.

Introduction Section of NCCI Musculoskeletal System Guidelines

Excerpt From the Musculoskeletal System Section of NCCI Guidelines

Physicians should report the HCPCS/CPT code that describes the procedure performed to the greatest specificity possible. A HCPCS/CPT code should be reported only if all services described by the code are performed. A physician should not report multiple HCPCS/CPT codes if a single HCPCS/CPT code exists that describes the services. This type of unbundling is incorrect coding.

Interpretation

If a single code encompasses the entire procedure, that code should be used, rather than separating parts of the procedure. This is true regardless of whether an edit exists in NCCI. If one CPT code includes the entire work performed, do not code separate components.

Example

The following CPT codes represent nasal fracture care:

21325 Open treatment of nasal fracture; uncomplicated

21335 Open treatment of nasal septal fracture, with concomitant open treatment of fractured septum

If a provider performs an uncomplicated open treatment of a nasal fracture and, during the same session, repairs the nasal septal fracture, there is one comprehensive code to reflect this operative session (CPT code 21335). Do not report CPT codes 21325 and 21336.

Evaluation and Management Services (99201-99499) and NCCI Guidelines

Evaluation and Management (E/M) services represent the medical encounter between a clinician and patient. Often there may be an E/M service provided at the same encounter as a procedure, so the NCCI guidelines provide instruction about when both an E/M CPT code and a procedure CPT code maybe be billed. Refer to Chapters 2 and 3 of this book for the complete discussion on E/M coding within the NCCI edit guidelines. However, we will offer a few musculoskeletal system examples here.

Example

A patient presents for a scheduled joint injection and has no other problems or complications. In this case, it is unlikely that a medical visit would be necessary or provided during the encounter. Only the joint injection should be coded.

Example

An elderly patient trips and falls down a long flight of stairs and has severe pain in his right wrist, hip, and shoulder; however, there are no visible injuries other than swelling over these joints. The patient's daughter takes him to an urgent care center, where they perform a complete history and examination and obtain radiographs. It is determined that the patient has:
- a severely bruised hip, for which they prescribe pain medication,
- a sprained wrist, for which they apply a splint, and
- a broken humerus, for which they immobilize the arm with a splint and refer the patient to an orthopaedic surgeon.

For this encounter, there would definitely be a necessary (as long as sufficiently documented) visit in addition to the splint applications.

Documentation Tip: *The physician must document suf-ficiently that a separate and distinct medical visit was needed (medical necessity) and was performed (work). If the visit exceeds what is considered normal preprocedure work, and that work is clearly documented, then a visit may be coded and a modifier 25 appended to the visit E/M code. Only the portion of the E/M that is beyond the preprocedure work should be included in the level assignment.*

Anesthesia (00100–01999) and NCCI Guidelines

As discussed extensively in Chapter 4, anesthesia provided by the physician performing the surgery or procedure is included in the surgeon's global fee for the surgery and not separately coded or paid.

Excerpt From the Musculoskeletal System Section of NCCI Guidelines[2(p4)]

Injections of local anesthesia for musculoskeletal pro-cedures (surgical or manipulative) are not separately reportable. For example, CPT codes 20526-20553 (therapeutic injection of carpal tunnel, tendon sheath, ligament, muscle trigger points) should not be reported for the administration of local anesthesia to perform another procedure. The NCCI guidelines contain many edits based on this principle. If a pro-cedure and a separate and distinct injection service unrelated to anesthesia for the former procedure are reported, the injection service may be reported with an NCCI-associated modifier if appropriate.

Interpretation

Local anesthetic is a part of the reimbursement for the procedure and not separately reportable. Often physicians performing minor procedures will inject some sort of anes-thetic (eg, lidocaine) to deaden the procedure site. One of the core policies within NCCI is that the reimbursement for the procedure includes anesthesia provided by the physi-cian performing the procedure. Therefore, local anesthetic is not separately coded. However, should there be an injec-tion for an unrelated condition performed during the same encounter as another procedure, both services are most likely appropriate to code. So, if a physician performed a

superficial bone biopsy and, prior to making the incision, injected a local anesthetic, the local anesthetic is bundled into the biopsy code and not separately reported.

Biopsy Services and NCCI Guidelines

Biopsies are the removing of samples of tissue for pathology examination.

Excerpt From the Musculoskeletal System Section of NCCI Guidelines[2(p4-5)]

Biopsy
A biopsy performed at the time of another more extensive procedure (e.g., excision, destruction, removal) is separately reportable under specific circumstances.

If the biopsy is performed on a separate lesion, it is separately reportable. This situation may be reported with anatomic modifiers or modifier -59.

If the biopsy is performed on the same lesion on which the more extensive procedure is performed, it is separately reportable only if the biopsy is utilized for immediate pathologic diagnosis prior to the more extensive procedure, and the decision to proceed with the more extensive procedure is based on the result of the pathologic examination. Modifier -58 may be reported to indicate that the biopsy and the more extensive procedure were planned or staged procedures.

If a biopsy is performed and submitted for patho-logic evaluation that will be completed after the more extensive procedure is performed, the biopsy is not separately reportable with the more extensive procedure.

Interpretation

Physicians must document clearly that either there are distinct anatomic sites for the biopsies versus the more extensive procedures or that they awaited the results of the pathology report prior to performing the more extensive procedures. Without sufficient documentation, only the more extensive procedure should be coded. Essentially, there are two ways to appropriately code a biopsy and another procedure. See Figure 6-2.

FIGURE 6-2 *Biopsy Coding Questions*

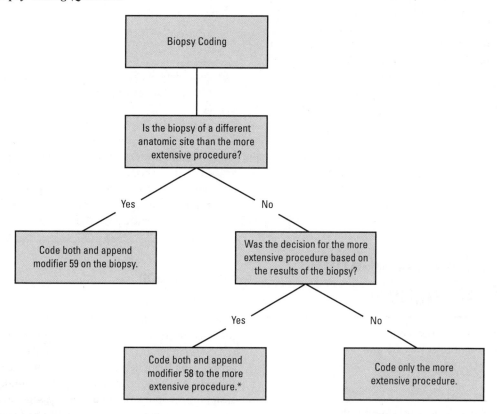

Arthroscopic Procedures Converted to Open Procedures Within NCCI Guidelines

Excerpt From the Musculoskeletal System Section of NCCI Guidelines[2(p5)]

If an arthroscopic procedure fails and is converted to an open procedure, only the open procedure is reportable. Thus, arthroscopic procedures are bundled into open procedures. If an arthroscopic procedure and open procedure are performed on different joints, the two procedures may be separately reportable with anatomic modifiers or modifier -59.

Interpretation

Providers want to approach a procedure with the greatest probability of success and the least trauma to the patient.

As a result, many times procedures are successfully completed using endoscopic methods avoiding the need for a more invasive method. However, on occasion during the procedure the provider determines that the success of the procedure will be improved by converting to an open procedure. This guideline in NCCI indicates that when a failed approach is followed during the same surgical session by a successful approach for a single procedure, only the successful procedure may be coded. Basically, only bills for one approach (the most successful one) will be paid for a single procedure.

An arthroscopy is an endoscopic joint examination done through a scope to view the joint cavity's interior structure. The following are common steps the provider follows during an arthroscopic procedure.
1. The scope is inserted through a small incision and the cavity is viewed.
2. Pictures are taken.
3. A biopsy is done.
4. Therapeutic services are performed, if necessary.

However, if different and distinct procedures are performed through different approaches, or on different joints, each procedure may be coded as long as other bundling issues are not relevant. Modifier 59 will likely be needed to indicate that separate and distinct services are supported by the documentation.

Therefore, when a physician attempts a rotator cuff repair through an arthroscopic approach but must convert to an open procedure to successfully perform the repair, only the open approach should be billed. The failed procedure is incidental to the successful procedure. Or, for a patient who presents for an arthroscopic rotator cuff repair and during the arthroscopic procedure, a distal claviculectomy is performed successfully, but when the rotator cuff is approached, the physician decides that the procedure needs to be performed via an open (incisional) approach and, therefore, does an open rotator cuff repair. In this example, both the arthroscopic claviculectomy with a modifier 59 and the open rotator cuff repair may be billed, because these are separate and distinct procedures.

Fractures and Dislocations and NCCI Guidelines

There are extensive guidelines within the NCCI policies regarding the coding of fracture care and dislocations.

Excerpt From the Musculoskeletal System Section of NCCI Guidelines[2(p5)]

The application of external immobilization devices (casts, splints, strapping) at the time of a procedure includes the subsequent removal of the device when performed by the same entity (e.g., physician, practice, group, employees, etc.). Providers should not report removal or repair CPT codes 29700-29750 for those services. These removal or repair CPT codes may only be reported if the initial application of the cast, splint, or strapping was performed by a different entity.

Interpretation

This guideline is consistent with the CPT codebook instructions that state that casting and strapping procedures include the removal of a cast or strapping. Because surgeries, including fracture repairs, include usual postoperative care, the removal of a cast by the original physician would be a part of the routine postoperative care paid as a part of the original surgery. These services should not be separately coded.

Excerpt From the Musculoskeletal System Section of NCCI Guidelines[2(p5)]

Casting/splinting/strapping should not be reported separately if a restorative treatment or procedure to stabilize or protect a fracture, injury, or dislocation and/or afford comfort to the patient is also performed. Additionally casting/splinting/strapping CPT codes should not be reported for application of a dressing after a therapeutic procedure.

Interpretation

Remember from our general NCCI coding edits discussion (see Chapter 2) that operative site closure and dressings are included in the global surgery reimbursement and should not be separately coded. Therefore, if a casting, strapping, or splinting is applied to the same anatomic site as another procedure to serve as dressing for the wound, the casting, strapping, or splinting should not be separately coded. However, if a cast is applied to a different anatomic location than another procedure performed during the same operative session, both services may be coded, and a modifier 59 might be needed.

As an example, a patient presents with an injured leg, and it is discovered that the femur is broken. The physician performs a closed reduction without manipulation of the fracture and applies a long-leg cast. In this scenario, the cast is included in the fracture repair and not separately reported, as it serves as an integral part of the fracture repair.

Another example would be a patient who presents to an urgent care center with multiple injuries. Lacerations on the right upper arm and face are sutured, a closed fracture on the right hand is immobilized by splinting, and the patient is referred immediately to an orthopedist.

In this scenario, the splint application may be coded in addition to the laceration repairs because it is of an independent site and injury. Also, note that there is no fracture repair being performed—only immobilization to protect the site until the patient presented to the orthopedist; therefore, splint application is appropriate coding.

Excerpt From the Musculoskeletal System Section of NCCI Guidelines[2(p6)]

CPT codes for closed or open treatment of fractures or dislocations include the application of casts, splints, or strapping.

Interpretation

This is merely reiterating that casting, strapping, and splinting are included in the payment for the fracture care and should not be coded separately (unless for an unrelated site).

Excerpt From the Musculoskeletal System Section of NCCI Guidelines[2(p6)]

If a physician treats a fracture, dislocation, or injury with a cast, splint, or strap as an initial service without any other definitive procedure or treatment and only expects to perform the initial care, the physician may report an evaluation and management (E&M) service, a casting/splinting/strapping CPT code, and a cast/splint/strap supply code (Q4001-Q4051).

Interpretation

This instruction from NCCI is exactly the same as that in the CPT codebook (boldface type added):

Excerpt From the CPT codebook[1(p126-127)] **on Casting and Strapping (CPT codes 29000-29799)**

The listed procedures apply when the cast application or strapping is a replacement procedure used during or after the period of follow-up care, **or when the cast application or strapping is an initial service performed without a restorative treatment or procedure(s) to stabilize or protect a fracture, injury, or dislocation and/or to afford comfort to a patient.** Restorative treatment or procedure(s) rendered by another physician following the application of the initial cast/splint/strap may be reported with a treatment of fracture and/or dislocation code.

If the physician applies the cast, splint, or strap only and has no intention of following the patient postapplication, the casting, strapping, and splinting codes may be used. As indicated in the policy, it is also likely that an E/M service would be applicable, but that would depend on the documentation for the encounter.

Example

A patient presents to an urgent care center with multiple injuries. Lacerations on the right upper arm and face are sutured, a closed fracture of the right hand is immobilized by splinting, and the is patient referred immediately to an orthopedist.

In this scenario, the urgent care center is not intending to follow the patient's fracture nor are they attempting repair. Their services are simply for immobilization to protect the site until the patient presents to the orthopedist; therefore, coding for splint application is appropriate.

Example

A patient presents to an emergency department (ED) with a broken finger. The ED clinician applies a cast and advises the patient to see an orthopaedic surgeon the following day.

It is clear that the ED physician does not expect to follow this patient postoperatively, as he is referring the patient to a surgeon. This would be coded as casting, along with an E/M code, if properly documented.

Example

A patient presents to the ED with a broken finger. The ED clinician manipulates the finger back into alignment and buddy-tapes the finger to an adjoining finger. He prescribes pain medication and advises the patient that he can return to the ED as needed or go to his primary care physician if necessary.

This example is a bit tricky, but, basically, the physician is performing restorative treatment, and this would be coded as fracture care, without adding a code for the taping. Also, it is likely that an E/M service would also be coded, depending on the level of documentation.

There are CPT codes (20670 and 20680) for removal of internal fixation devices (e.g., pin, rod). These codes are not separately reportable if the removal is performed as a necessary integral component of another procedure. For example, if a revision of an open fracture repair requires removal of a previously inserted pin, CPT code 20670 or 20680 is not separately reportable.

Similarly, if a superficial or deep implant (e.g., buried wire, pin, rod) requires surgical removal (CPT codes 20670 and 20680), it is not separately reportable if it is performed as an integral part of another procedure.

Interpretation

Throughout the NCCI edits we are reminded that when services are integral or incidental to another procedure, the incidental procedure should not be coded in addition to the other procedure. This guideline is no different. If removal of an implant is necessary in order to perform a more major procedure, do not code the implant removal. So, consider the case of a patient who had a history of a rod implantation in her right leg because of a fracture. Because of degenerative arthritis, her hip (adjacent to the previously implanted rod) required replacement, which necessitated removal of the original rod for insertion of the total hip prosthesis.

27130 Arthroplasty, acetabular and proximal femoral prosthetic replacement (total hip arthroplasty), with or without autograft or allograft

20670 Removal of implant; superficial (eg, buried wire, pin or rod) (separate procedure)

20680 deep (eg, buried wire, pin, screw, metal band, nail, rod or plate)

Because the implant removal is necessary in order to perform the hip replacement, the removal is integral to the arthroplasty and not separately reportable.

CPT Coding Tip: The deep implant removal (CPT code 20680) bundles into the hip replacement (see Table 6-1), but allows bypassing of the edit. That would be appropriate only if the implant removal was of a distinct (nonadjacent site).

1. *CPT 27130 is the hip arthroplasty.*
2. *CPT 20680 is the removal of a deep implant, which is bundled into the arthroplasty code.*

(continued)

TABLE 6-1 *Example of NCCI Edits for Implant Removal*

Column 1/Column 2 Edits

Column 1	Column 2	Modifier 0 = not allowed 1 = allowed 9 = not applicable
27130	C8950	1
2 1 30	C 2 52	3
2 30	C 45	
2 30	C 47	
2 30	C 51	
2 30	C 53	
2 30	C 54	
2 30	2 0	
27 30	20 45	
27130	20610	1
27130	20680	1
27130	20900	0
27130	20902	0
27130	27001	1
27130	27005	1
27130	27006	1

3. *NCCI edits allow the bundling of this code to be bypassed with modifier 59 only if the documentation supports that a separate and distinct site was involved.*

If a closed reduction procedure fails and is converted to an open reduction procedure at the same patient encounter, only the more extensive open reduction procedure is reportable.

Interpretation

This guideline follows the same logic as that of the failed endoscopies converted to open procedures (see earlier in this chapter) and reiterates CMS policy of paying for only the successful surgery when multiple attempts are performed within one operative session. Here, if a closed reduction repair of a fracture (noninvasive) is attempted and fails, and the provider converts to an open repair, only the open repair would be coded. To illustrate this guideline, take a surgeon who attempted a closed reduction repair on a broken humerus. However, the physician discovered that the manipulation was not aligning the bone properly and decided to access the fracture through an incision to expose the humerus and allow reduction of the fracture. The open repair was performed successfully.

Because the first procedure, the attempt at closed reduction, failed, only the open reduction is coded.

Excerpt From the Musculoskeletal System Section of NCCI Guidelines[2(p7)]

If interdental wiring (e.g., CPT code 21497) is necessary for the treatment of a facial or other fracture, arthroplasty, facial reconstructive surgery, or other facial/head procedure, the interdental wiring is not separately reportable. However, if interdental wiring is performed unrelated to another facial/head procedure, the interdental wiring may be separately reportable with modifier -59.

Interpretation

Again, throughout NCCI edits we are reminded that procedures incidental and integral to the performance of other more major procedures are not coded in addition to the procedure to which they are integral. If a patient is undergoing facial surgery utilizing interdental wiring, do not add a procedure code for the wiring. However, if the patient is undergoing interdental wiring and at the same time the patient is having an unrelated procedure, both should be appropriate to code. These two codes are the CPT codes for interdental wiring.

21497 Interdental wiring, for condition other than fracture

21110 Application of interdental fixation device for conditions other than fracture or dislocation, includes removal

The March 1997 *CPT Assistant*[5] also offered some guidance with the interdental wiring coding when it addressed the question of what is the difference between CPT codes 21110 and 21497?

CPT code 21110 represents a more complex service. The device described by this code is more permanent than wiring, and would have no removable parts. "Arch bars," an interdental fixation device that is bonded to the teeth to prevent teeth movement, is one example of a device illustrated by CPT code 21110.

Code 21497 refers to using wire between teeth, typically for stabilization procedures.

Example

A Le Fort I fracture is a fracture separating the palate and alveolus from the rest of the maxilla—a fracture that occurs above the roots of the teeth. This mobile maxillary segment moves like a loose denture. In repairing this type of fracture, it is not uncommon to need interdental wiring. The wiring should not be coded in addition to the Le Fort I fracture repair.

Excerpt From the Musculoskeletal System Section of NCCI Guidelines[2(p7)]

When it is necessary to perform skeletal/joint manipulation under anesthesia to assess range of motion, reduce a fracture or for any other purpose during another procedure in an anatomically related area, the corresponding manipulation code (e.g., CPT codes 22505, 23700, 27275, 27570, 27860) is not separately reportable.

Interpretation

It is common for a physician to manipulate a joint after anesthesia to determine the range of motion before proceeding to perform the primary procedure. This manipulation is not separately reported, as it does not add significantly to the overall procedure's complexity and is incidental to the performance of the procedure. For instance, a patient was prepared and ready for a shoulder rotator cuff repair. Once the patient was under general anesthesia, the provider assessed the shoulder's range of motion by manipulating the shoulder and noting the ranges. The physician then proceeded with the rotator cuff repair. The manipulation should not be coded in addition to the rotator cuff repair.

On the other hand, a patient might present with arthrofibrotic knees that do not improve with aggressive stretching and exercise in physical therapy. The physician decides to place the patient under anesthesia and break up and tear the restrictive, internal scar tissue within the joint by forcing the knee to fully bend and straighten. The surgeon accomplished this by way of strenuous, manual joint manipulation.

Because this is a specific, therapeutic procedure, the manipulation under anesthesia (MUA) may be coded as:

27570 Manipulation of knee joint under general anesthesia (includes application of traction or other fixation devices)

CPT Coding Tip: MUA is different from the manipulation done within fracture care (ie, reduction). MUA is when the physician takes a joint, such as a shoulder, and completes a range of motion, which involves manipulating the joint nearly full range to detect or repair adhesions as well as to stretch the muscles. This procedure is often performed immediately preceding a more therapeutic procedure and is incidental to the more therapeutic procedure unless for a separate condition.

The December 2001 *CPT Assistant*[6] offers further clarification on coding fractures not requiring manipulation. They posed the scenario:

My physician saw a patient for a nondisplaced tarsal bone fracture, which did not require manipulation. Rather than applying a cast, the physician gave the patient a prescription for a prefabricated short leg removable cast, which the patient filled elsewhere. My physician will be providing all follow-up fracture care and will check the fit of the removable cast at the first followup visit. Can this be reported as fracture care?

Yes. From a CPT coding perspective this would be reported using code 28450, *Treatment of tarsal bone fracture (except talus and calcaneus); without manipulation, each.* In this case, the physician has determined that there is a fracture, decided on the appropriate course of treatment, and is providing the associated follow-up fracture care, so he is meeting the requirements for reporting the fracture care code.

Medically Unlikely Edits in the NCCI Guidelines

Excerpt From the General Correct Coding Policies Section of NCCI Guidelines[3(p30)]

Medically Unlikely Edits (MUEs)
An MUE for a HCPCS/CPT code is the maximum number of units of service (UOS) under most circumstances allowable by the same provider for the same beneficiary on the same date of service.

Explanation

The following shows some examples of current CMS MUEs for musculoskeletal system services. CMS, Medicare administrative contractor, fiscal intermediary, and carrier Web sites should be checked for current MUEs.[7]

CPT Code	MUE	CPT Code Descriptor
24666 Simple repair of superficial wounds of scalp, neck, axillae, external genitalia, trunk and/or extremities (including hands and feet);	2	Open treatment of radial head or neck fracture, includes internal fixation or radial head excision, when performed; with radial head prosthetic replacement
27158	1	Osteotomy, pelvis, bilateral (eg, congenital malformation)
28002	3	Incision and drainage below fascia, with or without tendon sheath involvement, foot; single bursal space

General Policy Statements

Excerpt From the Musculoskeletal System Section of NCCI Guidelines[2(p8)]

If a tissue transfer procedure such as a graft (e.g., CPT codes 20900-20926) is included in the code descriptor of a primary procedure, the tissue transfer procedure is not separately reportable.

Interpretation

Obviously, whenever a code description includes component services, those services should never be coded separately. This would violate CPT and NCCI coding guidelines.

Example

23420 Reconstruction of complete shoulder (rotator) cuff avulsion, chronic (includes acromioplasty)

23130 Acromioplasty or acromionectomy, partial, with or without coracoacromial ligament release

The above CPT codes would not be coded together if performed during a single surgical session on the same shoulder. CPT code 23420 includes an acromioplasty, so it would be incorrect to add the acromioplasty to the rotator cuff reconstruction coding.

CPT code 20926 describes a graft of "other" tissues such as paratenon, fat, or dermis. Similar to other graft codes, this code may not be reported with another code where the code descriptor includes procurement of the graft. Additionally, CPT code 20926 may be reported only if another graft HCPCS/CPT code does not more precisely describe the nature of the graft.

Interpretation

There are really two points in this policy:
1. If the primary procedure CPT code includes the harvesting (procurement or obtaining) of the graft, the graft codes should not be added.
2. There are specific CPT codes for harvesting grafts (see the following excerpt). CPT code 20926 (other tissues graft) would be used only if there was not a specific code for the graft obtained.

Grafts (or Implants) (20900-20938)
Codes for obtaining autogenous bone, cartilage, tendon, fascia lata grafts, or other tissues through separate skin/fascial incisions **should be reported separately unless** the code descriptor references the harvesting of the graft or implant (eg, includes obtaining graft).

Some procedures routinely utilize monitoring of interstitial fluid pressure during the postoperative period (e.g., distal lower extremity procedures with risk of anterior compartment compression). CPT code 20950 (monitoring of interstitial fluid pressure) should not be reported separately for this monitoring.

Interpretation

When a physician is monitoring interstitial fluid pressure to diagnose muscle compartment syndrome, CPT code 20950 would be coded. However, if, as the previously mentioned policy indicates, the pressure is being monitored for postoperative follow-up, the code should not be added to the coding for the surgery itself. The monitoring is included in the surgery reimbursement.

20950   Monitoring of interstitial fluid pressure (includes insertion of device, eg, wick catheter technique, needle manometer technique) in detection of muscle compartment syndrome

If electrical stimulation is used to aid bone healing, bone stimulation codes (CPT codes 20974-20975) may be reported. CPT codes 64550-64595 describe procedures for neurostimulators which are utilized to control pain and should not be reported for electrical stimulation to aid bone healing. Similarly the physical medicine electrical stimulation codes (CPT codes 97014 and 97032) should not be reported for electrical stimulation to aid bone healing.

Interpretation

Generally, fractures heal normally with standard fracture care. However, on occasion, the healing process stops because of some type of risk or complication. For those occasions, electric current can stimulate bone growth and enhance the healing process.

There are several electrical bone growth stimulator CPT codes.

20974   Electrical stimulation to aid bone healing; noninvasive (nonoperative)

20975   invasive (operative)

20979   Low intensity ultrasound stimulation to aid bone healing, noninvasive (nonoperative)

The noninvasive type of stimulator is made up of coils or electrodes, which are placed on the skin near the fracture site. The invasive type includes percutaneous and implanted devices. The percutaneous type involves electrode wires inserted through the skin into the bone, whereas implanted devices include a generator placed under the skin or in the muscles near the gap between the ends of the bones that have not fused. The implanted devices are surgically placed and later surgically removed. The ultrasound fracture-healing device uses sound waves to heal bones. This device sends out low-frequency sound waves to promote faster healing of fresh fractures. An opening is created in the cast, and the device is applied to the skin. The device is typically used for twenty minutes each day.

These services are different from services using neurostimulators, which do not aid in bone healing. Rather, the neurostimulators serve to manage pain. The physical medicine simulators are modalities used to assist in regaining voluntary control over skeletal muscle—not for bone healing.

This NCCI guideline indicates that coders should make sure the code selected is appropriate for the procedure being performed.

Excerpt From the Musculoskeletal System Section of NCCI Guidelines[2(p9)]

Exploration of the surgical field is a standard surgical practice. Physicians should not report a HCPCS/CPT code describing exploration of a surgical field with another HCPCS/CPT code describing a procedure in that surgical field. For example, CPT code 22830 describes exploration of a spinal fusion. CPT code 22830 should not be reported with another procedure of the spine in the same anatomic area. However, if the spinal fusion exploration is performed in a different anatomic area than another spinal procedure, CPT code 22830 may be reported separately with modifier -59.

Interpretation

Throughout NCCI guidelines, we are instructed that exploration of an operative site is incidental to the primary procedure performed at that same site and should not be coded separately. However, if the site is different than the area of exploration, both services should be coded, with a modifier 59 appended to the exploration.

Excerpt From the Musculoskeletal System Section of NCCI Guidelines[2(p9)]

Debridement of tissue related to an open repair of a fracture or dislocation may be separately reportable with CPT codes 11010-11012. However, debridement of tissue in the surgical field integral to the successful completion of another musculoskeletal procedure is not separately reportable. For example, debridement of muscle and/or bone (CPT codes 11043-11044) associated with excision of a tumor of bone is not separately reportable. Similarly, debridement of tissue superficial (CPT codes 11040-11042, 11720-11721) to, but in the surgical field, of a musculoskeletal procedure is not separately reportable.

Interpretation

There are specific CPT codes for debridements performed at the same time at the same site as open repairs of fractures.

11010 Debridement including removal of foreign material associated with open fracture(s) and/or dislocation(s); skin and subcutaneous tissues

11011 skin, subcutaneous tissue, muscle fascia, and muscle

11012 skin, subcutaneous tissue, muscle fascia, muscle, and bone

These CPT codes may be billed in addition to the codes for the open repair of fractures. However, procedures other than open repairs of fractures would include the debridement as an integral part of the surgery and should not be coded in addition to the principal procedure if performed at the same anatomic site. As an example, a patient slid on gravel and fell, breaking her left tibia. The fracture site had a severe abrasion with significant debris at the site. The decision was made to perform an open fracture repair after debriding the site down to the subcutaneous tissue. In this scenario, both the fracture repair and debridement services may be coded.

However, a patient could present for a posttrauma finger amputation. Debridement is performed at the surgical site to clean necrotic tissue during the amputation. In this scenario, the debridement is incidental to the amputation and would not be coded additionally.

Excerpt From the Musculoskeletal System Section of NCCI Guidelines[2(p9)]

CPT codes 29874 (Surgical knee arthroscopy for removal of loose body or foreign body) and 29877 (Surgical knee arthroscopy for debridement/shaving of articular cartilage) should not be reported with other knee arthroscopy codes (29866-29889). HCPCS code G0289 (Surgical knee arthroscopy for removal of loose body, foreign body, debridement/shaving of articular cartilage at the time of other surgical knee arthroscopy in a different compartment of the same knee) may be reported.

Interpretation

CMS has specific guidelines for coding multiple knee arthroscopies performed on the same knee during a single surgical session. These guidelines indicate that if either procedure represented by CPT codes 29874 (removal of loose or foreign body) and 29877 (debridement of cartilage) are performed during the same session as other therapeutic knee arthroscopies, they may be coded only if performed in a different compartment. If the procedure is performed in a different compartment, HCPCS code G0289 should be used, rather than CPT code 29874 or 29877. So, basically, CPT codes 29874 and 29877 would never be used on the same Medicare claim as another knee arthroscopy CPT code (unless on different knees). However, G0289 could be billed for Medicare if a different compartment were involved for the removal of a loose or foreign body or cartilage debridement.

Additional Guidance from the August 2001 *CPT Assistant*[8] regarding Knee Arthroscopies:

… When both a diagnostic and surgical arthroscopy are performed, the diagnostic arthroscopy is an inclusive component of the surgical arthroscopy and would not be reported separately.

CPT codes for Knee Arthroscopy

29874 Arthroscopy, knee, surgical; for removal of loose body or foreign body (eg, osteochondritis dissecans fragmentation, chondral fragmentation)

Code 29874 describes a surgical knee arthroscopy performed to remove foreign bodies or loose bodies of the bone or cartilage within the knee joint. It may be necessary to enlarge the entry portal when large loose or foreign bodies need to be removed.

Please note that if a knee arthroscopy for removal of loose or foreign bodies (29874) is performed in the same knee compartment as procedures described by codes 29875-29881, then code 29874 should **not** be reported separately as this is considered to be an inclusive component of codes 29875-29881.

However, if a knee arthroscopy for removal of loose or foreign bodies (29874) is performed in a different knee compartment as the knee arthroscopy procedure codes 29875-29881, then code 29874 may be reported separately with modifier -59, *Distinct Procedural Service*, appended. For example, when smoothing down the cartilage and/or drilling holes to create microfractures is also performed in addition to removal of foreign bodies or loose bodies of the bone or cartilage within the knee joint, code 29879 may be reported in addition to code 29874 only if performed in a separate knee compartment. Modifier -59 should be appended to indicate that a separate compartment was involved.

29875 Arthroscopy, knee, surgical; synovectomy, limited (eg, plica or shelf resection) (separate procedure)

29876 synovectomy, major, two or more compartments (eg, medial or lateral)

Arthroscopic synovectomy is reported using codes 29875 and 29876. Limited synovectomy (29875) involves resection of the synovium and may include partial resection of the plica of one knee compartment. Major synovectomy (29876) involves removal of the synovium and plicae from two or more knee compartments.

Code 29875 is designated as a "separate procedure." Codes with the "separate procedure" designation normally would not be additionally reported when the procedure or service is performed as an **integral component** of another procedure or service. However, when a procedure or service designated as a separate procedure is carried out independently or is considered unrelated or distinct from the other procedure(s) or service(s) provided at that time, then it would be appropriate to report the code in conjunction with the other procedure(s) or service(s). Modifier -59, *Distinct Procedural Service*, should be appended to the separate procedure code to indicate that the procedure was distinct from the overall procedure. For example, if the knee arthroscopy with limited synovectomy were performed in a different knee compartment than another knee procedure, modifier -59 would be appended to code 29875 to indicate that a different compartment was involved.

It is important to note that both codes 29875 and 29876 should not be reported together, since the limited synovectomy (29875) is considered to be an inclusive component of the major synovectomy (29876), as the descriptor of code 29876 states that the major synovectomy involves two or more compartments.

29877   Arthroscopy, knee, surgical; debridement/shaving of articular cartilage (chondroplasty)

Code 29877 describes smoothing of roughened or damaged cartilage surrounding one or more of the articular ends of the bones in the knee joint by debridement or shaving. This code should be reported only one time, regardless of how many areas are debrided or shaved.[6]

Note: The *CPT Assistant* guidelines are slightly different from the NCCI guidelines, so different payors may have different requirements for these services.

Excerpt From the Musculoskeletal System Section of NCCI Guidelines[2(p9-10)]

The NCCI has an edit with column one CPT code of 24305 (tendon lengthening, upper arm and elbow, each tendon) and column two CPT code of 64718 (neuroplasty and/or transposition; ulnar nerve at elbow). When performing the tendon lengthening described by CPT code 24305, a neuroplasty of the ulnar nerve is not separately reportable, but a transposition of the ulnar nerve at the elbow is separately reportable. If a provider performs the tendon lengthening described by CPT code 24305 and performs an ulnar nerve transposition at the elbow, the NCCI edit may be bypassed by reporting CPT code 64718 appending modifier -59.

Explanation

Neuroplasty is the decompression or freeing of intact nerve from scar tissue. Transposition is forming a completely new tunnel for the nerve to be moved (transposed) out of the former tunnel and placed in the new tunnel.

So, this NCCI guideline instructs that a neuroplasty (freeing of the nerve) is incidental (does not add substantial work or time) to the tendon lengthening, but transposing the nerve is not. The transposition may be coded in addition to the tendon lengthening by appending a modifier 59 to the transposition service.

Excerpt From the Musculoskeletal System Section of NCCI Guidelines[2(p10)]

Some procedures (e.g., spine) frequently utilize intraoperative neurophysiology testing. Intraoperative neurophysiology testing (CPT code 95920) should not be reported by the physician performing an operative procedure since it is included in the global package. However, when performed by a different physician during the procedure, it is separately reportable by the second physician. The physician performing an operative procedure should not bill other 90000 neurophysiology testing codes for intraoperative neurophysiology testing (e.g., CPT codes 92585, 95822, 95860, 95861, 95867, 95868, 95870, 95900, 95904, 95925-95937) since they are also included in the global package.

Interpretation

This is a simple guideline: neurophysiology testing performed during the operative procedure is incidental to the surgery when performed by the surgeon and only coded separately when performed by a different physician than the surgeon. If the assistant surgeon performs the testing, that would still be considered incidental to the surgery and not separately reportable.

Excerpt From the Musculoskeletal System Section of NCCI Guidelines[2(p10)]

Spinal arthrodesis, exploration, and instrumentation procedures (CPT codes 22532-22865) include manipulation of the spine as an integral component of the procedures. CPT code 22505 (manipulation of spine requiring anesthesia, any region) should not be reported separately.

Interpretation

This restates an earlier guideline discussed in this chapter. When joint manipulation under anesthesia is necessary for any purpose during another procedure in an anatomically related area, the manipulation code is included in the other procedure and should not be separately billed.

Interpretation

The closure of a surgical incision is included in the primary procedure CPT code. It should not be coded additionally. This guideline indicates that the NCCI edits do not bundle repair codes in every potential surgery CPT code. Coders are still required to follow this guideline and to not add the closure CPT code to the primary surgery code. One example would be a surgeon performing a partial excision of a rib. In order to access the rib, the surgeon creates an incision down to the rib. On completion of the procedure, a layered closure of the skin is performed.

No additional code should be added for the closure. Only the rib excision procedure would be coded.

SUMMARY

- The entire Musculoskeletal Coding Policies Section of NCCI guidelines should be read.

- Fracture and/or Dislocation is the subsection that deals with repairing a fractured or dislocated site, and it is important because fracture repairs are such common procedures. This is the largest part of the NCCI edits for the musculoskeletal system.

- Guidelines in the general NCCI guidelines also apply to the codes in the musculoskeletal system guidelines.

- When arthroscopic or closed procedures fail and are converted to open procedures, only the open procedures are coded.

- Although NCCI policy states that *CPT Assistant* instructions are not always consistent with CMS guidelines, it is important to reference these guidelines when coding musculoskeletal procedures, as they offer great clarification on the coding.

- The initial repair includes the application and removal of the first cast. Do not add a code for cast application, because closure and dressing (eg, cast application) are part of the principal procedure. Cast removal is part of routine follow-up.

- When a fracture repair begins as a closed treatment but is converted to an open repair, code only the open repair.

- Watch for external fixation codes—many of these are not included in the fracture repair code and should be coded in addition to the primary fracture procedure.

Definitions and Acronyms

acromioplasty: Repair or partial repair of the acromion.

manipulation under anesthesia (MUA): Manipulation under anesthesia is when the physician will, after placing the patient under anesthesia, rotate a joint in varying directions to break up adhesions or scarring and provide more mobility for the joint.

synovectomy: Removal of the synovium.

CHAPTER EXERCISE

Review the following case information:

Operative Report

Postoperative diagnosis:
1. Popliteal cyst
2. Multiple osteochondral fragments through left knee
3. Chondromalacia, left patella
4. Mild degenerative meniscal tear, lateral compartment, left knee

Operative procedure:
1. Arthroscopic debridement, left knee
2. Removal of osteochondral fragments, left knee
3. Debridement, chondromalacia of the patella

The patient is brought to the operating room and placed supine on the operating table, and a general endotracheal anesthetic is given. A tourniquet is placed high on the left lower extremity, and the left lower extremity is prepped and draped in a sterile fashion. Through supermedial, inferomedial, and lateral portals, diagnostic arthroscopy is carried out. The suprapatellar pouch showed significant amounts of synovitis, mild to moderate, and there is grade II chondromalacia on the left patella laterally. There are several osteochondral fragments. The fragments are removed. Chondromalacia is eventually debrided, and some of the synovium is also taken down.

In the medial compartment, additional osteochondral fragments are identified and removed both with a shaver and with graspers. These measure at their largest size approximately 4 mm across. The meniscus is probed and without tear. The anterior cruciate ligament is photographed, probed, and found to be also without laxity or tear.

Laterally, the lateral meniscus shows some degenerative fraying, especially anteriorly into the lateral horn. This is removed using a shaver. Additional osteochondral fragments are then removed in the popliteal fossa. The knee is re-examined and drained and then irrigated out once again and then drained. The arthroscope is removed. The knee is injected with 12 mg Celestone and 20 cc of 0.25% Marcaine.

The portal sites are closed with subcuticular stitches of 4-0 Monocryl. The skin is repaired with Mastisol and half-inch Steri-Strips applied. Dressings of 4 × 4's, sterile Webril, and two 6-inch Ace wraps were taken from foot to upper thigh. They are held into position with surginette stockinet.

The patient tolerates the procedure well, and there are no complications. Final sponge, needle, and instrument counts are reported as correct.

What would be coded in this case and why?

ANSWERS TO CHAPTER EXERCISES

29870 Arthroscopy, knee, diagnostic, with or without synovial biopsy (separate procedure)

29874 Arthroscopy, knee, surgical; for removal of loose body or foreign body (eg, osteochondritis dissecans fragmentation, chondral fragmentation)

29875 Arthroscopy, knee, surgical; synovectomy, limited (eg, plica or shelf resection) (separate procedure)

29877 Arthroscopy, knee, surgical; debridement/shaving of articular cartilage (chondroplasty)

29881 Arthroscopy, knee, surgical; with meniscectomy (medial OR lateral, including any meniscal shaving)

Procedures Documented	Procedures Bundled	Comments
CPT 29870	Bundled	Diagnostic arthroscopies are always incidental to therapeutic arthroscopies per CPT guidelines.
CPT 29874×3	Code×1	Per CPT guidelines (see *CPT Assistant* August 2001 and NCCI edit guidelines), CPT 29874 is incidental to any other therapeutic surgeries performed within the same compartment. (For CMS claims, G0289 would be coded.)
CPT 29877	Bundled	Per CPT and NCCI guidelines, CPT 29877 is incidental to any other therapeutic surgeries within the same compartment.
CPT 29875	Bundled	Synovectomy is a separate procedure that is included in any other therapeutic knee arthroscopy billed.
CPT 29881	Code	…

REFERENCES

1. Centers for Medicare and Medicaid Services. "Chapter IV Surgery: Musculoskeletal System," NCCI Policy Manual for Medicare Services. www.cms.hhs.gov/NationalCorrectCodInitEd/01_overview.asp#TopOfPage. Accessed June 12, 2009.

2. American Medical Association. *Current Procedural Terminology CPT® 2009 Professional Edition*. Chicago, IL: American Medical Association; 2008.

3. Centers for Medicare and Medicaid Services. "Chapter I General Correct Coding Policies," NCCI Policy Manual for Medicare Services. www.cms.hhs.gov/NationalCorrectCodInitEd/01_overview.asp#TopOfPage. Accessed June 12, 2009.

4. American Medical Association. "Coding consultation, musculoskeletal system, 20692, 20693, 20694 (Q&A)," *CPT Assistant*. 2000;10(7):11.

5. American Medical Association. "Coding consultation, musculoskeletal, 21110, 21497 (Q&A)," *CPT Assistant*. 1997;7(3):10.

6. American Medical Association. "Coding consultation, musculoskeletal system, surgery, 28450 (Q&A)," *CPT Assistant*. 2001;11(12):7.

7. Centers for Medicare and Medicaid Services. "Practitioner – DME Supplier MUE Table." www.cms.hhs.gov/NationalCorrectCodInitEd/08_MUE.asp#TopOfPage. Accessed June 12, 2009.

8. American Medical Association. "Coding communication, arthroscopic knee procedures," *CPT Assistant*. 2001;11(8):5.

The Respiratory System

Chapter 7 provides background about the respiratory system, reviews the National Correct Coding Initiative (NCCI) coding guidelines for procedures performed on the respiratory system, and provides examples to reflect the logic behind the edits. As with the other chapters, an NCCI guideline is followed by our interpretation, an example, or both.

Respiratory System and NCCI Guidelines

Excerpt From the Respiratory System Section of NCCI Guidelines[1(p2)]

A. Introduction
The principles of correct coding discussed in Chapter I apply to the CPT codes in the range 30000-39999. Several general guidelines are repeated in this Chapter. However, those general guidelines from Chapter I not discussed in this chapter are nonetheless applicable.

Interpretation

The above instruction serves as a reminder that the general NCCI guidelines (introduced in Chapter 2 of this book) apply to each section of the CPT codebook even if they are not repeated within a chapter. The introductory guidelines were comprehensively covered in Chapter 2 of this book; those introductory guidelines that have clear application within the respiratory system are reiterated in this chapter.

Excerpt From the General Coding Policies Section of NCCI Guidelines[3(p6)]

Coding Based on Standards of Medical/Surgical Practice
Specific examples of services that are not separately reportable because they are components of more comprehensive services follow:

Surgical:
2. A "scout" bronchoscopy to assess the surgical field, anatomic landmarks, extent of disease, etc. is not separately reportable with an open pulmonary procedure such as a pulmonary lobectomy. By contrast, an initial diagnostic bronchoscopy is separately reportable. If the diagnostic bronchoscopy is performed at the same patient encounter as the open pulmonary procedure and does not duplicate an earlier diagnostic bronchoscopy by the same or another physician, the diagnostic bronchoscopy may be reported with modifier -58 to indicate a staged procedure. A cursory examination of the upper airway during a bronchoscopy with the bronchoscope should not be reported separately as a laryngoscopy.

Interpretation

NCCI guidelines provide a limited list of examples of the comprehensive/component code pairs. Although it is not a comprehensive list, it does provide some practical scenarios. Although all of the examples (see Chapter 2) are applicable to procedures performed within the respiratory system, bronchoscopies performed with lobectomies are specifically respiratory procedures.

For the bronchoscopy example, keep in mind that NCCI includes the identification of landmarks in the surgical approach (part of the standards of medical/surgical practice). A scout scope procedure is for landmark identification (looking at the lay of the land). However, the example that the Centers for Medicare and Medicaid Services (CMS) provides continues to distinguish a scout scope procedure from a diagnostic scope procedure, and this is an important principle in NCCI. If a truly diagnostic scope procedure is necessary before an open therapeutic procedure, the diagnostic scope procedure may be separately coded. As long as the scope procedure is truly diagnostic (the decision for the therapeutic open procedure is made based on the findings of the scope procedure). The physician's documentation must be very clear that the service is diagnostic. The scope procedure is not separately coded if the physician:

- knows prior to the scope procedure what therapeutic open procedure is going to be performed, or
- duplicates an earlier diagnostic bronchoscopy.

NCCI edits state that when the diagnostic scope procedure is performed prior to an open procedure, both procedures may be coded, and modifier 58 (staged procedure) should be appended to the diagnostic scope procedure code. CPT guidelines for modifier 58 indicate that this modifier should be appended to the code for the second (or later) procedure performed, rather than the code for the first procedure, which would be the open procedure. Usually, modifier 58 would be appended to the code for the second procedure; however, NCCI instructs to append modifier 58 to the diagnostic service code in this case.

Introduction Section of NCCI Respiratory System Guidelines

Excerpt From the Respiratory System Section of NCCI Guidelines[1(p2)]

Physicians should report the HCPCS/CPT code that describes the procedure performed to the greatest specificity possible. A HCPCS/CPT code should be reported only if all services described by the code are performed. A physician should not report multiple HCPCS/CPT codes if a single HCPCS/CPT code exists that describes the services. This type of unbundling is incorrect coding.

Interpretation

If a single code encompasses the entire procedure, use that code, rather than separating parts of the procedure into individual codes. This is true regardless of whether an edit exists in NCCI. If one CPT code includes the entire work performed, do not code separate components. For instance, during a single operative session, the physician removed two lobes of the lung, CPT code 32482 should be coded, as it encompasses both lobes. It would be incorrect to code 32480 twice. Because there are two lungs in normal anatomy, there is an MUE for CPT code 32480 that limits the services to two. Therefore, there is no edit to alert coders that billing two services for 32480 would be incorrect.

32480[2] Removal of lung, other than total pneumonectomy; single lobe (lobectomy)

32482 two lobes (bilobectomy)

Excerpt From the Respiratory System Section of NCCI Guidelines[1(p2)]

Open procedures of the thorax include the approach and exploration. CPT code 32100 (thoracotomy, major; with exploration and biopsy) should not be reported separately with open thoracic procedures to describe the approach and exploration. CPT code 32100 may be separately reportable with an open thoracic procedure if: (1) it is performed on the contralateral side; (2) it is performed on the ipsilateral side through a separate skin incision; or (3) it is performed to obtain a biopsy at a different site than the other open thoracic procedure.

Interpretation

Remember from the General Coding Guidelines discussion in Chapter 2 of this book that the surgical approach is included in the code for the primary procedure and should not be billed separately. This includes identification of anatomical landmarks, incision, evaluation of the surgical field, debridement of traumatized tissue, lysis of adhesions, and isolation of structures limiting access to the surgical field such as bone, blood vessels, nerves, and muscles, including stimulation for identification or monitoring.

Almost any procedure or service performed in order to gain successful access to the site for the root operation is incidental to that root operation and not billed separately. If the surgeon has to cut through adhesions just to access the site for the primary procedure, the lysis of adhesions is for access rather than for independent therapeutic reasons.

In the case of a surgery performed in the thoracic cavity (the area between the neck and abdomen), opening the chest (thoracotomy) in order to gain access for performing the procedure is incidental to that procedure. NCCI policy does offer that if a thoracotomy is performed at a different site from the anatomic site of the primary procedure, the thoracotomy may be added. Incising into a separate site obviously would not be necessary to access the site for the primary procedure. However, please note that the separately coded thoracotomy would need to be medically necessary and supported as a separate site within the documentation. This NCCI guideline provides an example within the respiratory system for the thoracotomy (incising into the thorax). If a procedure—for example, a lung resection—is performed on a patient, the thoracotomy becomes a part of the approach for the lung resection and should not be coded separately. However, if a patient has multiple gun shot wounds, and the surgeon performs an abdominal colectomy and a thoracotomy for exploration, because the thoracotomy was of a different anatomic site (abdomen vs thorax access), both may be coded.

Respiratory Services (30000-32999) and NCCI Guidelines

Excerpt From the Respiratory System Section of CCI Guidelines[1](p4-5)

The nose and mouth have mucocutaneous margins. Numerous procedures (e.g., biopsy, destruction, excision) have CPT codes that describe the procedure as an integumentary procedure (CPT codes 10000-19999), a nasal procedure (CPT codes 30000-30999), or an oral procedure (CPT codes 40000-40899). If a procedure is performed on a lesion at or near a muco-cutaneous margin, only one CPT code which best describes the procedure may be reported. If the code descriptor of a CPT code from the respiratory system (or any other system) includes a tissue transfer service (e.g., flap, graft), the CPT codes for such services (e.g., transfer, graft, flap) from the integumentary system (e.g., CPT codes 14000-15770) should not be reported separately.

Interpretation

This is a tricky guideline to understand, so we will dissect it one piece at a time:

a. The nose and mouth have mucocutaneous margins. Dorland's dictionary within *CodeManager*[4] defines mucocutaneous as: mu•co•cu•ta•ne•ous (mu"ko-ku-tacne-ms)[*muco-+cutaneous*] pertaining to or affecting the mucous membrane and the skin.

b. Numerous procedures have CPT codes that describe the procedure as integumentary, nasal, or oral. If a procedure is performed on a lesion at or near a mucocutaneous margin, only one CPT code may be reported.

Because the CPT codebook captures surgeries performed on the integumentary, nasal, or oral systems, if a single procedure is performed on a single anatomic site, and that site includes mucocutaneous tissue, do not code separately for the integumentary portion (cutaneous) from the nasal or oral services. Choose the code best describing the service performed.

c. If the code descriptor of a CPT code from the respiratory system includes a tissue transfer service, the CPT codes for the tissue transfer from the integumentary system should not be reported. Do not add a code for tissue transfer if that service is included in the description of the primary procedure CPT code. This would constitute unbundling.

The following CPT codes illustrate a variety of services coded within the respiratory system.

31610   Tracheostomy, fenestration procedure with skin flaps

This code indicates *with skin flaps*; therefore, it would be incorrect to code a skin flap procedure additionally.

31820   Surgical closure tracheostomy or fistula; without plastic repair

31825   with plastic repair

CPT code 31825 indicates *with plastic repair*. Coding a skin repair code in addition to this code would be unbundling services. Also, note that choosing CPT code 31820 and a skin repair code would also be incorrect because there is a comprehensive code (CPT code 31825) that includes both elements of the procedure.

30400   Rhinoplasty, primary; lateral and alar cartilages and/or elevation of nasal tip (For obtaining tissues for graft, see 20900-20926, 21210)

For the rhinoplasty services, the CPT codebook shows that we can add codes from the musculoskeletal system for obtaining tissue grafts.

Excerpt From the Respiratory System Section of NCCI Guidelines[1(p5)]

A biopsy performed in conjunction with a more extensive nasal/sinus procedure is not separately reportable unless the biopsy is examined pathologically prior to the more extensive procedure, and the decision to proceed with the more extensive procedure is based on the result of the pathologic examination.

Example: If a patient presents with nasal obstruction, sinus obstruction and multiple nasal polyps, it may be reasonable to perform a biopsy prior to, or in conjunction with, polypectomy and ethmoidectomy. A separate biopsy code (e.g., CPT code 31237 for nasal/sinus endoscopy) should not be reported with the removal nasal/sinus endoscopy code (e.g., CPT code 31255) because the biopsy tissue is procured as part of the surgery, not to establish the need for surgery.

Interpretation

As pointed out in Chapter 2 of this book, this guideline is a very important one in NCCI. Essentially, the NCCI policy states that if a biopsy is truly diagnostic and helps determine the need for a second procedure, both services should be coded. In this case, the second procedure should have a modifier 58 (staged procedure) appended to bypass the bundling edit. However, if a biopsy incidentally results from an excision and does not represent a separate and distinct diagnostic procedure, do not code the biopsy separate from the excision.

See Figure 7-1 for a decision tree for coding biopsies.

FIGURE 7-1 *Decision Tree for Coding Biopsies Performed With More Extensive Procedures*

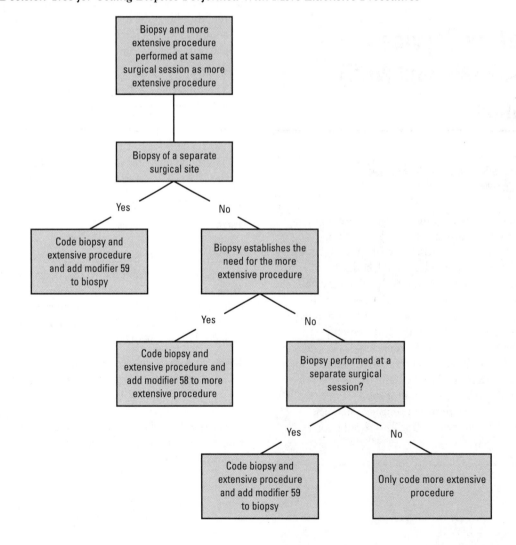

When a diagnostic or surgical endoscopy of the respiratory system is performed, it is a standard of practice to evaluate the access regions. A separate HCPCS/CPT code should not be reported for this evaluation of the access regions. For example, if an endoscopic anterior ethmoidectomy is performed, a diagnostic nasal endoscopy should not be reported separately simply because the approach to the ethmoid sinus is transnasal. Similarly, fiberoptic bronchoscopy routinely includes a limited examination of the nasal cavity, pharynx, and larynx. A separate HCPCS/CPT code should not be reported with the bronchoscopy HCPCS/CPT code for this latter examination whether it is ("cursory") or complete.

If medically reasonable and necessary endoscopic procedures are performed on two regions of the respiratory system with different types of endoscopes, both procedures may be separately reportable.

Interpretation

This is a common directive throughout NCCI guidelines—do not code diagnostic endoscopies performed during a therapeutic endoscopic procedure. Further, endoscopies performed through natural orifices (eg, nasal cavity, mouth, anus) follow an anatomic path that allows for exploring the structures along that path. Procedures performed on any structures along the path of the endoscopic examination should not be separately coded, even if there is a distinct CPT code for the service. If, however, a distinct and separate endoscopy was performed (different endoscope inserted), both services may be coded if the procedure is documented and medically necessary.

For example, a physician performs a nasal endoscopy, nasopharyngoscopy, and laryngoscopy during a single patient encounter. According to NCCI edits, the nasopharyngoscopy is never coded in addition to the nasal endoscopy (the edit cannot be bypassed). However, the nasal endoscopy and laryngoscopy may both be coded, with a modifier 59 appended to the nasal endoscopy code, if, according to the American Academy of Otolaryngology,

"… the surgeon's medical records provide clear documentation explaining the necessity of using two different endoscopes on the same date of service. A provider should NOT report both codes of a code pair edit if the nasal endoscopy can be performed with the same flexible endoscope utilized for the laryngoscopy."[5]

If the findings of a diagnostic endoscopy lead to the performance of a non-endoscopic surgical procedure at the same patient encounter, the diagnostic endoscopy may be reported separately. However, if a "scout" endoscopic procedure to evaluate the surgical field (e.g., confirmation of anatomic structures, confirmation of adequacy of surgical procedure such as tracheostomy) is performed at the same patient encounter as an open surgical procedure, the endoscopic procedure is not separately reportable.

Interpretation

This guideline is thoroughly reviewed within Chapter 2 and repeated here with an example from the respiratory system section. To repeat our interpretation of this guideline from Chapter 2, if an endoscopic procedure that precedes an open procedure is truly diagnostic, the diagnostic endoscopy may be coded in addition to the open procedure. The documentation within the record is critical here, because it must clearly support that the endoscopy was diagnostic and not merely for land-marking the surgical site.

CPT Coding Tip: When coding, see if the preoperative diagnosis differs from the postoperative diagnosis, as this could be an indication of whether the endoscopy is truly diagnostic. If there is a symptom, or a rule-out diagnosis preoperatively, then that helps support the endoscopy as being diagnostic.

There should be a procedure indications section at the beginning of the operative note. This too can help clarify whether the endoscopy is diagnostic or not.

Physicians should clearly document whether the endoscopy is diagnostic or not.

NCCI edits state that when the diagnostic scope procedure is performed prior to an open procedure, it may be coded by adding modifier 58 (staged procedure) to the diagnostic scope procedure code. CPT guidelines for modifier 58 indicate that this modifier should be appended to the second (or later) procedure performed, rather than to the first procedure. This would indicate that modifier 58 should be appended to the open procedure. As mentioned earlier, the usual coding methodology is to append modifier 58 to the second performed procedure; however, the NCCI guidelines specifically instruct coders to append the modifier to the diagnostic service. Documentation within the record is critical and must clearly support that the endoscopy was diagnostic and not merely for land-marking the surgical site.

Therefore, a patient presents with persistent throat pain and earaches. The physician performs a nasal endoscopy, and through a different scope, going through the mouth, the physician also performs a laryngoscopy. If it were documented clearly that different scopes and different orifices were involved, both procedures may be coded, with a modifier 59 appended to the nasal endoscopy code.

Excerpt From the Respiratory System Section of NCCI Guidelines[1(p6)]

If an endoscopic procedure fails and is converted into an open procedure, the endoscopic procedure is not separately reportable with the open procedure.

Interpretation

This is another standard guideline, with NCCI policies stating that failed approaches, or approaches that are converted to different approaches, are incidental to successful approaches, and only the successfully approached procedure should be coded. This was covered in depth in Chapter 2.

A wonderful clarification within this policy is the example offered by CMS within the NCCI policy manual.[3(p6)] In the example that follows, CMS clarifies that code for the diagnostic endoscopy (if the procedure were truly diagnostic) may be added to the code for the successful, open procedure, even when the open procedure follows a failed (not coded) therapeutic endoscopy. Remember, diagnostic endoscopies are always incidental to therapeutic endoscopies. So if there is a diagnostic endoscopy that precedes a therapeutic endoscopy, the diagnostic service is not coded separately *unless* the therapeutic endoscopy fails, and the provider converts to a successful open procedure.

Here is the example offered from NCCI[3(p6)]:

Example: A patient presents with aspiration of a foreign body. A bronchoscopy is performed identifying lobar foreign body obstruction, and an attempt is made to remove this obstruction bronchoscopically. It would be inappropriate to report CPT codes 31622 (diagnostic bronchoscopy) and 31635 (surgical bronchoscopy with removal of foreign body). Only the "surgical" endoscopy, CPT code 31635, may be reported. **In this example, if the endoscopic effort is unsuccessful and a thoracotomy is performed, the diagnostic bronchoscopy may be reported separately in addition to the thoracotomy** (emphasis added). Modifier -58 may be used to indicate that the diagnostic bronchoscopy and the thoracotomy are staged or planned

procedures. However, the CPT code for the surgical bronchoscopy to remove the foreign body is not separately reportable because the procedure was converted to an open procedure. If the surgeon decides to repeat the bronchoscopy after induction of general anesthesia to confirm the surgical approach to the foreign body, this confirmatory bronchoscopy is not separately reportable although the initial diagnostic bronchoscopy may still be reportable.

Excerpt From the Respiratory System Section of NCCI Guidelines[1(p6-7)]

When a sinusotomy is performed in conjunction with a sinus endoscopy, only one service may be reported. *CPT Manual* instructions indicate that surgical sinus endoscopy includes a sinusotomy (if appropriate) and a diagnostic sinus endoscopy. However, if the medically necessary procedure is a sinusotomy and a sinus endoscopy is performed to evaluate adequacy of the sinusotomy and visualize the sinus cavity for disease, it may be appropriate to report the sinusotomy HCPCS/CPT code rather than the sinus endoscopy HCPCS/CPT code.

Interpretation

This guideline elaborates on the CPT codebook guideline in which sinusotomies are included in the sinus endoscopies when performed together. The NCCI policy takes this one step further by adding that if the primary procedure is the sinusotomy, and the endoscopy is a follow-up step to determine the success of the sinusotomy, then the endoscopy becomes incidental to the sinusotomy, rather than the other way around.

Excerpt From the Respiratory System Section of NCCI Guidelines[1(p7)]

Control of bleeding is an integral component of endoscopic procedures and is not separately reportable. For example, control of nasal hemorrhage (CPT code 30901) is not separately reportable for control of bleeding during a nasal/sinus endoscopic procedure. However, if bleeding occurs in the postoperative period and requires return to the operating room for treatment, a HCPCS/CPT code for control of the bleeding may be reported with modifier -78 indicating that the procedure was a complication of a prior procedure requiring treatment in the operating room.

Interpretation

Bear in mind that postoperative complications are not coded in addition to the surgery unless they require a return to the operating room. Also, if a physician must control bleeding of the surgical site (internal or external) in concert with the procedure, no additional code should be added to the primary procedure, as control of bleeding is included in the global package of the main surgery.

Excerpt From the Respiratory System Section of NCCI Guidelines[1(p7)]

If laryngoscopy is required for elective or emergency placement of an endotracheal tube, the laryngoscopy is not separately reportable.

If laryngoscopy is required for placement of a tracheostomy, the tracheostomy (CPT codes 31600-31610) may be reported. The laryngoscopy is not separately reportable.

Interpretation

Laryngoscopies are included in the CPT codes for placement of an endotracheal tube or for creating a tracheostomy if the laryngoscopy is used to assist in the primary procedures. The laryngoscopy is not for a separately identifiable purpose or of a different anatomic site.

Coding Tip: *A laryngoscopy is an examination of the back of the throat, including the voice box (larynx) and vocal cords. A laryngoscopy examination is either indirect or direct.*

Indirect laryngoscopy: *Indirect laryngoscopy is done in a doctor's office using a small hand mirror held in the mouth at the back of the throat, a head mirror worn by the doctor, and a light source. The mirror worn by the doctor reflects light into the mouth. Some doctors now use headgear equipped with a bright light. Indirect laryngoscopy has been largely replaced by newer direct fiberoptic laryngoscopic techniques that provide better views and greater comfort during the examination.*

Direct fiberoptic (flexible or rigid) laryngoscopy: *Direct laryngoscopy uses a fiberoptic scope that allows the doctor to see deeper into the throat than during indirect laryngoscopy. The laryngoscope is either flexible or rigid. Fiberoptic scopes provide better views and are better tolerated than older, rigid scopes. Rigid scopes are still used in surgery. Direct rigid laryngoscopy may be used to perform surgical procedures, including removing foreign*

objects that may get caught in the throat, collecting tissue samples (biopsy), removing polyps from the vocal cords, or performing laser treatment. Direct rigid laryngoscopy may also be used to help diagnose cancer of the voice box (larynx).

- *Direct, operative: General anesthesia is employed for the visualization of the larynx by passing a rigid or fiberoptic endoscope through the mouth and pharynx to the larynx.*
- *Tracheoscopy: The insertion of a bronchoscope to examine the trachea.*

Excerpt From the Respiratory System Section of NCCI Guidelines[1]

CPT code 31500 describes an emergency endotracheal intubation procedure and should not be reported when an elective intubation is performed.

Interpretation

Be careful when reading CPT code nomenclature, as CPT code 31500 specifies emergency intubation and should not be used except with an emergency procedure. Often, emergency intubations are performed during critical care services, and the intubation may be coded in addition to the adult (or nonneonatal) critical service (CPT 99291-99292); however, the time used for the intubation should be subtracted from the total critical care time billed. If the time to intubate were included in the total time for the critical care, this would be double coding of that time. The emergency intubation is included in neonatal critical care (CPT codes 99468-99476) and not separately coded. The neonatal codes are per day codes; therefore, time to provide critical care is not used in determining coding.

Elective intubation is usually performed as a necessary part of other care and is included in the CPT code for the primary service.

Excerpt From the Respiratory System Section of NCCI Guidelines[1(p7-8)]

The descriptor for CPT code 31600 (Tracheostomy, planned (separate procedure)) includes the "separate procedure" designation. Therefore, pursuant to the CMS "separate procedure" policy, a tracheostomy is not separately reportable with laryngeal surgical procedures that frequently require tracheostomy (e.g., laryngotomy, laryngectomy, laryngoplasty).

Interpretation

This guideline is straightforward, but it is a key reminder that CPT codes that are designated as *separate procedures* are not coded in addition to other procedures performed during the same operative session on the same surgical site.

Excerpt From the Respiratory System Section of NCCI Guidelines[1(p8)]

CPT code 92511 (nasopharyngoscopy with endoscope) should not be reported separately when performed as a cursory examination with other respiratory endoscopic procedures.

Interpretation

Although the nasopharyngoscopy does not fall within the respiratory system section of the CPT codebook surgery systems, there is still an important guideline regarding this service when it is performed during the same session as other respiratory endoscopies. The nasopharyngoscopy is an endoscopic examination of the area behind the soft palate to the nasopharyngeal wall. This service is incidental to the nasal endoscopy as well as the laryngoscopy and bronchoscopy. The CPT code nomenclature designates this service as a separate procedure, which, remember, would mean that it is not coded in addition to a more major procedure of the same or adjacent anatomic site when performed during a single encounter. NCCI edits bundle CPT code 92511 into most other respiratory endoscopic procedures; however, for laryngoscopies, a modifier 59 may be appended to the nasopharyngoscopy code if there is documented support that different encounters or approaches are used for each procedure. The documentation would also need to support why distinct services were necessary.

Excerpt From the Respiratory System Section of NCCI Guidelines[2(p8)]

A surgical thoracoscopy is not separately reportable with an open thoracotomy procedure, the latter being the more extensive procedure. However, if the clinical findings of a diagnostic thoracoscopy lead to the decision to perform an open thoracotomy, the diagnostic thoracoscopy may be separately reportable. A thoracoscopy to evaluate anatomic landmarks or assess extent of disease in a previously diagnosed patient is not separately reportable with an open thoracotomy.

Interpretation

This guideline instructs that if both an endoscopic and open procedure are performed for the same treatment, only the open (or more extensive) procedure should be coded. However, if a diagnostic endoscopy and an open procedure of the same body area are performed on a single date of service (regardless of whether they are within the same procedure session), both may be coded. Important here is that the endoscopy (thoracoscopy) must be diagnostic. A diagnostic endoscopic procedure will often help determine if and which therapeutic procedure should be performed. The more major procedure (or open procedure) is based, at least in part, on the results of the diagnostic endoscopy. Modifier 58 (staged or related procedure) would be appended to the open (or later) procedure code.

Additional Comment and Interpretation

An article in the *CPT Assistant*[6] agrees with the NCCI guidelines except regarding failed endoscopic procedures converted to open surgeries. The *CPT Assistant* article indicates that the coder should code both services with a modifier 52 on the endoscopy code, whereas NCCI guidelines instruct to bundle the endoscopy into the open surgery code. Not all payers follow NCCI guidelines, so understanding CPT coding guidelines is very critical to ensuring that appropriate reimbursement is received. For CMS claims (or other payers who follow NCCI policy), the failed endoscopy would not be separately coded unless it represented a true diagnostic service.

A case in point would be a patient who presents after a motor vehicle accident with a small, open wound to the chest. The surgeon performs a thoracoscopy to determine the extent of damage. The thoracoscopy reveals that the patient has a traumatic injury that can be repaired through the thoracoscopy.

Correct coding is as follows:

32654   Thoracoscopy, surgical; with control of traumatic hemorrhage

In the same scenario, the surgeon discovers during the thoracoscopy that the injury cannot be repaired through the endoscopic approach, so he performs an open thoracotomy repair.

Correct coding is as follows:

32110   Thoracotomy, major; with control of traumatic hemorrhage and/or repair of lung tear

32601   Thoracoscopy, diagnostic (separate procedure); lungs and pleural space, without biopsy

A modifier 58 should be appended to the thoracotomy code.

Excerpt From the Respiratory System Section of NCCI Guidelines[2(p8)]

A tube thoracostomy (CPT code 32020 (32551 in 2008)) may be performed for drainage of an abscess, empyema, or hemothorax. The code descriptor for CPT code 32020 (32551 in 2008) defines it as a "separate procedure." It is not separately reportable when performed at the same patient encounter as another open procedure on the ipsilateral side of the thorax.

Interpretation

As discussed in prior chapters, separate procedures are not billable when they are performed during a single operative session on the same anatomic site. This guideline reiterates that instruction. In the case of tube thoracostomies, they would be billable only if they were performed:

• without another procedure of the thorax or
• on a different side from another procedure of the thorax.

Excerpt From the Respiratory System Section of NCCI Guidelines[2(p8)]

CPT code 92502 (otolaryngologic examination under general anesthesia) is not separately reportable with any other otolaryngologic procedure performed under general anesthesia.

Interpretation

An otolaryngologic examination performed under anesthesia is incidental to any other otolaryngologic procedure, as it becomes not separately distinguishable (see Chapter 2 of this book) from the other procedures performed. Services that are not separately distinguishable are when the component service is essentially a critical part of the comprehensive procedure, and the component should not be separately coded. For example, a patient has a diagnostic otolaryngologic examination performed under anesthesia (CPT code 92502) followed by a tonsillectomy (CPT code 42825). In this case, the otolaryngologic examination is bundled into the tonsillectomy and is not separately billed. This edit may not be bypassed with a modifier.

Medically Unlikely Edits

Excerpt From the General Correct Coding Policies Section of NCCI Guidelines[3(p30)]

Medically Unlikely Edits (MUEs)
An MUE for a HCPCS/CPT code is the maximum number of units of service (UOS) under most circumstances allowable by the same provider for the same beneficiary on the same date of service.

Explanation

The following shows some examples of current MUEs for respiratory system services. CMS, Medicare administrative contractor, fiscal intermediary, and carrier Web sites should be checked for current MUEs.[7]

CPT Code		MUE	CPT Code Descriptor
30100	Simple repair of superficial wounds of scalp, neck, axillae, external genitalia, trunk and/or extremities (including hands and feet);	3	Biopsy, intranasal
31292		2	Nasal/sinus endoscopy, surgical; with medial or inferior orbital wall decompression
31365		1	Laryngectomy; total, with radical neck dissection

SUMMARY

• The entire respiratory section from the NCCI manual should be read.

• All approaches are bundled into root operation procedures and should not be billed separately.

• Diagnostic endoscopic procedures performed on adjacent structures along the path of an endoscopy all bundle into the endoscopy of the farthest site, unless different accesses or endoscopes are involved.

Definitions and Acronyms

American Academy of Otolaryngology: This is the specialty society for physicians who provide ENT-related services.

bronchoscopy: Examination of the bronchi through a bronchoscope.

Centers for Medicare and Medicaid Services (CMS): This is a branch of the Department of Health and Human Services (HHS) responsible for overseeing the Medicare and Medicaid federal health care programs. Information may be found at www.cms.hhs.gov.

contralateral: Situated on, pertaining to, or affecting the opposite side, as opposed to ipsilateral.

dermoid cyst: An epidermal cyst, usually present at birth, representing a disorder of embryologic development, generally occurring along lines of embryonic fusion, with middorsal, midventral, and branchial cleft locations, most often involving the head, especially around the eyes, and the neck, and lined with stratified squamous epithelium containing cutaneous appendages, including hair.

ethmoidectomy: Excision of the ethmoid cells or of a portion of the ethmoid bone.

ipsilateral: Situated on, pertaining to, or affecting the same side, as opposed to contralateral.

laryngoscopy: Examination of the interior of the larynx, especially that performed with the laryngoscope.

lobectomy: Excision of a lobe, as of the thyroid, liver, brain, or lung.

mediastinoscopy: Examination of the mediastinum by means of an endoscope inserted through an anterior incision in the suprasternal notch, permitting direct inspection and biopsy of tissue in the anterior superior mediastinum.

mucocutaneous: Pertaining to or affecting the mucous membrane and the skin.

pneumonectomy: The excision of lung tissue, especially of an entire lung.

sinusotomy: Incision into a sinus.

thoracotomy: Surgical incision into the pleural space through the wall of the chest.

CHAPTER EXERCISE

Review the following case information:

Operative Report

Preoperative diagnosis:
1. Chronic hyperplastic rhinosinusitis
2. Allergies
3. Asthma
4. Status post polypectomy and sinus surgery

Postoperative diagnosis: Same

Operative procedure:
1. Left sinusotomy 3 or more sinuses to include:
   - Nasal and sinus endoscopy
   - Endoscopic intranasal polypectomy
   - Endoscopic total ethmoidectomy
   - Endoscopic sphenoidotomy
   - Endoscopic nasal antral windows, middle meatus, and inferior meatus
   - Endoscopic removal of left maxillary sinus contents

2. Right sinusotomy three or more sinuses to include:
   - Nasal and sinus endoscopy
   - Endoscopic intranasal polypectomy
   - Endoscopic total ethmoidectomy
   - Endoscopic sphenoidotomy
   - Endoscopic nasal antral windows, middle meatus, and inferior meatus
   - Endoscopic removal of right maxillary sinus contents

Anesthesia: General endotracheal

Estimated blood loss: 250 cc

Fluids replaced: 1200 cc

Complications: None

Drains/packs: Bilateral Gelfilm in the middle meatus. Bilateral Telfa gauze impregnated with bacitracin. Bilateral Vaseline gauze between the folds of Telfa.

Findings: Complete nasal obstruction by polyps with obscuring of all of the normal landmarks. The right middle turbinate was found and preserved. The residual node of the left middle turbinate was found and preserved. There was thickened hyperplastic mucosa throughout the sinuses with some polyps in the sinuses, and the majority of the sinus cavities were filled with inspissated glue-like mucopurulent debris. At the end of the case there were no visible polyps, the airway was clear, and the debris had been removed.

Procedure: The patient is taken to the operating room and placed in the supine position, and general endotracheal anesthesia adequately obtained. A pharyngeal pack is placed. The nose is infiltrated with Xylocaine with epinephrine and Cottonoids soaked in 4% cocaine are placed. The procedure is performed in a similar manner on the left and right sides. The Cottonoids are removed.

The 30 degree wide angle sinus telescope with EndoScrub and the Stryker Hummer device are used to remove the polyps starting anteriorly and working posteriorly. This leads to visualization of the middle turbinates. The middle meatus disease is removed. The area of the uncinate process and infundibulum is shaved away, and forceps are used to remove portions of bone particle. Using blunt dissection, the agger nasi cells, ethmoid, and spheroid sinuses are entered and the contents removed with forceps and suction. The inferior turbinates are infractured, and a mosquito clamp is placed through the lateral nasal wall into the maxillary sinuses through the inferior meatus. That opening is opened with forward and backward biting forceps, sinus endoscopy is performed, and inspissated mucus and debris are cleaned out of the sinuses.

In a similar manner, the sinuses are opened from the middle meatus and the sinuses cleaned. In the above manner, the ethmoid, spheroid, and maxillary sinuses are cleaned of debris and inspissated mucus suctioned from the frontal recesses.

The patient is then suctioned free of secretions, adequate hemostasis noted. Gelfilm is soaked, rolled, and placed in the middle meatus. Telfa gauze is impregnated with Bacitracin, folded, and placed in the nose. Vaseline gauze is placed between the folds of Telfa. The pharyngeal pack is removed. The patient is suctioned free of secretions, adequate hemostasis noted, and the procedure terminated. The patient tolerates it well and leaves the operating room in satisfactory condition.

What would be coded in this case and why?

ANSWERS TO CHAPTER EXERCISES

The following services were documented and all were performed bilaterally:

31237 Nasal/sinus endoscopy, surgical; with biopsy, polypectomy or debridement (separate procedure)

31255 Nasal/sinus endoscopy, surgical; with ethmoidectomy, total (anterior and posterior)

31267 Nasal/sinus endoscopy, surgical, with maxillary antrostomy; with removal of tissue from maxillary sinus

31276 Nasal/sinus endoscopy, surgical with frontal sinus exploration, with or without removal of tissue from frontal sinus

31288 Nasal/sinus endoscopy, surgical, with sphenoidotomy; with removal of tissue from the sphenoid sinus

Final coding and comments for this exercise:

Procedures Documented	Procedures Bundled	Comments
CPT codes 31237-50	Bundled	Per NCCI guidelines, a biopsy in conjunction with a more extensive procedure is coded only when the biopsy determines the need for the more extensive procedure.
CPT codes 31255-50	Okay to Code	
CPT codes 31267-50	Okay to Code	
CPT codes 31276-50	Okay to Code	
CPT codes 31288-50	Okay to Code	

REFERENCES

1. Centers for Medicare and Medicaid Services. "Chapter V Surgery: Respiratory, Cardiovascular, Hemic and Lymphatic Systems," NCCI Policy Manual for Medicare Services. www.cms.hhs.gov/NationalCorrectCodInitEd/01_overview.asp#TopOfPage. Accessed June 12, 2009.

2. American Medical Association. *Current Procedural Terminology CPT® 2009 Professional Edition.* Chicago, IL: American Medical Association; 2008.

3. Centers for Medicare and Medicaid Services. "Chapter I General Correct Coding Policies," NCCI Policy Manual for Medicare Services. www.cms.hhs.gov/NationalCorrectCodInitEd/01_overview.asp#TopOfPage. Accessed June 12, 2009.

4. American Medical Association. *CodeManager 2009: A complete medical coding software solution.* Chicago, IL: American Medical Association; 2009.

5. American Academy of Otolaryngology. *Reporting Nasal Endoscopy and Laryngoscopy CPT Codes on the Same Date of Service.* American Academy of Otolaryngology—Head and Neck Surgery. www.entnet.org/Practice/upload/Reporting-CPT-Code-Nasal-Endoscopy-and-Laryngoscopy-Codes.pdf. Accessed February 16, 2009.

6. American Medical Association. "Thoracic surgery coding," *CPT Assistant.* 1994;4(3):1.

7. Centers for Medicare and Medicaid Services. "Practitioner – DME Supplier MUE Table." www.cms.hhs.gov/NationalCorrectCodInitEd/08_MUE.asp#TopOfPage. Accessed June 12, 2009.

The Cardiovascular System

Chapter 8 provides background about the cardiovascular system, reviews the National Correct Coding Initiative (NCCI) coding guidelines for procedures performed on the cardiovascular system, and provides examples to reflect the logic behind the edits. This chapter provides an NCCI guideline followed by an interpretation, an example, or both. In prior chapters, the general NCCI guidelines (those applying to all services) have been thoroughly reviewed. This chapter will address only those guidelines directly applicable to cardiovascular *Current Procedural Terminology* (CPT®)[1] coding.

Introduction to the Cardiovascular System and NCCI Guidelines

Excerpt From the Cardiovascular System Section of NCCI Guidelines[2(p2)]

A. Introduction
The principles of correct coding discussed in Chapter I apply to the CPT codes in the range 30000-39999. Several general guidelines are repeated in this Chapter. However, those general guidelines from Chapter I not discussed in this chapter are nonetheless applicable.

Interpretation

This instruction serves as a reminder that the general NCCI guidelines (introduced in Chapter 2 of this book) apply to each section of the CPT codebook, even if they are not repeated within a specific chapter. The introductory guidelines were reviewed comprehensively in Chapter 2 of this book, and those general guidelines that

have clear application within the cardiovascular system sections will be recapped in this chapter.

Excerpt From the General Coding Policies Section of NCCI Guidelines[3(p4)]

Coding Based on Standards of Medical/Surgical Practice
Most HCPCS/CPT code defined procedures include services that are integral to them. Some of these integral services have specific CPT codes for reporting the service when not performed as an integral part of another procedure. (For example, CPT code 36000 (introduction of needle or intracatheter into a vein) is integral to all nuclear medicine procedures requiring injection of a radiopharmaceutical into a vein. CPT code 36000 is not separately reportable with these types of nuclear medicine procedures. However, CPT code 36000 may be reported alone if the only service provided is the introduction of a needle into a vein.)

Interpretation

Within the General Coding guidelines of NCCI, we are instructed to include all integral services for a procedure in the code for the primary procedure and not bill integral services separately. In other words, any service or procedure that is a necessary part of the primary procedure should not be coded in addition to the primary procedure—it is included in the work for the primary procedure. A case in point would be the NCCI example of the introduction of a needle or catheter into a vein for a radiopharmaceutical procedure. The introduction of the needle or catheter is a fundamental part of the radiopharmaceutical procedure because the injection is for the pharmaceutical. The same would be true of infusion therapy. In order to perform infusion therapy, the provider must insert a needle into the patient's vein; therefore, the needle insertion is an integral part of the infusion therapy.

The April 2003 *CPT Assistant*[4] addresses some questions about the Cardiovascular System/Surgery codes 36000, 90780, and 90781.

Is it appropriate to report codes 36000, *Introduction of needle or intracatheter, vein*, and 90780, *Intravenous infusion for therapy/diagnosis, administered by physician or under direct supervision of physician; up to one hour*, separately, or would the introduction of the needle be included in procedure code 90780?

Answer: Codes 90780 and 90781 include placement of an intravenous catheter. Therefore, it would not be appropriate to report code 36000, *Introduction of needle or intracatheter, vein* in addition to code(s) 90780-90781.

Excerpt From the General Coding Policies Section of NCCI Guidelines[3(p7)]

Many invasive procedures require vascular and/or airway access. The work associated with obtaining the required access is included in the pre-procedure or intra-procedure work. The work associated with returning a patient to the appropriate post-procedure state is included in the post-procedure work.

Intravenous access (e.g., CPT codes 36000, 36400, 36410) is not separately reportable when performed with many types of procedures (e.g., surgical procedures, anesthesia procedures, radiological procedures requiring intravenous contrast, nuclear medicine procedures requiring intravenous radiopharmaceutical).

Interpretation

In order to perform many invasive procedures, vascular or airway access must be gained. This procedure is not coded in addition to the surgery, anesthesia, or other procedure being performed. If, however, the procedure does not usually require vascular or airway access, there is a potential opportunity to code the access additionally.

Two points to consider:

1. If the procedure *usually* requires the *type* of airway or vascular access provided, the access should not be coded in addition to the procedure for which it was used.

2. If the procedure does not usually require the type of airway or vascular access provided, the access may be coded additionally, only if the provider clearly documents why the procedure required the access.

Documentation Tip: *This is an opportunity to remind providers that they must clearly document in the medical record if vascular access is an exception and why the access was necessary for the procedure. This helps support the billing of the access in addition to the primary procedure.*

For procedures performed under general anesthesia, services include vascular access throughout a procedure. The vascular access when used for the anesthesia is not separately coded, as it is integral to the anesthesia. Also, computed tomographic angiographies (CTA) have codes that include injection of intravenous (IV) contrast. For these codes, the injection is an integral component of the procedure and should not be coded separately.

70496 Computed tomographic angiography, head, with contrast material(s), including noncontrast images, if performed, and image postprocessing

Injection of contrast material is part of the "with contrast" CTA procedure; therefore, it is not appropriate to separately report the code for the administration of contrast. The supply of contrast, however, may be reported separately with CPT code 99070, *Supplies and materials provided by the physician over and above those usually included with the office visit or other services rendered (list drugs, trays, supplies, or materials provided)*, or with the appropriate HCPCS Level II code for the contrast material used.

Excerpt From the General Coding Policies Section of NCCI Guidelines[3(p8)]

After vascular access is achieved, the access must be maintained by a slow infusion (e.g., saline) or injection of heparin or saline into a "lock." Since these services are necessary for maintenance of the vascular access, they are not separately reportable with the vascular access CPT codes or procedures requiring vascular access as a standard of medical/surgical practice. CPT code 37201 (Transcatheter therapy, infusion for thrombolysis other than coronary) should not be reported for use of an anticoagulant to maintain vascular access.

Interpretation

In order to maintain the patency of a vascular access, substances are administered directly into the IV line or catheter to keep them open and flowing freely. The examples offered are saline or heparin locks. If these are strictly for the maintenance of the vascular access and not for a therapeutic reason, the maintenance procedures are not separately coded. However, if there is transcatheter infusion therapy performed, the appropriate CPT code (eg, CPT code 37201 or other appropriate code) may be billed in addition to other services performed.

Determine from the documentation whether the infusion is for maintenance or therapy. If it cannot be determined, ask the provider to clarify.

CPT Coding Tip: Some payers require at least 15 minutes of infusion time documented before CPT 37201 may be used. Although the CPT guidelines do not impose such a requirement (see excerpt from CPT Assistant below). Check with your payer and check documentation. A common time frame for thrombolytic infusion is 60 minutes; however, advancements in technology have been able to reduce successful infusion times so a minimum measure would be reasonable at 15 minutes.

The February 1997 issue of *CPT Assistant*[5] addressed the issue of coding the Treatment of a Thrombosed Arteriovenous Fistula:

> If treating a thrombosed arteriovenous fistula … by means of thrombolytic infusion, report code 37201 for the infusion of the thrombolytic agent (ie, urokinase or streptokinase). These agents work to dissolve a clot or thrombus.

Time Element and the Relative Value

A common misconception about code 37201 is that it should only be reported for infusions that last 24 to 48 hours. The descriptor of code 37201 does not contain a time increment and was never intended to be time dependent.

Therefore, it is appropriate to use code 37201 to report a 24 to 48 hour infusion, as well as to report a 1 hour infusion. The relative value of this service is weighted to encompass both short and long infusions. This is because the intensity of the service is considerably greater in shorter infusions, while in longer infusions, the patient is cared for outside the operating suite. In this case, the physician is allowed to report the evaluation and management services provided outside the suite. Return visits, at which time the catheter may be exchanged and/or repositioned, are also reported separately. During shorter, more intense infusions, physicians do not generally provide repositioning or evaluation and management services.

Special Note: CPT 37201 indicates infusion, which usually bears a requirement of at least 15 minutes of infusion. Physicians should document the time of infusion to make sure the code is supported.

Excerpt From the General Coding Policies Section of NCCI Guidelines[3(p8)]

When a procedure requires more invasive vascular access services (e.g., central venous access, pulmonary artery access), the more invasive vascular service is separately reportable if it is not typical of the procedure, and the work of the more invasive vascular service has not been included in the valuation of the procedure.

Insertion of a central venous access device (e.g., central venous catheter, pulmonary artery catheter) requires passage of a catheter through central venous vessels and, in the case of a pulmonary artery catheter, through the right atrium and ventricle. These services often require the use of fluoroscopic guidance.

Separate reporting of CPT codes for right heart catheterization, selective venous catheterization, or pulmonary artery catheterization is not appropriate when reporting a CPT code for insertion of a central venous access device. Since CPT code 75998 describes fluoroscopic guidance for central venous access device procedures, CPT codes for more general fluoroscopy (e.g., 76000, 76001, 77002) should not be reported separately.

Interpretation

There are three different elements in this principle:

1. All services that are usual, integral to, or incidental to primary procedures are not separately reported. However, those services not usual for a procedure may usually be reported in addition to the primary procedure. In this policy, CMS indicates that if a particular patient's clinical scenario requires more invasive vascular access than what is usual for the procedure, the more invasive access may be coded in addition to the procedure.

2. When central venous access is necessary and separately coded in addition to the primary procedure, do not code the central venous access as if it was a heart catheterization, selective catheterization, or pulmonary artery catheterization. To code placement of a central line as anything else would be incorrect coding.

3. Given that there is a specific code for fluoroscopic guidance for central line placement, other fluoroscopy codes would be unsuitable.

The Cardiovascular System (33010-37799) and NCCI Guidelines

Excerpt From the Cardiovascular System Section of NCCI Guidelines[2(p8-9)]

Cardiovascular System
When a coronary artery bypass procedure is performed, the most comprehensive code describing the procedure should be reported.

Interpretation

Keep in mind, NCCI directs coders to follow the CPT codebook guidelines when coding. The CPT codebook instructs that procurement of the saphenous vein is included in the CPT code for the coronary artery bypass graft (CABG). Careful review of the CPT codebook guidelines when coding CABG procedures will help ensure correct and optimal coding.

Example

A physician performs a quadruple CABG using one venous and three artery grafts. The venous graft was from the saphenous vein.

33510 Coronary artery bypass, vein only; single coronary venous graft

33517 Coronary artery bypass, using venous graft(s) and arterial graft(s); single vein graft (List separately in addition to code for primary procedure)

33533 Coronary artery bypass, using arterial graft(s); single arterial graft

33534 two coronary arterial grafts

33535 three coronary arterial grafts

For a patient with a combined venous-arterial CABG, CPT codes 33517 (venous) + 33535 (3 arteries) are used. The saphenous vein procurement is included in the code for the venous graft (CPT code 33517) and is not separately billed per the CPT codebook guidelines.

Read the instructions in the CPT codebook carefully to ensure proper coding of these procedures.

Excerpt From the Cardiovascular System Section of NCCI Guidelines[2(p9)]

During venous or combined arterial venous coronary artery bypass grafting procedures (CPT codes 33510-33523), it is occasionally necessary to perform epi-aortic ultrasound. This procedure may be reported with CPT code 76998 (ultrasonic guidance, intraoperative) appending modifier -59. CPT code 76998 should not be reported for ultrasound guidance utilized to procure the vascular graft.

Interpretation

Atherosclerosis poses a significant risk of stroke for patients undergoing CABG procedures. The epiaortic ultrasound is a diagnostic tool to help surgeons measure the risk during the procedure. If a medically necessary epiaortic ultrasound is performed to monitor or diagnose this risk, a code may be added for this service. CPT code 76998 with modifier 59 may be added to the CABG procedure codes. Modifier 59 is necessary because CPT code 76998 bundles into the CABG CPT codes.

If an ultrasound is performed to procure a graft, CPT 76998 should not be coded in addition to the CABG procedure, as it then becomes an integral part of the surgery.

Here is the difference:

- If the ultrasound is a diagnostic tool, it would be coded in addition to the CABG.
- If the ultrasound serves to locate and retrieve a graft vessel, it is an inherent part of the CABG and should not be coded separately.

Excerpt From the Cardiovascular System Section of NCCI Guidelines[2(p9)]

Many of the code descriptors in the CPT code range 36800-36861 (hemodialysis access, intervascular cannulation, shunt insertion) include the "separate procedure" designation. Pursuant to the CMS "separate procedure" policy, these "separate procedures" are not separately reportable with vascular revision procedures at the same site/vessel.

Interpretation

As a reminder of basic CPT coding guidelines, any CPT codes designated as separate procedures should not be coded in addition to other, more major procedures performed at the same anatomic operative site during the same surgical session. This NCCI policy highlights the fact that many of the CPT codes in the Hemodialysis Access, Intervascular Cannulation for Extracorporeal Circulation, or Shunt Insertion range of codes are designated as separate procedures. Therefore, if another, more major procedure is performed on the same vessel, the separate procedure CPT code should not be coded.

This guideline applies throughout the CPT codebook and is not limited to those services highlighted by the NCCI policies. Take the example of a physician performing a thromboendarterectomy with a patch graft on a patient's subclavian artery, along with an AV fistula on the same vessel.

35301 Thromboendarterectomy, including patch graft, if performed; carotid, vertebral, subclavian, by neck incision

36831 Thrombectomy, open, arteriovenous fistula without revision, autogenous or nonautogenous dialysis graft (separate procedure)

Note that CPT code 35301 includes a thrombectomy and, therefore, reporting CPT code 36831 in addition to code 35301 would be incorrect, unless the procedures were performed on different vessels.

CPT code 36831 is designated as a separate procedure, which indicates that different vessels must be involved for this code to be added to the primary procedure code.

The following is an excerpt from the *CodeManager's* Clinical Vignette of Procedure for CPT code 35301 (emphasis added). Note that this service includes a shunt insertion as well.

CodeManager's Clinical Vignette of Procedure (35301)[6]

The neck is incised along the anterior border of the sternocleidomastoid muscle, and the soft tissue is dissected away from the carotid sheath. The common carotid, internal carotid, and external carotid arteries are exposed, mobilized, and encircled, with care taken not to injure the vagus or hypoglossal nerves. Systemic anticoagulation is administered, the arteries are clamped, and the common carotid artery is opened longitudinally. This incision is carried across the bifurcation, onto the internal carotid artery, and beyond the terminus of the obstructive plaque. Intraoperative electroencephalography recording is sometimes used in this portion of the operation to follow brain function during blood flow interruption. A shunt may be inserted for cerebral perfusion if required.

Using magnification loupes, the surgeon dissects the plaque from the common, external, and internal carotid arteries. The endarterectomy site is inspected carefully, searching for residual remnants of plaque, which are removed. Fine sutures are used to tack down any distal shelf at the endpoint of the endarterectomy in the internal carotid. When the surgeon is confident that no loose segments of plaque remain within the vessel, the arteriotomy is closed. **Often a diamond-shaped synthetic or venous patch is incorporated in this arterial suture line to increase the diameter of the artery.** If a shunt has been used, it is removed just prior to completion of the arterial closure. Vascular clamps are released with reinitiation of blood flow, and hemostasis of the suture line is achieved. The incision is closed in three layers.

Tip: Read the CPT clinical vignettes (located in the CodeManager 2009[7] software for many CPT codes) to understand many of the components that are integral or inherent in procedures. CodeManager is a coding reference software offered by the AMA. It includes the entire CPT, HCPCS, ICD-9-CM code sets, Medicare reimbursement information, and Dorland's dictionary. In addition, CPT Assistant and the Insider's View may also be used as added reference components. CodeManager 2009 may be purchased from the AMA bookstore at www.amabookstore.com.

Excerpt From the Cardiovascular System Section of NCCI Guidelines[2(p9-10)]

An aneurysm repair may require direct repair with or without graft insertion, thromboendarterectomy, and/or bypass. When a thromboendarterectomy is performed at the site of an aneurysm repair or graft insertion, the thromboendarterectomy is not separately reportable. If a bypass procedure requires an endarterectomy to insert the bypass graft, only the code describing the bypass may be reported. The endarterectomy is not separately reportable. If both an aneurysm repair (e.g., after rupture) and a bypass are performed at separate non-contiguous sites, the aneurysm repair code and the bypass code may be reported with an anatomic modifier or modifier -59. If a thromboendarterectomy is medically necessary, due to vascular occlusion in a different vessel, the appropriate code may be reported with an anatomic modifier or modifier -59 indicating that the procedures were performed in non-contiguous vessels.

Interpretation

An aneurysm repair involves removal of the aneurysm (a weakened area of an artery). Given that blood clots (thrombi) commonly occur in aneurysms, the repair might also require a thrombectomy. Because an aneurysm represents a weakened section of artery, a graft may be necessary to repair the site. These (thrombectomy and bypass) services are included in the aneurysm repair codes and are not separately reportable because they are common components of the repair.

By simply reading the CPT codes for aneurysm repairs, one can see that the necessary excisions and graft insertions are included in the repairs. See this code as an example:

35001   Direct repair of aneurysm, pseudoaneurysm, or excision (partial or total) and graft insertion, with or without patch graft; for aneurysm and associated occlusive disease, carotid, subclavian artery, by neck incision

Note that the code description includes excision and graft insertion.

If, however, different sites or vessels that are not contiguous are being operated on and, if one vessel has an aneurysm repaired and the other vessel has a bypass graft inserted, both services may be coded because they are of different sites. For example, a patient presents for open repair of an abdominal aorta aneurysm (AAA). The surgeon cuts into the aorta at the site of the aneurysm and, after clamping the artery on either side of the aneurysm, cuts into the

weakened area and removes thrombus from the site. Once all the thrombus is removed, the surgeon inserts a graft.

35081   Direct repair of aneurysm, pseudoaneurysm, or excision (partial or total) and graft insertion, with or without patch graft; for aneurysm, pseudoaneurysm, and associated occlusive disease, abdominal aorta

This code includes all aspects of the surgeon's work and would be the only code assigned. Another example would be that of a patient who presents for open repair of an abdominal aorta aneurysm (AAA). The surgeon cuts into the aorta at the site of the aneurysm and, after clamping the artery on either side of the aneurysm, cuts into the weakened area and removes the thrombus from the site. Once all the thrombus is removed, the surgeon inserts a graft. On the carotid artery, the patient has a thrombus that is going to be excised with a patch graft.

35081   Direct repair of aneurysm, pseudoaneurysm, or excision (partial or total) and graft insertion, with or without patch graft; for aneurysm, pseudoaneurysm, and associated occlusive disease, abdominal aorta

35301   Thromboendarterectomy, including patch graft, if performed; carotid, vertebral, subclavian, by neck incision

This code includes all aspects of the surgeon's work for the abdominal aorta aneurysm (AAA), but would not include any work on the carotid artery so CPT code 35301 with a modifier 59 would be coded as well.

Excerpt From the Cardiovascular System Section of NCCI Guidelines[2(p10)]

At a given site, only one type of bypass (venous, non-venous) code may be reported. If different vessels are bypassed with different types of grafts, separate codes may be reported. If the same vessel has multiple obstructions and requires bypass with different types of grafts in different areas, separate codes may be reported. However, it is necessary to indicate that multiple procedures were performed by using an anatomic modifier or modifier -59.

Interpretation

Only one bypass code may be used per anatomic site. Note that this policy allows for multiple coding if separate vessels are bypassed or if multiple obstructions are at different sites in a single vessel. Documentation here is crucial. It must be clearly supported that distinct sites were repaired. So, for example, a 70-year-old woman undergoes a left subclavian-to-vertebral artery bypass operation with an interposed saphenous vein graft because of severe stenosis of the vertebral artery bilaterally, CPT 35515 would be the only code necessary; however, a modifier LT (left) could be added for greater specificity.

35515 Bypass graft, with vein; subclavian-vertebral

If, however, the surgeon continues the operation by creating a femoral-popliteal bypass using the saphenous vein, the surgery should be coded with CPT codes 35515 and 35556:

35515 Bypass graft, with vein; subclavian-vertebral

35556 Bypass graft, with vein; femoral-popliteal

Procurement of the saphenous vein is included in the vein bypass graft codes per the CPT codebook.

Excerpt From the Cardiovascular System Section of NCCI Guidelines[2(p10)]

When an open vascular procedure (e.g., thrombo-endarterectomy) is performed, the repair and closure are included components of the vascular procedure. CPT codes 35201-35286 (repair of blood vessel) are not separately reportable in addition to the primary vascular procedure.

Interpretation

Recall within the NCCI introductory guidelines, specifically, the Standards of Medical/Surgical Practice section, necessary surgical closure and dressing is included in the code for the primary procedure and should not be coded separately from the root operation. As a necessary component of a primary procedure, the surgical closure is what the physician had to perform the component in order to successfully accomplish the comprehensive service. It should not be separated from the comprehensive service when being coded.

When a thromboendarterectomy (excision of a thrombus and a part of the arterial lining) is performed, it is necessary to close or repair the vessel on which the excision was done.

Take the case of a patient presenting for a thrombo-endarterectomy of the popliteal artery (CPT code 35303). On completion of the procedure, the physician sutures the popliteal artery for closure of the wound site.

It would be incorrect to add a code for repairing a lower extremity blood vessel (CPT code 35226) in addition to the thromboendarterectomy unless a separate site was involved.

Excerpt From the Cardiovascular System Section of NCCI Guidelines[2(p10)]

If an unsuccessful percutaneous vascular procedure is followed by an open procedure by the same physician at the same patient encounter (e.g., percutaneous transluminal angioplasty, thrombectomy, embolectomy, etc., followed by a similar open procedure such as thromboendarterectomy), only the HCPCS/CPT code for the successful procedure, which is usually the more extensive, open procedure may be reported. If a percutaneous procedure is performed on one lesion, and a similar open procedure is performed on a separate lesion, the HCPCS/CPT code for the percutaneous procedure may be reported with modifier -59 only if the lesions are in distinct and separate anatomically defined vessels. If similar open and percutaneous procedures are performed on different lesions in the same anatomically defined vessel, only the open procedure may be reported.

Interpretation

As mentioned in prior chapters, when planning surgical procedures, physicians want to use the least invasive and/ or most effective approach. On occasion, the planned approach is insufficient to the overall success of the procedure and the surgeon must convert to a different approach during the procedure. Failed approaches, or approaches that are converted to different approaches, are incidental to successful approaches and only the successfully approach procedure should be coded. However, if separate and distinct sites are corrected by different approaches, both may be coded with a modifier 59 appended to the less invasive approach. An example of this would be a patient presenting for a percutaneous transluminal angioplasty of the right iliac artery (CPT code 35473) which fails. During the procedure, the physician determines that an open procedure might be more successful and continues the procedure via an open approach (CPT code 35454). In this scenario, only the open angioplasty should be coded. However, if the right iliac artery was successfully repaired via a percutaneous approach and the left iliac vessel necessitated an open approach, both services should be coded with a modifier 59 appended to the percutaneous vessel service code.

Note, the NCCI guidelines direct coders to use modifier 59 although other payers may prefer the lateral modifiers (RT and LT) as more specific.

These codes fall under the Mutually Exclusive edits within NCCI but do allow bypassing the edits when the procedures are performed on contralateral sides.

When a non-coronary percutaneous intravascular interventional procedure is performed on the same vessel at the same patient encounter as diagnostic angiography (arteriogram/venogram), only one selective catheter placement code for the vessel may be reported.

Interpretation

If the same access site is used for both a diagnostic and a therapeutic service during the same session, the access is coded only once. If multiple vascular access sites are necessary, then each access site is coded separately. If different vascular families are accessed, each may be separately coded. So, a bilateral renal arteriogram and right renal artery stent deployment are performed on a patient during a single surgical session. In this case, because both the diagnostic and therapeutic services are performed on the same anatomic site, the selective catheter placement should be coded only one time.

Diagnostic angiograms performed on the same date of service as a percutaneous intravascular interventional procedure should be reported with modifier -59. If a diagnostic angiogram (fluoroscopic or computed tomographic) was performed prior to the date of the percutaneous intravascular interventional procedure, a second diagnostic angiogram cannot be reported on the date of the percutaneous intravascular interventional procedure unless it is medically reasonable and necessary to repeat the study to further define the anatomy and pathology. Report the repeat angiogram with modifier -59. If it is medically reasonable and necessary to repeat only a portion of the diagnostic angiogram, append modifier -52 to the angiogram CPT code.

Interpretation

If a diagnostic angiography precedes a therapeutic interventional radiologic procedure, add a code for the diagnostic study with a modifier 59 only if a decision for therapy has not already been made and the angiography is for completely diagnostic purposes. If a prior diagnostic study has been performed for the same vessel, the documentation should substantiate changes in patient's history or other information that would clearly support an additional diagnostic study. An example would be a bilateral renal arteriogram and right renal artery stent deployment performed on a patient during a single encounter. If there was no prior diagnostic study and the physician clearly indicated that the arteriogram was for diagnostic purposes and the decision to continue onto the stent placement was made in part on the results of the diagnostic study, both the arteriogram and stent deployment may be coded with a modifier appended to the stent deployment code.

If a median sternotomy is utilized to perform a cardiothoracic procedure, the repair of the sternotomy is not separately reportable. CPT codes 21820-21825 (treatment of sternum fracture) should not be reported for repair of the sternotomy.

If a cardiothoracic procedure is performed after a prior cardiothoracic procedure with sternotomy (e.g., repeat procedure, new procedure, treatment of postoperative hemorrhage), removal of embedded wires is not separately reportable.

Interpretation

Remember from the General Coding Guidelines discussion in Chapter 2 of this book, the surgical approach and closure are included in the code for the primary procedure and should not be billed separately.

In the case of a surgery performed in the thoracic cavity (the area between the neck and abdomen), accessing the site through the sternum via incision and separating of the sternum (sternotomy) and closure of that surgically created sternum wound are both incidental to that procedure. Do not code either of these in addition to the primary procedure performed at that access site.

If removal of embedded wires or other previously placed foreign bodies is necessary in order to perform a more major procedure, do not code the wire removal as it then becomes part of the access or approach for the current procedure.

Tip: If removal of the embedded wire becomes very complicated and adds significantly to the procedure, there might be an opportunity to append a modifier 22 (increased procedural service) to the primary procedure.

The documentation must support that the work involved in the procedure was increased significantly over the usual work.

The CPT code 33945 is for a heart transplant, and in order to perform a heart transplant, the surgeon would have to open the patient's sternum (sternotomy) and on conclusion of the procedure, the sternum would be closed. Neither the sternotomy nor closure should be coded in addition to the transplant service because they are necessary and integral components to the root operation.

Excerpt From the Cardiovascular System Section of NCCI Guidelines[2(p12)]

If a superficial or deep implant (e.g., buried wire, pin, rod) requires surgical removal (CPT codes 20670 and 20680), it is not separately reportable if it is performed as an integral part of another procedure. For example, if a reoperation for coronary artery bypass or valve procedure requires removal of previously inserted sternal wires, removal of these wires is not separately reportable.

Interpretation

Throughout the NCCI edits we are reminded that any services that are integral or incidental to another procedure should not be coded in addition to the other procedure. This guideline is no different. If removal of an implant is necessary in order to perform a more major procedure, do not code the implant removal.

Example

A patient has a history of a triple bypass procedure and presents for a CABG reoperation. The prior sternotomy site has been closed with embedded straight wires, which the surgeon removes during the access for the reoperation. The wires are removed solely to access the site for the reoperation. Because the wire removal is necessary in order to perform the reoperation, the removal is not separately reportable.

Excerpt From the Cardiovascular System Section of NCCI Guidelines

CPT codes 36500 (venous catheterization for selective organ blood sampling) or 75893 (venous sampling through catheter with or without angiography…) may be reported for venous blood sampling through a catheter placed for the sole purpose of venous blood sampling. CPT code 75893 includes concomitant venography if performed. If a catheter is placed for a purpose other than venous blood sampling with or without venography (CPT code 75893), it is a misuse of CPT codes 36500 or 75893 to report them in addition to CPT codes for the other venous procedure(s).

Interpretation

If a patient has a catheter previously placed for other reasons (infusion therapy, for example), obtaining specimens through that catheter would not be separately reported. CPT code 36500 is for the placement of the catheter for the exclusive purpose of specimen sampling. It would be incorrect to use this code for a sampling through an earlier-placed catheter. If the catheter is placed solely for the purpose of sampling, it would be appropriate to report CPT code 36500. Basically, if the catheter was already in the patient, do not add CPT code 36500 when the specimen is taken.

Excerpt From the Cardiovascular Section of NCCI Guidelines[2(p12)]

Peripheral vascular bypass CPT codes describe bypass procedures with venous and other grafting materials (CPT codes 35501-35683). These procedures are mutually exclusive since only one type of bypass procedure may be performed at a site of obstruction. If multiple sites of obstruction are treated with different types of bypass procedures at the same patient encounter, multiple bypass procedure codes may be reported with anatomic modifiers or modifier -59.

Interpretation

The codes referenced in this guideline (CPT codes 35501-35683) include bypass grafts using veins, other than veins, and composite grafts. This guideline indicates that the different types of grafts are mutually exclusive because only one obstruction is being treated. Therefore, if one site is treated, only one code should be used. If multiple sites are treated, multiple codes may be billed. A case in point would be that of a patient having a vein bypass graft of the carotid-brachial vessel. The coding would be:

35556 Bypass graft, with vein; femoral-popliteal

If CPT code 35656 (Bypass graft, with other than vein; femoral-popliteal) was also coded, there would be a conflict because only a single obstructed site is being treated (femoral-popliteal). Different sites would have different codes.

Excerpt From the Cardiovascular System Section of NCCI Guidelines[2(p12)]

When percutaneous angioplasty of a vascular lesion is followed at the same session by a percutaneous or open atherectomy, generally due to insufficient improvement in vascular flow with angioplasty alone, only the most comprehensive atherectomy that was performed (generally the open procedure) is reported.

Interpretation

Again, failed procedures are incidental to successful procedures regardless of approach. This guideline illustrates that if an attempted procedure is unsuccessful because of insufficient improvement in flow, and the physician performs a different procedure of the same site, the failed procedure is not coded.

Example

Table 8-1 illustrates the column 1/column 2 bundling edits for CPT code 35480 (Transluminal peripheral atherectomy, open; renal or other visceral artery).

As one can see, CPT code 35490 (Transluminal peripheral atherectomy, percutaneous; renal or other visceral artery) bundles into CPT code 35480 as an inherent component.

TABLE 8-1 *Column 1/Column 2 Bundling Edits for CPT Code 35480*

Column 1	Column 2	Modifier 0=not allowed 1=allowed 9=not applicable
35480	C8950	1
35480	C8952	1
35480	G0345	1
35480	G0347	1
35480	G0351	1
35480	G0353	1
35480	G0354	1
35480	01924	0
35480	34820	1
35480	34834	1
35480	35490	1
35480	36000	1
35480	36002	1
35480	36410	1
35480	37202	1

Excerpt From the Cardiovascular System Section of NCCI Guidelines[2(p13)]

Many Pacemaker/Pacing Cardioverter-Defibrillator procedures (HCPCS/CPT codes 33202-33249, G0297-G0300) and Intracardiac Electrophysiology procedures (CPT codes 93600-93662) require intravascular placement of catheters into coronary vessels or cardiac chambers under fluoroscopic guidance. Physicians should not separately report cardiac catheterization or selective vascular catheterization CPT codes for placement of these catheters. A cardiac catheterization CPT code is separately reportable if it is a medically reasonable, necessary, and distinct service performed at the same or different patient encounter. Fluoroscopy codes are not separately reportable with the procedures described by HCPCS/CPT codes 33202-33249, G0297-G0300, and 93600-93662. Similarly, ultrasound guidance is not separately reportable with these CPT codes. Physicians should not report CPT codes 76942, 76998, 93318, or other ultrasound procedural codes if the ultrasound procedure is performed for guidance during one of the procedures described by HCPCS/CPT codes 33200-33249, G0297-G0300, or 93600-93662.

Interpretation

Services that are the standard of care in the performance of other procedures are not coded in addition to the primary procedure being performed. (See Chapter 2 for complete interpretation of standard of care.)

When a physician places a pacemaker or cardiac defibrillator or performs a diagnostic electrophysiology study, a usual component of these services is the placing of a catheter. When performed in conjunction with and as a part of the pacemaker placement, cardiac defibrillator placement, or electrophysiology study, the catheter placement is not separately coded.

Electrophysiology studies are somewhat invasive. The study is performed with the patient under local anesthesia and conscious sedation. The procedure involves inserting a catheter attached to electricity monitoring electrodes into a blood vessel, often through a site in the groin or neck, and winding the catheter wire up into the heart. The journey from entry point to heart muscle is navigated using images created by a fluoroscope to provide continuous images of the catheter and heart muscle. Once the catheter reaches the heart, electrodes at its tip gather data and a variety of electrical measurements are made. These data pinpoint the location of the faulty electrical site. During this "electrical mapping," the electrophysiologist may instigate, through pacing (the use of tiny electrical impulses), some of the very arrhythmias that are the crux of the problem. The events are safe, given the range of expertise and resources close at hand and are necessary to ensure the precise location of the problematic tissue.

The CPT codebook instructions also indicate that the catheters are a component of the CPT code and are not to be coded separately.

Excerpt From the Cardiovascular System Section of NCCI Guidelines[2(p13-14)]

CPT code 37202 (transcatheter therapy, infusion other than for thrombolysis, any type …) describes an arterial infusion of a non-chemotherapeutic medication for a purpose other than thrombolysis. This code should not be utilized to report intravenous infusions, arterial push injections (CPT code 90773), or chemotherapy infusions.

Interpretation

Transcatheter therapy, represented by CPT code 37202, is for the continuous catheter-directed infusion of a therapeutic medication (eg, papaverine, verapamil, vasopressin).

The NCCI guideline indicates that this code should not be used when the procedure performed is represented by more specific codes.

The following codes have very specific application and would be used instead of CPT code 37202 as appropriate.

Intravenous Infusions

96360 Intravenous infusion, hydration; initial, 31 minutes to 1 hour

96361 each additional hour (List separately in addition to code for primary procedure)

96365 Intravenous infusion, for therapy, prophylaxis, or diagnosis (specify substance or drug); initial, up to 1 hour

96366 each additional hour (List separately in addition to code for primary procedure)

Chemotherapy Infusions

96409 Chemotherapy administration; intravenous, push technique, single or initial substance/drug

+ 96411 intravenous, push technique, each additional substance/drug (List separately in addition to code for primary procedure)

96413 Chemotherapy administration, intravenous infusion technique; up to 1 hour, single or initial substance/drug

+ 96415 each additional hour (List separately in addition to code for primary procedure)

The following is a *CPT Assistant*[6] description of CPT code 37202 and additional comment on bundling as it applies to this code.

Code 37202 was first intended and developed to describe prolonged infusions into peripheral arteries. Transcatheter infusion/injection of intracoronary drugs (eg, nitrates, calcium channel blockers) during cardiac catheterization procedures have become routine and are considered an integral part of both the diagnostic catheterization codes (93501-93556) and the coronary intervention codes (92980-92996). Cardiologists may, however, report code 37202 in unusual circumstances by appending the -59 modifier (distinct procedural service) and providing adequate documentation.

Excerpt From the Cardiovascular System Section of NCCI Guidelines[2(p14)]

CPT code 37215 describes a percutaneous transcatheter placement of intravascular stent(s) in the cervical carotid artery utilizing distal embolic protection. It includes all ipsilateral selective carotid arterial catheterization, all diagnostic imaging for ipsilateral cervical and cerebral carotid arteriography, and all radiological supervision and interpretation (RS&I). Physicians should not unbundle the RS&I services. For example, a provider should not report CPT code 75962 (RS&I for transluminal balloon angioplasty of a peripheral artery) for angioplasty of the cervical carotid artery which is an included service in the procedure defined by CPT code 37215. Additionally since the carotid artery is not a peripheral artery, it is a misuse of CPT code 75962 to describe a carotid artery procedure. These same principles would apply to CPT code 37216, but it is currently a noncovered service code on the Medicare Physician Fee Schedule.

Interpretation

As required by the CPT codebook instructions and NCCI principles, do not code any selective carotid catheterizations, or diagnostic cervical or cerebral arteriographies, or related supervision and interpretation codes when they are performed on the same side (ipsilateral) as the stent placement. So, if a provider places a stent through a catheter into a patient's left common carotid artery and the physician selectively placed a catheter into the cervical carotid artery, the only code billed would be CPT 37215.

Do not add a code for the selective placement (CPT 36215) or the angiography (CPT 75676) as they are included in the payment for the stent placement.

If, however, the stent was placed on the left side and a separate angiography through selective catheter placement was performed on the right side, the stent placement (CPT code 37215), the selective catheter placement (CPT 36215), and the angiography (CPT 75676) may be coded. Appropriate lateral modifiers (LT – left, RT – right) should be appended to help bypass the bundling edits.

Excerpt From the Cardiovascular System Section of NCCI Guidelines[2(p15)]

Operative ablation procedures (CPT codes 33250-33266) include cardioversion as an integral component of the procedures. CPT codes 92960 or 92961 (elective cardioversion) should not be reported separately with the operative ablation procedure codes unless an elective cardioversion is performed at a separate patient encounter on the same date of service. If electrophysiologic study with pacing and recording is performed during an operative ablation procedure, it is integral to the procedure and should not be reported separately as CPT code 93624 (electrophysiologic follow-up study with pacing and recording to test effectiveness of therapy…).

Interpretation

Cardioversion is the process of an electrical shock being delivered to the heart to convert an abnormal heart rhythm back to a normal rhythm. Electrophysiology (EP) studies analyze the electrical system of the heart to determine details of abnormal heartbeats. Both of these are considered integral to the operative ablation surgeries.

If either were performed in a separate encounter, the operative ablation and cardioversion or EP study could be coded with a modifier 59 appended to the otherwise bundled code. Note, the cardioversion is also incidental to the EP studies, so if these two procedures were performed during the same session, only the EP study should be coded.

- ⊙ **92960** Cardioversion, elective, electrical conversion of arrhythmia; external

- ⊙ **92961** internal (separate procedure)

Note the internal cardioversion is designated as a separate procedure code.

CPT Assistant[7] explains that CPT code

92961 is designated as a separate procedure. Internal elective cardioversion is not separately reported when performed as an integral component of another procedure/service as in an electrophysiological study or cardiac catheterization. However, if the internal elective cardioversion is performed independently, unrelated or distinct from other procedure(s)/service(s) provided at that time, then it would be appropriate to separately report the internal cardioversion. The parenthetical note that follows the code indicates that it is not appropriate to report internal cardioversion in conjunction with codes 93618-93652 (from the intracardiac electrophysiological procedures series of codes) and codes 93741-93744 (from the series of codes describing other vascular studies).

Medically Unlikely Edits (MUEs)

Excerpt From the General Correct Coding Policies Section of NCCI Guidelines[3(p30)]

Medically Unlikely Edits (MUEs)

An MUE for a HCPCS/CPT code is the maximum number of units of service (UOS) under most circumstances allowable by the same provider for the same beneficiary on the same date of service.

Explanation

The following shows some examples of current MUEs for cardiovascular system services. CMS, Medicare administrative contractor, fiscal intermediary, and carrier Web sites should be checked for current MUEs.

CPT Code	MUE	CPT Descriptor
35190	2	Repair, acquired or traumatic arteriovenous fistula; extremities
35226	3	Repair blood vessel, direct; lower extremity
35509	1	Bypass graft, with vein; carotid-contralateral carotid

SUMMARY

- The entire cardiovascular services section from the NCCI manual should be read.

- The CPT codebook instructions should be read when these procedures are coded. Many of the NCCI edit principles directly follow the CPT codebook guidelines.

- Usually, multiple procedures performed on a single vessel are bundled into the most complex procedure performed. When the provider is treating a single condition at a single site with multiple procedures, the NCCI policies should be reviewed to determine whether multiple codes may be used.

Definitions and Acronyms

cardioversion: The restoration of normal rhythm of the heart by electrical shock.

computed tomographic angiography (CTA): This procedure uses contrast media and special radiographic equipment to produce detailed vascular pictures.

contralateral: Situated on, pertaining to, or affecting the opposite side, as opposed to ipsilateral.

coronary artery bypass graft (CABG): This is a surgery to bypass narrowed or blocked coronary arteries.

electrophysiology (EP) study: The mechanisms, functions, and performance of the electrical activities of specific regions of the heart; the term is usually used in describing studies of such phenomena by invasive (intracardiac) recording of spontaneous activity as well as of cardiac responses to programmed stimuli. The studies are performed to assess complex arrhythmias, elucidate symptoms, evaluate abnormal electrocardiograms, assess risk, and design treatment; they increasingly include therapeutic methods in addition to diagnostic and prognostic procedures.

intravenous (IV): *Intra* meaning *within* and *venous* meaning *vein*, *intravenous* means within a vein. Usually used for administering substances (eg, intravenous infusion of medications).

ipsilateral: Situated on, pertaining to, or affecting the same side, as opposed to contralateral.

percutaneous transluminal angioplasty: This is a minimally invasive procedure that uses balloons that are inserted and manipulated through a vessel to mechanically widen an obstructed (or narrowed) blood vessel.

percutaneous transluminal coronary angioplasty (PTCA): As defined above, a percutaneous angioplasty is a minimally invasive procedure using balloons inserted through a vessel to widen a blood vessel. In PTCA, the vessels are coronary vessels.

radiopharmaceutical: A radioactive pharmaceutical, nuclide, or other chemical used for diagnostic or therapeutic purposes.

sternotomy: The operation of cutting through and separating the sternum.

thrombolysis: Lysis (to cause or produce disintegration) of a thrombus or thrombi.

thrombus: A stationary blood clot along the wall of a blood vessel, frequently causing vascular obstruction. Some authorities differentiate thrombus formation from simple coagulation or clot formation.

CHAPTER EXERCISE

Indication: Bilateral leg pain

Procedures: Aortogram with runoff, angioplasty and stent right external iliac artery

Details: The patient's left groin was sterilely prepped and draped in the usual fashion. Via retrograde left femoral arterial approach, a 5Fr vascular sheath was inserted. 5Fr pigtail catheter was introduced into the abdominal aorta. An abdominal aortogram was obtained. The catheter was pulled down into the distal abdominal aorta and a bilateral runoff arteriogram was obtained.

Findings: There are single renal arteries present bilaterally. The left renal artery was previously stented. The renal arteries appear widely patent bilaterally. The abdominal aorta demonstrates atherosclerotic calcification, but no significant stenosis. The common iliac arteries demonstrate atherosclerotic calcification, but no significant stenosis. The internal iliac arteries are patent bilaterally with atherosclerotic calcification present.

Mild to moderate stenoses are present within the internal iliac arteries bilaterally. There is an 80% diameter reducing stenosis involving the right external iliac artery in its mid portion. The left external iliac artery demonstrates moderate atherosclerotic disease, but no significant stenosis. The common femoral arteries are patent bilaterally. There is atherosclerotic calcification and plaquing within both superficial femoral arteries. Moderate atherosclerotic disease is present on the right side with no area of stenosis greater than 50% identified. On the left side there are two areas of very high grade stenosis present in the proximal and mid left superficial femoral arteries. The previously stented portion of the left superficial femoral artery remains patent with good flow within it. No significant stenosis in this stented portion of the left superficial femoral artery is identified. The popliteal arteries demonstrate some mild atherosclerotic disease, but no significant stenosis. There is significant trifurcation disease present with primarily perioneal runoff on the right side.

The anterior tibial artery has an occlusion in its proximal extent with reconstitution of the anterior tibial artery which then continues through the level of the ankle and into the foot. On the left side there is peroneal and anterior tibial runoff which is continuous.

It was felt the patient would benefit from improvement of inflow on the right side. A 7Fr Balkan sheath was then inserted and advanced into the right external iliac artery. With the sheath in place in the external iliac artery, a catheter and guidewire were advanced across the external iliac artery into the common femoral artery. An Amplatz guidewire was left in place. A 9mm x 30mm Luminex stent was deployed across the area of stenosis in the distal external iliac artery.

The area was then balloon dilated to 8mm diameter with an 8mm x 2cm long angioplasty balloon. There was a good angiographic result. The sheath was pulled back and there was a moderate stenosis which was in the 60% range in the very proximal external iliac artery. This was balloon dilated to 8mm diameter with an 8mm x 2cm long angioplasty balloon. There was a good response to angioplasty of the right external iliac artery proximally. There was a high grade stenosis present at the origin of the right internal iliac artery which remained patent after balloon dilatation of the external iliac artery. The catheter and sheath were then removed and hemostasis was obtained with a perclose suture device.

Impression: Previously stented left renal artery remains widely patent with no significant stenosis in the right renal artery.

Atherosclerotic calcification throughout the arterial system from the aorta through the trifurcation vessels.

No significant stenosis identified within the aorta or common iliac arteries bilaterally although atherosclerotic calcification and plaquing is present.

High grade stenosis right internal iliac artery at its origin. 60% diameter reducing stenosis right external iliac artery at its origin as well as a very high grade stenosis in the mid to distal right external iliac artery.

These responded well to angioplasty proximally and angioplasty and stenting in the distal portion. A good angiographic result was obtained.

The left external iliac artery demonstrates moderate atherosclerotic disease, but no significant stenosis.

Atherosclerotic plaquing in the superficial femoral artery in the right side with no area of high grade stenosis identified.

High grade stenosis in the proximal and mid left superficial femoral artery with the previously stented portion of the left superficial femoral artery remaining widely patent.

If the patient has a good symptomatic response on the right side after angioplasty of the external iliac artery and remains symptomatic on the left side, angioplasty of the left superficial femoral artery could be undertaken.

Popliteal arteries demonstrate no significant stenosis bilaterally.

Sort segment occlusion right anterior tibial artery in its mid portion with moderate atherosclerotic disease in the right perioneal artery. These are the two dominant runoff vessels to the right foot.

Anterior tibial and peroneal runoff on the left side with no significant atherosclerotic stenosis present. Atherosclerotic plaquing in the superficial femoral artery in the right side with no area of high grade stenosis identified.

High grade stenosis in the proximal and mid left superficial femoral artery with the previously stented portion of the left superficial femoral artery remaining widely patent.

If the patient has a good symptomatic response on the right side after angioplasty of the external iliac artery and remains symptomatic on the left side, angioplasty of the left superficial femoral artery could be undertaken. Popliteal arteries demonstrate no significant stenosis bilaterally.

Sort segment occlusion right anterior tibial artery in its mid portion with moderate atherosclerotic disease in the right peroneal artery. These are the two dominant runoff vessels to the right foot.

What portion(s) of this procedure can be coded and why?

ANSWERS TO CHAPTER EXERCISES

5Fr pigtail catheter was introduced into the abdominal aorta (36200 for aorta placement).

An abdominal aortogram (75625 for aortography) was obtained. The catheter was pulled down into the distal abdominal aorta (No code for placement but does change the way angiography will be coded) and a bilateral runoff arteriogram was obtained (75716 for extremity angiography…cannot determine how far down the angiography was performed).

A 7Fr Balkan sheath was then inserted and advanced into the right external iliac artery (36246 for common femoral – lose 36200 unless there was a separate insertion). A 9mm x 30mm Luminex stent was deployed (37205 + 75960) across the area of stenosis in the distal external iliac artery. The area was then balloon dilated (do not code as angioplasty was for deployment) to 8mm diameter with an 8mm x 2cm long angioplasty balloon.

Final Coding

36246 (+36200 if separate insertion site)

75625

75716-59

75960

37205

REFERENCES

1. American Medical Association. *Current Procedural Terminology CPT® 2009 Professional Edition.* Chicago, IL: American Medical Association; 2008.

2. Centers for Medicare and Medicaid Services. "Chapter V Surgery: Respiratory, Cardiovascular, Hemic and Lymphatic Systems," NCCI Policy Manual for Medicare Services. www.cms.hhs.gov/NationalCorrectCodInitEd/01_overview.asp#TopOfPage. Accessed June 12, 2009.

3. Centers for Medicare and Medicaid Services. "Chapter I General Correct Coding Policies," NCCI Policy Manual for Medicare Services. www.cms.hhs.gov/NationalCorrectCodInitEd/01_overview.asp#TopOfPage. Accessed June 12, 2009.

4. American Medical Association. *CPT Assistant.* "Coding Consultation: Questions and Answers, Cardiovascular System/Surgery, 36000, 90780, 90781 (Q&A)." 2003;13(4):26.

5. American Medical Association. *CPT Assistant.* "Thrombolytic Therapy: Coding the Treatment of a Thrombosed Arteriovenous Fistula." 1997;7(2):1.

6. American Medical Association. *CodeManager®* 2008.

7. Centers for Medicare and Medicaid Services. "Practitioner – DME Supplier MUE Table." www.cms.hhs.gov/NationalCorrectCodInitEd/08_MUE.asp#TopOfPage. Accessed June 12, 2009.

8. American Medical Association. *CPT Assistant.* "Coding Communication: Cardioversion: External vs. Internal." 2000;10(11):9.

The Hemic and Lymphatic Systems

Chapter 9 provides background about the hemic and lymphatic systems, reviews the National Correct Coding Initiative (NCCI) coding guidelines for procedures performed on these systems, and provides examples to reflect the logic behind the edits. As with the other chapters, this chapter provides an NCCI guideline followed by our interpretation, an example, or both.

Introduction to the Hemic-Lymphatic System and NCCI Guidelines

Excerpt From the Hemic-Lymphatic System Section of NCCI Guidelines[2(p2)]

A. Introduction
The principles of correct coding discussed in Chapter I apply to the CPT codes in the range 30000-39999. Several general guidelines are repeated in this Chapter. However, those general guidelines from Chapter I not discussed in this chapter are nonetheless applicable.

Interpretation

The above instruction serves as a reminder that the general NCCI guidelines (introduced in Chapter 2 of this book) apply to each section of the *Current Procedural Terminology* (CPT®)[1] codebook even if they are not repeated within a chapter. The introductory guidelines were covered comprehensively in Chapter 2 of this book and will not be repeated here.

Excerpt From the Hemic-Lymphatic System Section of NCCI Guidelines[2(p15)]

When bone marrow aspiration is performed alone, the appropriate code to report is CPT code 38220. When a bone marrow biopsy is performed, the appropriate code is CPT code 38221 (bone marrow biopsy). This code cannot be reported with CPT code 20220 (bone biopsy).

Interpretation

This NCCI guideline is a reminder to coders to be careful when coding and make sure the most correct code is applied, based on the documentation.

CPT code 38220 is coded when bone marrow is aspirated (small amount of bone marrow fluid and cells through a needle inserted into the bone). CPT code 38221 is coded when the needle or trocar removes the soft tissue inside the bone. CPT code 20220 is coded when a bone (not the marrow) is biopsied.

38220 Bone marrow; aspiration only

38221 biopsy, needle or trocar

20220 Biopsy, bone, trocar, or needle; superficial (eg, ilium, sternum, spinous process, ribs)

CPT Assistant[3] explains these guidelines through the following excerpt:

From a CPT coding perspective, if multiple aspirations are obtained at the same insertion site, then code 38220 should be reported one time. However, if a separately distinct needle site was aspirated (eg, iliac and sternum), then it would be appropriate to report code 38220 appended by modifier '59,' *Distinct procedural service*, for the additional site. Supporting documentation should be reflected in the medical record to provide an adequate description and need for the additional aspiration site(s).

CPT codes 38220 and 38221 may only be reported together if the two procedures are performed at separate sites or at separate patient encounters. Separate sites include bone marrow aspiration and biopsy in different bones or two separate skin incisions over the same bone.

When both a bone marrow biopsy (CPT code 38221) and bone marrow aspiration (CPT code 38220) are performed at the same site through the same skin incision, do not report the bone marrow aspiration, CPT code 38220, in addition to the bone marrow biopsy (CPT code 38221). HCPCS/CPT code G0364 may be reported to describe the bone marrow aspiration performed with bone marrow biopsy through the same skin incision on the same date of service.

Interpretation

38220 Bone marrow; aspiration only

38221 biopsy, needle or trocar

G0364 Bone marrow aspiration performed with bone marrow biopsy through the same incision on the same date of service

The Centers for Medicare and Medicaid Services (CMS) created a Healthcare Common Procedure Coding System (HCPCS) code (G0364) to report the aspiration service when a bone marrow biopsy and aspiration are performed at the same site during a single encounter. So, if both an aspiration and biopsy are performed at a single anatomic site, CPT code 38221 and HCPCS code G0364 should be coded.

Sometimes the bone marrow is aspirated prior to a biopsy being performed, and the documentation might note that the needle was repositioned or perhaps a different site altogether was biopsied. For both services to be coded, the documentation would need to clearly support separate sites and that both an aspirate and biopsy were medically necessary.

If distinct sites were biopsied and aspirated, the CPT codes 38221 and 38220 would be billed. A modifier 59 would be needed when CPT codes 38221 and 38220 were coded together to indicate separate sites. It should be noted that the medically unlikely edits (MUEs) for each of these codes is limited to two, meaning that each code has a unit of service limitation of two.

For example, a medical oncologist performs bone marrow aspirations on a patient's pelvis. Three samples are extracted from the site. A local anesthetic is injected, and a bandage is applied.

CPT code 38220x1 would be appropriate for this encounter. Because there is no documentation that the multiple samples were extracted from distinct sites, only one service may be billed.

On the other hand, consider a patient with Hodgkin's lymphoma has a bone marrow biopsy with aspiration on the right iliac crest through the same incision. To ensure adequacy of the specimen, the left iliac crest is also biopsied.

CPT codes 38221-50 would be appropriate for this encounter because bilateral biopsies were performed. The aspiration would be coded G0364 because it involved the same site as the biopsy. G0364 does not bundle into CPT code 38221, so modifier 59 would not be required. G0364 is mutually exclusive with CPT code 38220 (aspiration of a different site). It would be incorrect to code both G0364 and CPT code 38220 together for the same site, because they both represent aspirations.

Medically Unlikely Edits for the Hemic and Lymphatic Systems

An MUE for a HCPCS/CPT code is the maximum number of units of service (UOS) under most circumstances allowable by the same provider for the same beneficiary on the same date of service.

Explanation

Table 9-1 shows some examples of current MUEs for hemic-lymphatic system services. CMS, Medicare administrative contractor, fiscal intermediary, and carrier Web sites should be checked for current MUEs.

TABLE 9-1 *Medically Unlikely Edit (MUE) Examples for the Hemic/Lymphatic System*

CPT Code	MUE	CPT Code Descriptor
38100	1	Splenectomy; total (separate procedures)
38724	2	Cervical lymphadenectomy (modified rodical neck dissection)

SUMMARY

Read the entire hemic/lymphatic section from the NCCI manual.

Definitions and Acronyms

bone marrow aspiration: Extraction of a small amount of bone marrow fluid and cells through a needle put into a bone.

bone marrow biopsy: Extracting soft tissue from inside the bone through a needle or trocar.

Healthcare Common Procedure Coding System (HCPCS): These are the code sets used for filing Medicare bills consisting of Level I CPT codes and Level II HCPCS codes.

lymph: fluid that enters the lymph nodes through filtration then empties into the subclavian vein to mix back with blood.

lymphocytes: Type of white blood cells.

Resource-Based Relative Value Scale (RBRVS): RBRVS is Medicare's fee schedule for paying professional fee services (eg, physicians, non-physician providers) and includes coverage criteria for HCPCS coding billed by those practitioners.

CHAPTER EXERCISE

Review the following case information:

Diagnosis: Splenomegaly of unknown origin, rule out lymphoma or other malignancy.

Procedures: 1. Open splenectomy. 2. Mesenteric lymph node biopsy.

Anesthesia: General

Findings: The spleen was quite large, as expected. Additionally, there were what appeared to be extensive retroperitoneal and mesenteric lymph nodes consistent with probable lymphoma. There was a small amount of ascites. The liver was without obvious masses. The small bowel and colon were without obvious abnormality. The gallbladder was without abnormality.

Operation: The patient was identified in preoperative holding and taken to the operating room, where he was placed supine on the operating table. After general anesthesia was induced, the abdomen was prepped and draped in the usual sterile fashion. Time out for patient identification was performed. A midline celiotomy incision was made from a few centimeters below the xiphoid to an infraumbilical position. The skin was divided with a scalpel, followed by cautery for the remaining layers. The fascia was elevated and entered with cautery until it was clear that we were within the abdomen. At this point, we extended the

incision the rest of the way using cautery. A very large spleen could be seen at this point. Attempts to medialize the spleen were thwarted by some adhesions at the superior pole to the diaphragm. These were divided with cautery, and then we were able to pull the spleen down and medial to begin dissection. We began in the inferior pole near the splenorenal ligament and divided this with a combination of cautery and clamps with ties. Next, we moved superiorly and took down short gastrics. This freed up the superior pole of the spleen nicely, opening it up so that we could visualize the hilar structures. Dissection using serially applied clamps and either suture ligature or stick ties as appropriate was then performed to divide the remaining vessels. Separate divisions of the superior and inferior pole vessels were performed. The spleen was then passed off the field as the specimen. Hemostasis was obtained using additional stick ties where necessary and argon beam cautery on the raw areas of prior spleen to retroperitoneal attachments and the diaphragmatic attachments to the spleen. After hemostasis, we thoroughly irrigated the wound. Next, we did a mesenteric lymph node biopsy. Prior, we had done a complete exploration of the abdomen, and the only abnormality noted was what appeared to be extensive nodal disease within the retroperitoneum and the mesentery of the small bowel and colon. A representative lymph node area was then dissected out sharply, and the small bowel mesentery, and hemostasis was obtained. This lymph node was passed off the field as a separate specimen. We assured hemostasis once again and then began closure. The fascia was closed with a double-looped #1 Maxon suture. The subcutaneous tissue was thoroughly irrigated, and the skin was closed with staples. Dry gauze dressings were applied, and then the patient was brought out of anesthesia, extubated, and returned to the recovery area in stable condition.

What would be coded for this case and why?

ANSWERS TO CHAPTER EXERCISES

CPT codes 38100, Splenectomy; total (separate procedure), *and 38500,* Biopsy or excision of lymph node(s); open, superficial *represent the entire service provided.*

REFERENCES

1. American Medical Association. *Current Procedural Terminology (CPT®) 2009 Professional Edition.* Chicago, IL: American Medical Association; 2008.

2. American Medical Association. *CPT Assistant.* "Coding communication: surgery: hemic and lymphatic system, 38220 (Q&A)." 2007;17(6):10.

3. American Medical Association. *CPT Assistant.* "Coding communication: surgery: hemic and lymphatic system, 38220 (Q&A)." 2004;14(1):26.

The Digestive System

Chapter 10 provides background about the digestive system, reviews the National Correct Coding Initiative (NCCI) coding guidelines for procedures performed on the digestive system, and provides examples to reflect the logic behind the edits. As with the other chapters, an NCCI guideline is followed by our interpretation, an example, or both.

Introduction Section of NCCI Digestive System Guidelines

Excerpt From the Digestive System Section of NCCI Guidelines[1(p2)]

A. Introduction
The principles of correct coding discussed in Chapter I apply to the CPT codes in the range 40000-49999. Several general guidelines are repeated in this Chapter. However, those general guidelines from Chapter I not discussed in this chapter are nonetheless applicable.

Interpretation

This instruction directs that the overall NCCI guidelines apply to each section of the CPT codebook, and, even if they are not repeated within a chapter, they are nonetheless a guideline to be followed. The introductory guidelines were covered comprehensively in Chapter 2 of this book; those introductory guidelines that have a clear application within the digestive system are reiterated in this chapter.

Excerpt From the General Coding Policies Section of NCCI Guidelines[2(p6)]

Coding Based on Standards of Medical/Surgical Practice
    Specific examples of services that are not separately reportable because they are components of more comprehensive services follow:

Surgical:
Since a colectomy requires exposure of the colon, the laparotomy and adhesiolysis to expose the colon are not separately reportable.

Interpretation

NCCI guidelines provide a limited list of examples of the comprehensive/component code pairs. Although it is not a comprehensive list, there are some practical scenarios. Although most of the examples (see Chapter 2) are applicable to procedures performed within the digestive system, colectomies are specifically digestive procedures.

There are often adhesions blocking the surgeon's access for procedures. For an open colectomy (performed through a laparotomy) in which adhesions were blocking the surgeon's ability to access the colon, lysis of those adhesions is a likely part of the procedure. Remember that NCCI includes the "surgical approach including identification of anatomical landmarks, incision, evaluation of the surgical field, debridement of traumatized tissue, lysis of adhesions, and isolation of structures limiting access to the surgical field" (part of the standards of medical/surgical practice).

So, the laparotomy and lysis of adhesions are all part of the standard practice of performing a colectomy. However, if the lysis of adhesions was complicated, and the physician documents well the complexity or extensiveness of the lysis, there might be an opportunity to append a modifier 22 to the colectomy code.

Excerpt From the General Correct Coding Policies Section of NCCI Guidelines[2(10)]

> For endoscopic biopsies, multiple biopsies of a single or multiple lesions are reported with one unit of service of the biopsy code.

Interpretation

The CPT codes for endoscopic biopsies include multiple biopsy sites during a single endoscopic examination. Therefore, regardless of how many different polyps or sites are biopsied, code the biopsy only once. The CPT code description for these services clearly indicates that one code is used, regardless of the number of biopsies. Please see in the following example that the CPT code for a procto-sigmoidoscopy with biopsy includes multiple biopsies.

45305 Proctosigmoidoscopy, rigid; with biopsy, single or multiple

For example, during a proctosigmoidoscopy, if the physician takes multiple biopsy samples of the sigmoid colon, rectum, and descending colon, code 45305 should be reported because CPT code 45305 includes one or more biopsies in the description. Therefore, code 45305 is the only code necessary and only report it once.

Excerpt From the General Coding Policies Section of NCCI Guidelines[2(p10)]

> Exposure and exploration of the surgical field is integral to an operative procedure and is not separately reportable. For example, an exploratory laparotomy (CPT code 49000) is not separately reportable with an intra-abdominal procedure.

Interpretation

NCCI guidelines provide a limited list of examples of the comprehensive/component code pairs (see Chapter 2 of this book). Although it is not a comprehensive list, it does provide some practical scenarios. Keep in mind that NCCI includes the "surgical approach including identification of anatomical landmarks, incision, evaluation of the surgical field, debridement of traumatized tissue, lysis of adhesions, and isolation of structures limiting access to the surgical field ..." (part of the standards of medical/surgical practice). An exploratory laparotomy is an incision into the abdomen (laparotomy) and evaluation of the field (exploratory), which would be a standard part of performing open

abdominal procedures. Exploratory laparotomies should not be billed in addition to open abdominal procedures.

NCCI has not established an edit for every potential open abdominal procedure to bundle the CPT code for exploratory laparotomy (CPT code 49000). It is important to review and understand the guidelines to avoid unbundling the laparotomy from the primary surgery CPT code.

An open appendectomy includes the approach and access through the abdomen as well as the surgeon's evaluation of the surgical field. When an appendectomy is performed, do not code the laparotomy in addition to the appendectomy CPT code.

 CPT Coding Tip: *On occasion, trauma surgeons must perform an extensive laparotomy to determine the extent of a patient's injuries. Once the laparotomy is complete, the surgeon may perform other major procedures. In these cases, if the trauma surgeon (or other provider) documents the extensiveness of the laparotomy and how it impacted the overall surgery (eg, time involved, findings from exploration, decision making process), there is a potential opportunity for appending a modifier 22 (increased procedural service) to the primary procedure performed through the laparotomy incision.*

Endoscopic Services and NCCI Guidelines

Excerpt From the Digestive System Section of NCCI Guidelines[1(p4)]

> Services that are an integral component of an endoscopic procedure are not separately reportable. These services include, but are not limited to, venous access (e.g., CPT code 36000), infusion/injection (e.g., CPT codes 90760-90775), non-invasive oximetry (e.g., CPT codes 94760 and 94761), and anesthesia provided by the surgeon.

Note: Although the CMS NCCI guidelines still include references to CPT codes 90760 through 90775, those codes have been deleted and replaced with CPT codes 96360 through 96375.

Interpretation

NCCI instructs that all services *clinically* integral to the performance of a service (CPT code) should not be separately billed, regardless of whether a CPT code exists for the integral (included) service.

Although CMS provides examples (see the previous excerpt) of integral services, a digestive-system-specific example can be used to clarify this policy:

A patient presents for a colonoscopy, which is performed with the patient under conscious sedation provided by the physician performing the colonoscopy. The conscious sedation is introduced via intravenous access, and a heparin lock is inserted to maintain the catheter's patency. Additionally, the patient is monitored with oximetry. The colonoscopy is performed, as is a hot biopsy polypectomy.

Only the colonoscopy with hot biopsy (CPT code 45384) would be billed. The conscious sedation via intravenous access, heparin lock, and oximetry are all included services in the colonoscopy code. Note that CPT code 45384 includes moderate sedation when the sedation is administered by the operating provider. The symbol, ☉, is placed before this code in the CPT codebook. See Chapter 4 for additional information on conscious sedation.

> **Excerpt From the Digestive System Section of NCCI Guidelines[1(p4)]**
>
> Per *CPT Manual* instructions, surgical endoscopy includes diagnostic endoscopy. A diagnostic endoscopy HCPCS/CPT code should not be reported with a surgical endoscopy code.

Interpretation

Remember that we must follow CPT codebook instructions, and CPT guidelines state that all diagnostic endoscopies are incidental to the surgical endoscopy when they are performed during the same session and along the same anatomic pathway.

Before each endoscopic CPT code range, instructions that "Surgical endoscopy always includes diagnostic endoscopy," and, as long as the procedure is of a single endoscopic pathway, only the surgical service would be coded. Two different pathways (upper gastrointestinal (GI) tract accessed through an endoscope being placed through the mouth vs lower GI tract accessed through an endoscope placed through the anal canal) are coded separately.

The diagnostic endoscopy CPT codes are designated as *separate procedure* codes; therefore, they would not be coded in addition to other, more major procedures performed during the same surgical session on the same anatomic pathway. See Chapter 2 for further discussion on separate procedures.

So, to reinforce this guideline with an example, take a diagnostic esophagogastroduodenoscopy (EGD) and a therapeutic colonoscopy that are performed during the same encounter.

These two services are different anatomic pathways— one is for the upper GI tract, and the other is for the lower GI tract. Because they are of different anatomic pathways, both may be coded. According to NCCI edits, the EGD and colonoscopy do not bundle together, which makes sense because they are clearly separate anatomic sites. Therefore, a modifier to bypass these edits should not be necessary.

Another example would be when a diagnostic EGD is performed, followed by a hot biopsy removal of a polyp on the lower esophagus.

According to NCCI guidelines and CPT codebook instruction, only the hot biopsy removal code would be billed, and the diagnostic study is included in the removal code.

> **Excerpt From the Digestive System Section of NCCI Guidelines[1(p4)]**
>
> If multiple endoscopic services are performed, the most comprehensive code describing the service(s) rendered should be reported. If multiple services are performed and not adequately described by a single HCPCS/CPT code, more than one code may be reported. The multiple procedure modifier -51 should be appended to the secondary HCPCS/CPT code. Only medically necessary services may be reported. Incidental examination of other areas should not be reported separately.

Interpretation

There are many different principles within this guideline.

1. Do not code component CPT codes if there is a comprehensive code that includes all the components.
2. If there is no comprehensive code, the component codes may be used. Modifier 51 may be necessary on the lesser procedures.
3. Whenever multiple codes are billed, each service must be medically necessary.
4. Incidental examinations of other areas are included in the primary services bill. *Incidental* here means that the examination requires an insignificant amount of additional work.

For example, if a patient presents for a colonoscopy and the physician performs a diagnostic colonoscopy and discovers multiple polyps. One polyp is removed via hot biopsy, and all others are removed via a snare technique.

Given that there is no comprehensive code including both the hot biopsy and snare removal services, two codes are required (CPT codes 45384 and 45385).

45384 Colonoscopy, flexible, proximal to splenic flexure; with removal of tumor(s), polyp(s), or other lesion(s) by hot biopsy forceps or bipolar cautery

⊙ **45385** Colonoscopy, flexible, proximal to splenic flexure; with removal of tumor(s), polyp(s), or other lesion(s) by snare technique

Modifier 59 would be needed on one of the codes to inform the payer that the removals were of distinct polyps.

Another example would be if during a complete colonoscopy, the physician also examines the rectum and sigmoid areas of the large intestine.

Those examinations are incidental to the colonoscopy. See this excerpt from the CPT codebook as to what a proctosigmoidoscopy, sigmoidoscopy, and colonoscopy include. Note that the colonoscopy comprises examination of the entire colon, including the rectum and sigmoid colon.

Excerpt From the CPT Codebook Discussing Endoscopy[3(p207)]

Endoscopy (45300-45392)
Definitions
Proctosigmoidoscopy is the examination of the rectum and sigmoid colon.

Sigmoidoscopy is the examination of the entire rectum, sigmoid colon and may include examination of a portion of the descending colon.

Colonoscopy is the examination of the entire colon, from the rectum to the cecum, and may include the examination of the terminal ileum.

45303 Proctosigmoidoscopy, rigid; with dilation (eg, balloon, guide wire, bougie)

45378 Colonoscopy, flexible, proximal to splenic flexure; diagnostic, with or without collection of specimen(s) by brushing or washing, with or without colon decompression (separate procedure)

The CPT code for the colonoscopy would include both a proctosigmoidoscopy and a sigmoidoscopy, because they are all along the same pathway (lower GI tract).

Excerpt From the Digestive System Section of NCCI Guidelines[1(4)]

If the same endoscopic procedure (e.g., polypectomy) is performed multiple times at a single patient encounter in the same region as defined by the *CPT Manual* narrative, only one CPT code may be reported with one unit of service.

Interpretation

The CPT codes for endoscopic procedures are "per endoscopy per procedure methodology," meaning that if a single endoscopy (eg, colonoscopy) is performed, and one type of procedure (eg, hot biopsy) is performed multiple times during the single endoscopy, the procedure is coded only once. However, if, during a single endoscopy, different procedure methodologies were performed at distinct sites, each method could be coded. See Table 10-1 for a quick check of how to code digestive system endoscopies.

As long as there are different procedures and distinct sites, multiple services may be coded.

As an example, if during an EGD, the physician performs multiple snare polypectomies along the entire route of the EGD, CPT code 43251 would be coded one time, as the description includes multiple polypectomies.

However, if during an EGD, the physician performs snare polypectomies of three distinct polyps and also performs a biopsy of a different site, then both a snare polypectomy and biopsy code may be billed, because distinct sites and different methods were involved. CPT codes 43251 and 43239 would also be coded.

⊙ **43239** Upper gastrointestinal endoscopy including esophagus, stomach, and either the duodenum and/or jejunum as appropriate; with biopsy, single or multiple

⊙ **43251** Upper gastrointestinal endoscopy including esophagus, stomach, and either the duodenum and/or jejunum as appropriate; with removal of tumor(s), polyp(s), or other lesion(s) by snare technique

CPT code 43239 bundles into CPT code 43251, according to NCCI edits. These bundle because biopsy services bundle into excisions when they are performed on the same polyp. Because the biopsy in this circumstance was on a different polyp, modifier 59 would be appropriately appended to CPT code 43239.

TABLE 10-1 *Multiple Endoscopy Coding*

Example Scenario	How to Code	Why
One polyp treated with one method	One CPT code	There is only one procedure performed.
One polyp treated with two methods	One CPT code	There was only one site involved. This should be coded by the most extensive procedure only.
Two polyps treated with one method	One CPT code	There was only one method involved and the digestive endoscopy codes include one or more sites within a single code's description.
Two polyps each treated with different methods	Two CPT codes	There were two sites and two methods, both are coded.

Excerpt From the Digestive System Section of NCCI Guidelines[1(p5)]

Gastroenterologic tests included in CPT code range 91000-91299 are frequently complementary to endoscopic procedures. Esophageal and gastric washings for cytology when performed are integral components of an upper gastrointestinal endoscopy (CPT code 43235). Therefore, CPT codes 91000 (esophageal intubation and collection of washings for cytology ...) and 91055 (gastric intubation, washings, and preparing slides for cytology ...) should not be separately reported when performed as part of an upper gastrointestinal endoscopic procedure. Provocative testing (CPT code 91052) may be expedited during gastrointestinal endoscopy (e.g., procurement of gastric specimens). When performed concurrent with an upper gastrointestinal endoscopy, CPT code 91052 should be coded with modifier -52 indicating a reduced level of service was performed.

Interpretation

43235 Upper gastrointestinal endoscopy including esophagus, stomach, and either the duodenum and/or jejunum as appropriate; diagnostic, with or without collection of specimen(s) by brushing or washing (separate procedure)

91000 Esophageal intubation and collection of washings for cytology, including preparation of specimens (separate procedure)

91052 Gastric analysis test with injection of stimulant of gastric secretion (eg, histamine, insulin, pentagastrin, calcium and secretin)

91055 Gastric intubation, washings, and preparing slides for cytology (separate procedure)

Because CPT code 43235 includes specimen collection by brushing or washing (see previous), it would be duplicating the specimen collection portion of the procedure to add a code for collection of washings by using either CPT code 91000 or 91055.

CPT codes 91000 and 91055 are also designated as separate procedures and are bundled into any other related, more major procedure performed during the same patient encounter. CPT code 91052 (gastric analysis) is not designated as a separate procedure code, but the NCCI guidelines ask that a modifier 52 (reduced service) be appended to this code when the service is performed in conjunction with an upper endoscopy. Because the specimen collection is an inherent part of both the endoscopy and the gastric analysis, not reducing the code with modifier 52 would be double coding the specimen collection.

It would be difficult to know to use modifier 52 if the NCCI guidelines were not read, as there is no NCCI edit of CPT code 91052 when that code is billed with CPT code 43235. It is crucial to review and understand the guidelines to ensure proper coding of services.

Table 10-2 shows the NCCI edits for an EGD. Note that both CPT codes 91000 and 91055 bundle into CPT code 43235 (EGD) and do not allow a modifier to bypass the edit.

Excerpt From the Digestive System Section of NCCI Guidelines[1(p5)]

If an endoscopy or enteroscopy is performed as a common standard of practice when performing another service, the endoscopy or enteroscopy is not separately reportable. For example, if a small intestinal endoscopy or enteroscopy is performed during the creation or revision of an enterostomy, the small intestinal endoscopy or enteroscopy is not separately reportable.

TABLE 10-2 NCCI Edits for EGD With Esophageal and Gastric Intubation

Column 1	Column 2	Modifier 0 = not allowed 1 = allowed 9 = not applicable
43235	90772	1
43235	90774	1
43235	90775	1
43235	90780	1
43235	90781	1
43235	90782	0
43235	90783	0
43235	90784	0
43235	91000	0
43235	91055	0
43235	91105	1
43235	92511	0
43235	93000	1
43235	93005	1

Interpretation

This is a tough one, because this coding requires knowing the standard of practice, which coders are not often privy to. A few thoughts to make this easier:

1. For nonclinical coders, meet with the provider(s) of the services and ask whether there are any documented standards for the most commonly performed procedures within the practice.

2. Inquire through the specialty societies to determine whether they have any published standards.

3. Read the operative reports carefully and remember all the NCCI guidelines, especially those in Chapter 2 (the general guidelines):

   a. Services integral to other services are not separately reportable. If the operative report reads as if the endoscopy is a standard part of the primary surgery, ask the surgeon what the normal practice would be for the surgery. Research the surgery.

   b. Remember, NCCI guidelines state that only one approach to perform a procedure should be coded (reread Chapter 2). If the endoscopy seems to be for visualization of the surgery site, do not code the endoscopy.

   c. If the endoscopy is for a diagnostic purpose prior to performing an open or percutaneous procedure, the endoscopy is likely to be coded.

   d. If the endoscopy is for a distinct and separate therapeutic reason, the endoscopy is likely to be appropriately coded.

A "scout" endoscopy to assess anatomic landmarks or assess extent of disease preceding another surgical procedure at the same patient encounter is not separately reportable. However, an endoscopic procedure for diagnostic purposes to decide whether a more extensive open procedure needs to be performed is separately reportable. In the latter situation, modifier -58 may be utilized to indicate that the diagnostic endoscopy and more extensive open procedure were staged procedures.

Interpretation

NCCI guidelines include identification of landmarks as a part of the surgical approach (as noted in the standards of medical/surgical practice). A scout scope procedure is for landmark identification (looking at the lay of the land) and not for diagnosing or treating. Scout scope procedures are complementary components of the primary procedure. CMS distinguishes a scout scope procedure from a *diagnostic* scope procedure, which is an important principle in NCCI. If a truly diagnostic scope procedure is necessary before an open therapeutic procedure, the diagnostic scope procedure may be separately coded, as long as the scope procedure is truly diagnostic (the decision for the therapeutic open procedure is made based on the findings of the scope procedure). The physician's documentation must be very clear that the service is supported as diagnostic. The scope procedure is not separately coded if the physician:

- knows prior to the scope procedure that therapeutic open procedure is going to be performed or has already performed a diagnostic scope procedure or goes on to perform a therapeutic scope procedure.

NCCI edits state that when the *diagnostic* scope procedure is performed prior to an open procedure, both procedures may be coded, and modifier 58 (staged procedure) should be appended. If an endoscopic procedure that precedes an open procedure is truly diagnostic, the diagnostic endoscopy may be coded in addition to the open procedure. The documentation within the record is critical here, because it must clearly support that the endoscopy was diagnostic and not merely for land-marking the surgical site.

For instance, an EGD is performed to diagnose the cause of a patient's dysphagia. The physician discovers that the patient had achalasia. He proceeds to perform an esophagomyotomy via an open technique.

In this case, both the diagnostic endoscopy (EGD) and the therapeutic open procedure (esophagomyotomy) may be billed, and modifier 58 should be appended to indicate the staged service.

CPT Coding Tip: When coding, see if the preoperative diagnosis differs from the postoperative diagnosis, as this could be an indication of whether the endoscopy is truly diagnostic. If there is a symptom or a rule-out diagnosis preoperatively, that helps support the endoscopy as being diagnostic.

There should always be a procedure indications section at the beginning of the operative note. This too can help clarify whether the endoscopy was diagnostic or not.

Physicians should clearly document whether the endoscopy was diagnostic or not.

Excerpt From the Digestive System Section of NCCI Guidelines[1](p5)

If esophageal dilation as described by CPT codes 43450-43458 is unsuccessful and followed by an endoscopic esophageal dilation procedure, only the endoscopic esophageal dilation procedure may be reported. The physician should not report the unsuccessful procedure.

Interpretation

NCCI guidelines (see Chapter 2 of this book) state that "if a procedure utilizing one approach fails and is converted to a procedure utilizing a different approach, only the successful procedure may be reported." When planning surgical procedures, physicians want to use the least invasive and most effective approach. On occasion, the planned approach is insufficient to the overall success of the procedure, and the surgeon must convert to a different approach during the procedure. Failed approaches, or approaches that are converted to different approaches, are incidental to successful approaches, and only the successfully approach procedure should be coded.

Excerpt From the Digestive System Section of NCCI Guidelines[1](p6)

Intubation of the gastrointestinal tract (e.g., percutaneous placement of G-tube) includes subsequent removal of the tube. CPT codes such as 43247 (upper gastrointestinal endoscopic removal of foreign body) should not be reported for routine removal of previously placed therapeutic devices.

Interpretation

Often, the removal is not performed on the same date as the insertion, so this policy could also be seen to address more global surgery rather than bundling issues; however, it is worth noting that the CPT codebook states that CPT code 43247 should not be coded when the procedure to remove the percutaneous endoscopic gastrostomy (PEG) tube is performed by the same physician and is simply part of the follow-up to the placement of the tube. However, if removal of the tube is necessary because of a problem the patient is having with the tube, this code may be used.

For example, a patient who is undergoing radiation therapy has a PEG tube placed for feeding, and at the conclusion of treatment, the PEG is removed. In this case, the removal is a standard part of the insertion and should not be coded.

On the other hand, a patient who is undergoing dysphagia treatment and has a PEG tube placed; two weeks later, an infection started in the tube, and the physician has to remove the tube in the GI suite. In this case, the removal may be coded.

Excerpt From the Digestive System Section of NCCI Guidelines[1](p13)

A biopsy performed at the time of another more extensive procedure (eg, excision, destruction, removal) is separately reportable under specific circumstances.

If the biopsy is performed on a separate lesion, it is separately reportable.

Interpretation

If a biopsy of a site was obtained and a more extensive procedure was performed on a separate site, both services may be coded. A modifier 59 may be needed, depending on the situation. Two different anatomic locations must be involved to allow billing for both services. Therefore, if a patient presents for a biopsy of the liver and a hemorrhoidectomy. These are two distinct anatomical sites, and both services may be coded. However, if a patient presents for a colonoscopy, and the provider performs biopsies of several polyps and a snare excision of a biopsied polyp, only the most extensive procedure for that anatomic site, the snare procedure (CPT code 45385), may be coded, but the biopsy of that site could not be coded. However, because there were other polyps that were biopsied without being excised, those biopsies (CPT code 45380) may be reported in addition to the snare polypectomy. These would be reported:

⊙ **45380**   Colonoscopy, flexible, proximal to splenic flexure; with biopsy, single or multiple

⊙ **45385**   Colonoscopy, flexible, proximal to splenic flexure; with removal of tumor(s), polyp(s), or other lesion(s) by snare technique

A modifier 59 must be appended to the biopsy code because it bundles into the polypectomy code.

Excerpt From the Digestive System Section of NCCI Guidelines[1(p13)]

If a biopsy is performed on the same lesion on which the more extensive procedure is performed, it is separately reportable only if the biopsy is utilized for immediate pathologic diagnosis prior to the more extensive procedure, and the decision to proceed with the more extensive procedure is based on the result of the pathologic examination. Modifier -58 may be reported to indicate that the biopsy and the more extensive procedure were planned or staged procedures.

Interpretation

As discussed in Chapter 5 of this book, notice that the decision for the more major procedure is based, at least in part, on the results of the biopsy. In this scenario, the biopsy is clearly a diagnostic service driving the decision for the therapeutic service. Modifier 58 (staged or related procedure) is appended to the second, more extensive procedure, rather than modifier 59. To review an example, take a patient who presents for a biopsy of a liver mass. During the biopsy procedure, the tissue sample is sent for frozen section, and the surgeon awaits the pathology results. The results indicate a diagnosis that results in the physician deciding to perform a partial lobectomy, which was performed during the same surgical setting.

Appropriate coding would be to code the biopsy and the lobectomy with a modifier 58 appended to the lobectomy code.

Explanation: The biopsy was truly an independent diagnostic step in the procedure and drove the treatment decision. Therefore, both services may be coded. Remember to use modifier 58, not modifier 59.

CPT Coding Tip: *Code biopsies in addition to more extensive procedures only when the biopsy was done:*
- *to establish the need for a more extensive service or*
- *on a different anatomic site or*
- *during a separate operative session.*

Excerpt From the Digestive System Section of NCCI Guidelines[1(p6)]

Control of bleeding is an integral component of endoscopic procedures and is not separately reportable. If it is necessary to repeat an endoscopy to control bleeding at a separate patient encounter on the same date of service, the HCPCS/CPT code for endoscopy for control of bleeding is separately reportable with modifier -78 indicating that the procedure required return to the operating room (or endoscopy suite) for a related procedure during the postoperative period.

Interpretation

Bear in mind that postoperative complications are not coded in addition to the surgery unless they require a return to the operating room. Also, if a physician must control bleeding of the surgical site (internal or external) in concert with the procedure, no additional code should be added to the primary procedure, as control of bleeding is included in the global package of the main surgery. This is true regardless of whether the procedure is endoscopic or nonendoscopic (see general guidelines). If the control of bleeding was performed during a separate surgical encounter in which the patient had to be returned to the operating room or the endoscopy suite, the service may be coded with a modifier 78.

There are endoscopy codes for control of bleeding:

45382   Colonoscopy, flexible, proximal to splenic flexure; with control of bleeding (eg, injection, bipolar cautery, unipolar cautery, laser, heater probe, stapler, plasma coagulator)

This would be coded when the primary purpose of the procedure was to control bleeding. If a polypectomy was performed, and bleeding from the wound site resulted, no code is used because control of bleeding would be a usual part of the polypectomy. So, the guidelines for coding of the control of bleeding would be:
- If the control of bleeding is the primary reason for the procedure, code it.
- If the control of bleeding is to cauterize a site at which another procedure was performed, do not code the bleeding control, as it becomes a part of reimbursement for the first procedure.

> **Excerpt From the Digestive System Section of NCCI Guidelines[1(p6)]**
>
> If an endoscopic procedure fails and is converted into an open procedure at the same patient encounter, only the open procedure is reportable.

Interpretation

As mentioned in prior chapters of this book, when planning procedures, physicians want to use the least invasive and most effective approach. On occasion, the planned approach is insufficient to the overall success of the procedure, and the surgeon must convert to a different approach during the procedure. Failed approaches, or approaches that are converted to different approaches, are incidental to successful approaches, and only the successfully approached procedure should be coded.

For example, a patient presents for a cholecystectomy, and the physician attempts to perform the procedure laparoscopically but cannot complete the procedure successfully through the laparoscope. The physician converts the procedure to an open cholecystectomy and completes the procedure effectively.

Only the successful procedure may be coded: the open cholecystectomy.

> **Excerpt From the Digestive System Section of NCCI Guidelines[1(p6)]**
>
> If a transabdominal colonoscopy via colostomy (CPT code 45355) and/or standard sigmoidoscopy or colonoscopy is performed as a necessary part of an open procedure (e.g., colectomy), the endoscopic procedure(s) is (are) not separately reportable. However, if either endoscopic procedure is performed as a diagnostic procedure upon which the decision to perform the open procedure is made, the endoscopic procedure may be reported separately. Modifier -58 may be utilized to indicate that the diagnostic endoscopy and the open procedure were staged or planned services.

Interpretation

As a standard policy within NCCI, services that are a necessary component to another procedure are not coded independently from the primary procedure for which they are performed. If the physician had to perform the component in order to successfully accomplish the comprehensive service, that component should not be separated from the comprehensive service in coding. If the endoscopic procedure served as a separate diagnostic study (see prior discussion within this chapter), both services may be coded, with a modifier 58 appended to the second procedure. Take, for example, a physician who plans to do a partial open colectomy but needs to isolate the area of disease more concretely, the physician may perform a colonoscopy in conjunction with the colectomy.

The colonoscopy is not diagnostic but rather an incidental component to the colectomy. The colonoscopy would not be coded separately.

> **Excerpt From the Digestive System Section of NCCI Guidelines[1(p6-7)]**
>
> If the larynx is viewed through an esophagoscope or upper gastrointestinal endoscope during endoscopy, a laryngoscopy CPT code cannot be reported separately. However, if a medically necessary laryngoscopy is performed with a separate laryngoscope, both the laryngoscopy and esophagoscopy (or upper gastrointestinal endoscopy) CPT codes may be reported with NCCI-associated modifiers.

Interpretation

Often a laryngoscopy can be performed during an upper GI endoscopic examination without adding significant work to the procedure. When the laryngoscopy is incidental to the upper GI endoscopy, it should not be coded separately. In order to code a laryngoscopy in addition to an upper GI endoscopy, the documentation must support that the laryngoscopy was performed through a separate endoscope.

Table 10-3 shows an example from the NCCI edits for an esophagoscopy and laryngoscopy. The diagnostic laryngoscopy codes bundle into the esophagoscopy codes. Please note that the indirect (CPT code 31505) and flexible fiberoptic (CPT code 31575) laryngoscopies may not be coded in addition to the upper GI endoscopy (CPT codes 43200, 43235, etc). Only the direct (CPT code 31525) laryngoscopy bundling edit may be bypassed with modifier 59.

TABLE 10-3 *Example From NCCI Edits Regarding Esophagoscopies and Laryngoscopies*

Column 1	Column 2	Modifier 0 = not allowed 1 = allowed 9 = not applicable
43200	00740	0
43200	00810	0
43200	31505	0
43200	31525	1
43200	31575	0
43200	36000	1
43200	36005	1
43200	36010	1
43200	36011	1

> Please note that the indirect (CPT code 31505) and flexible fiberoptic (CPT code 31575) laryngoscopies may not be coded in addition to the upper GI endoscopy (CPT codes 43200, 43235, etc.). Only the direct (CPT code 31525) laryngoscopy bundling edit may be bypassed with modifier 59.

Abdominal Procedures (49000-49801) and NCCI Guidelines

Excerpt From the Digestive System Section of NCCI Guidelines[1(p7)]

Hepatectomy procedures (e.g., CPT codes 47120-47130, 47133-47142) include removal of the gallbladder based on anatomic considerations and standards of practice. A cholecystectomy CPT code is not separately reportable with a hepatectomy CPT code.

Interpretation

When the liver is resected, the gallbladder is usually removed (especially if the resection is on the right side of the liver). Therefore, as the procedure is standard practice, the gallbladder removal (cholecystectomy) would not be coded separately. NCCI edits bundle the gallbladder removal in with the liver resection codes. The edit may not be bypassed with a modifier. These surgeries would not be performed in separate sessions on the same day. If the liver or a portion of the liver was removed, and the gallbladder was also removed, do not code the cholecystectomy.

Excerpt From the Digestive System Section of NCCI Guidelines[1(p7)]

A medically necessary appendectomy may be reported separately. However, an incidental appendectomy of a normal appendix during another abdominal procedure is not separately reportable.

Interpretation

Appendectomies are often performed during other abdominal procedures. Do not code the appendectomy when it is performed during other abdominal procedures, unless there is disease present creating the independent need for removal of the appendix. This is an NCCI and CPT codebook guideline. The CPT codes were established to use when appendectomies are appropriately coded in addition to other abdominal surgeries. See the description of CPT code 44955, which follows.

44950   Appendectomy;

+ 44955   when done for indicated purpose at time of other major procedure (not as separate procedure) (List separately in addition to code for primary procedure)

44960   for ruptured appendix with abscess or generalized peritonitis

Therefore, for a patient who has a planned partial colectomy during which the surgeon also removes the appendix, the appendectomy should not be coded in addition to the colectomy. However, if a patient has an emergency colectomy during which the surgeon notes that the appendix is inflamed and infected and proceeds to remove the appendix as well, the appendectomy may be coded with CPT code 44955 because there is a therapeutic reason for performing both procedures.

Excerpt From the Digestive System Section of NCCI Guidelines[1(p7)]

If a hernia repair is performed at the site of an incision for an open abdominal procedure, the hernia repair (CPT codes 49560-49566) is not separately reportable. The hernia repair is separately reportable if it is performed at a site other than the incision and is medically reasonable and necessary. An incidental hernia repair is not medically reasonable and necessary and should not be reported separately.

Interpretation

Hernia repairs at the site of an incision for an abdominal procedure are not coded in addition to the open abdominal procedure. The hernia repair becomes incidental to the open abdominal surgery. Recall from Chapter 2 of this book that "if a definitive surgical procedure requires access through diseased tissue, a separate service for this access is not separately reportable."

Even though the hernia was repaired, the procedure was not separately distinguishable from the access for the major procedure.

Excerpt From the Digestive System Section of NCCI Guidelines[1(p7)]

If a recurrent hernia requires repair, a recurrent hernia repair code may be reported. A code for incisional hernia repair should not be reported in addition to the recurrent hernia repair code unless a medically necessary incisional hernia repair is performed at a different site.

Interpretation

Recurrent hernia: a hernia at the site of a previous hernia repair.

Incisional hernia: a hernia in the area of an old abdominal scar.

Many times these hernias (incisional and recurrent) are defined as one in the same, but they are not the same for CPT coding. Incisional means there was another

non-hernia surgery performed at the site where a current hernia exists, and the incision of the prior surgery is the site of the current hernia. A recurrent hernia distinguishes that the hernia is at the site of a prior hernia repair. If the hernia being repaired is a recurrent hernia, use the appropriate recurrent hernia repair CPT code. If the hernia repaired is an incisional hernia, use the incisional hernia codes.

Excerpt From the Digestive System Section of NCCI Guidelines[1(p7-8)]

Removal of excessive skin and subcutaneous tissue (panniculectomy) at the site of an abdominal incision for an open procedure including hernia repair is not separately reportable. CPT code 15830 should not be reported for this type of panniculectomy. However, an abdominoplasty which requires significantly more work than a panniculectomy is separately reportable.

A panniculectomy is the removal of skin only, whereas an abdominoplasty involves the muscles as well. If a panniculectomy is performed at the same time as an open abdominal procedure (NCCI points out hernia repairs), the panniculectomy is incidental to the more major procedure and should not be coded separately. If the more extensive procedure of an abdominoplasty is performed with another open abdominal procedure, the abdominoplasty may be coded in addition to the other abdominal procedure.

The trick here is in the coding: Abdomenoplasties are coded with CPT code 15830 (panniculectomy) and CPT code 15847 (add-on code for abdominoplasty). There is not one code that encompasses all components of an abdominoplasty surgery. Therefore, in order to bill the abdominoplasty in addition to the hernia repair, use CPT code 15830-59 (to bypass the bundling edit) and CPT code 15847 in addition to the hernia repair CPT codes.

Excerpt From the Digestive System Section of NCCI Guidelines[1(p8)]

CPT code 49568 is an add-on code describing implantation of mesh or other prosthesis for incisional or ventral hernia repair. This code may be reported with incisional or ventral hernia repair CPT codes 49560-49566. Although mesh or other prosthesis may be implanted with other types of hernia repairs, CPT code 49568 should not be reported with these other hernia repair codes.

Interpretation

CPT codebook guidelines as well as this NCCI policy indicate that the mesh insertions, when performed with hernia repairs, may be coded in addition to the hernia repair only for incisional or ventral hernias. Do not code the mesh insertion when it is performed for any other type of hernia. If there are multiple hernias being repaired and one is an incisional or ventral hernia with mesh insertion and the other hernias are nonincisional or nonventral, all hernia repairs may be coded as well as the mesh insertion, with a modifier 59 appended to the mesh insertion code.

So, take a physician performing an incisional hernia repair (open approach) who uses mesh for the repair. In this scenario, the mesh code may be added to the incisional hernia repair code. However, for a physician who performs an umbilical hernia repair (open approach) and uses mesh for the repair, the mesh code should not be added to the umbilical hernia repair code.

 CPT Coding Tip: In CPT 2009[3], additional laparoscopic hernia repair codes were added, and the mesh insertion is incidental to all laparoscopic hernia repairs. Do not add a code for mesh insertion when the procedure is performed with laparoscopic repairs.

Excerpt From the Digestive System Section of NCCI Guidelines[1(p8)]

Open enterolysis (CPT code 44005) and laparoscopic enterolysis (CPT code 44200) are defined by the *CPT Manual* as "separate procedures." They are not separately reportable with other intra-abdominal or pelvic procedures. However, if a provider performs an extensive and time-consuming enterolysis in conjunction with another intra-abdominal or pelvic procedure, the provider may append modifier -22 to the CPT code describing the latter procedure. The local carrier will determine whether additional payment is appropriate.

Interpretation

In prior chapters we have discussed that lysis of adhesions is a component of the surgical approach (gaining access to the site of the surgery) and should not be coded separately. The CPT codes for this lysis are designated as separate procedures, meaning they are incidental to other procedures performed during the same session at the same anatomic location. This guideline further explains that if the surgeon had to lyse extensive adhesions and documents how the procedure was more difficult, took more time, or otherwise increased the effort for the surgery, a modifier 22 may be appended to address the extensive lysis of adhesions. See the earlier explanation of modifier 22 in this chapter. To illustrate this point, consider a physician performing an open gastrectomy procedure and on incising the abdomen discovers dense adhesions. The surgeon documents that an additional 45 minutes were required in a usual 1-hour operation because of the need to lyse the adhesions. In this case, a modifier 22 is most likely supported for the lysis of adhesions.

Excerpt From the Digestive System Section of NCCI Guidelines[1(p8)]

Per *CPT Manual* instructions, a diagnostic laparoscopy (CPT code 49320) is not separately reportable with a surgical laparoscopy.

Interpretation

This is a reminder that we must follow CPT codebook instructions, and CPT guidelines state that all diagnostic laparoscopies are incidental to the surgical laparoscopies when performed during the same session. Before each endoscopic CPT code range, instruction that "Surgical laparoscopy always includes diagnostic laparoscopy." Also, the diagnostic laparoscopy CPT codes (see CPT code 49320) are designated as separate procedure codes; therefore, they would not be coded in addition to other, more major procedures performed during the same surgical session through the same approach.

Other General Thoughts From NCCI Guidelines Regarding the Digestive System

Excerpt From the Digestive System Section of NCCI Guidelines[1(p10)]

The vagotomy CPT codes 43635-43641 and 64752-64760 are not separately reportable with esophageal or gastric procedures that include vagotomy as part of the service. For example, the esophagogastrostomy procedure described by CPT code 43320 includes a vagotomy if performed. The vagotomy procedures are mutually exclusive, and only one vagotomy procedure code may be reported at a patient encounter.

Interpretation

A vagotomy is the cutting of the vagus nerve to reduce acid secretion in the stomach. The vagotomy is commonly performed in conjunction with other procedures. If a CPT code description includes vagotomy, a separate vagotomy code should not be billed. If the vagotomy is performed to assist in the work of another procedure and not for a separate and distinct service, do not code the vagotomy.

Excerpt From the Digestive System Section of NCCI Guidelines[1(p10)]

If closure of an enterostomy or fistula involving the intestine requires resection and anastomosis of a segment of intestine, the resection and anastomosis of the intestine are not separately reportable.

Interpretation

44620 Closure of enterostomy, large or small intestine;

44625   with resection and anastomosis other than colorectal

44626   with resection and colorectal anastomosis (eg, closure of Hartmann type procedure)

Throughout the NCCI edits we are reminded that when any services that are integral or incidental to another procedure are performed, the incidental procedure should not be coded in addition to the other procedure. This guideline is no different. If resection and anastomosis are necessary in order to close an enterostomy or fistula, choose the CPT code that includes these services (either CPT code 44625 or 44626), rather than coding the resection and anastomosis separately.

 CMS Tip: *The resection with anastomosis (CPT code 44120) bundles into the enterostomy closure (see the following) but allows bypassing of the edit. That would be appropriate only if the resection was of a distinct (nonadjacent site) or perhaps rarely in a separate operative session. See Table 10-4 for the NCCI edits.*

1. CPT code 44625 is the code for the enterostomy closure.
2. CPT code 44120 is the code for the resection and anastomosis that is bundled into the enterostomy code.
3. NCCI edits allow the bundling of this code to be bypassed with modifier 59 *only* if the documentation supports that a separate and distinct site/session was involved.

TABLE 10-4 *Anastomosis and Enterostomy Bundling Edits*

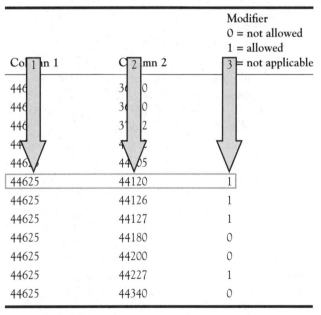

Column 1	Column 2	Modifier 0 = not allowed 1 = allowed 3 = not applicable
446__	36__0	
446__	36__0	
446__	3__2	
44__	4__	
446__	44_05	
44625	44120	1
44625	44126	1
44625	44127	1
44625	44180	0
44625	44200	0
44625	44227	1
44625	44340	0

Excerpt From the Digestive System Section of NCCI Guidelines[1(p10)]

If multiple services are utilized to treat hemorrhoids at the same patient encounter, only one HCPCS/CPT code describing the most extensive procedure may be reported. If an abscess is drained during the treatment of hemorrhoids, the incision and drainage is not separately reportable unless the incision and drainage is at a separate site unrelated to the hemorrhoids. In the latter case, the incision and drainage code may be reported appending an anatomic modifier or modifier -59.

Interpretation

Only one code for hemorrhoidectomy is reported; the most extensive procedure necessary to successfully accomplish the hemorrhoidectomy would be appropriate. In addition, any incidental drainage of an abscess at the same site would be included in the hemorrhoidectomy code and not separately reported.

Excerpt From the Digestive System Section of NCCI Guidelines[1(p10)]

The *CPT Manual* contains groups of codes describing different approaches or methods to accomplish similar results. These codes are generally mutually exclusive of one another. For example, CPT codes 45110-45123 describe different proctectomy procedures and are mutually exclusive of one another. Other examples include groups of codes for colectomies (CPT codes 44140-44160), gastrectomies (CPT codes 43620-43635), and pancreatectomies (CPT codes 48140-48155).

Interpretation

Part one of this guideline addresses when a surgeon utilizes multiple approaches in the surgery. As mentioned earlier in this chapter as well as in Chapter 2, surgical approaches are incidental to the primary procedure and not separately reportable; therefore, never add a code for an approach. There are certain surgeries that may be performed through a variety of approaches (colectomies, cholecystectomies) unless the CPT codebook directs differently. Because approaches are incidental to the procedure, using additional CPT codes based solely on multiple approaches

would be overcoding the surgery. Therefore, if two approaches are used to accomplish a single procedure, both approaches are still incidental to the primary procedure.

Within the digestive system, when multiple approaches are used it usually signifies that one approach was unsuccessful and was converted to a different approach. Part two of this guideline addresses cases in which the surgeon incorporates multiple methods of completing procedures.

NCCI policies remind us that the CPT codebook often describes groups of similar codes differing in the complexity of the service. Unless services are performed at separate patient encounters or at separate anatomic sites, the less complex service is included in the more complex service and is not separately reportable. Only the most complex procedure performed during a single encounter on a single anatomic site may be coded. The lesser services are incidental to the more complex procedure. This guideline is consistent with the other guidelines within NCCI, for example, failed procedures are incidental to successful procedures when performed during the same surgical session. To reiterate this point, the following are the CPT codes for the various types of pancreatectomy procedures. Only one of these procedures could be coded during a single surgical session. The choice of code is dependent on:

1. total versus subtotal excision,
2. area of resection (if subtotal), and
3. associated procedures.

48140 Pancreatectomy, distal subtotal, with or without splenectomy; without pancreaticojejunostomy

48145   with pancreaticojejunostomy

48146 Pancreatectomy, distal, near-total with preservation of duodenum (Child-type procedure)

48148 Excision of ampulla of Vater

48150 Pancreatectomy, proximal subtotal with total duodenectomy, partial gastrectomy, choledochoenterostomy and gastrojejunostomy (Whipple-type procedure); with pancreatojejunostomy

48152   without pancreatojejunostomy

48153 Pancreatectomy, proximal subtotal with near-total duodenectomy, choledochoenterostomy and duodenojejunostomy (pylorus-sparing, Whipple-type procedure); with pancreatojejunostomy

48154   without pancreatojejunostomy

48155 Pancreatectomy, total

Excerpt From the Digestive System Section of NCCI Guidelines[1(p10)]

If an excised section of intestine includes a fistula tract, a fistula closure code should not be reported separately. Closure of the fistula is included in the excision of intestine.

Interpretation

If a diseased site is repaired as a part of a more major procedure, the repair becomes incidental to the more major procedure, as it does not add significant effort on the part of the surgeon. This is a bit different than the earlier guideline stating that closure of an enterostomy or fistula includes the resection. The coding of fistula closure versus resection should be driven by the root operation the surgeon is pursuing. So, if the fistula is the primary concern, code the fistula closure. If the resection is the point of the procedure, code the resection. An example of this would be, if a section of intestine is removed due to disease, and within the excised area, a fistula is connected to another organ. The intestinal excision incorporates the fistula repair as a part of the overall procedure. And, the repair of the fistula is incidental to the entire section that is excised. It does not require substantial additional effort.

Excerpt From the Digestive System Section of NCCI Guidelines[1(p11)]

The mouth and anus have mucocutaneous margins. Numerous procedures (e.g., biopsy, destruction, excision) have CPT codes that describe the procedure as an integumentary procedure (CPT codes 10000-19999) or as a digestive system procedure (CPT codes 40000-49999). If a procedure is performed on a lesion at or near a mucocutaneous margin, only one CPT code which best describes the procedure may be reported. If the code descriptor of a CPT code from the digestive system (or any other system) includes a tissue transfer service (e.g., flap, graft), the CPT codes for such services (e.g., transfer, graft, flap) from the integumentary system (e.g., CPT codes 14000-15770) should not be reported separately.

Interpretation

This guideline asks that documentation be worded to clearly indicate whether the integumentary or digestive system codes should be used. If the procedure is performed on the skin of the lips, use the codes from the integumentary system. If the procedure is performed on tissue (mucous, etc) deeper than the skin, the code should be from the digestive system. Always use the most specific code. Additionally, several codes within the digestive system include the reconstruction. Do not add the integumentary reconstruction codes to the digestive codes, because reconstruction is included in the CPT code description for the digestive system services.

The following codes for lip procedures include the repair. Do not code two codes (the excision and repair) from integumentary system codes if the more appropriate coding is a single comprehensive code from digestive system codes.

40520	Excision of lip; V-excision with primary direct linear closure
40525	full thickness, reconstruction with local flap (eg, Estlander or fan)
40810	Excision of lesion of mucosa and submucosa, vestibule of mouth; without repair
40812	with simple repair
40814	with complex repair
40816	complex, with excision of underlying muscle

SUMMARY

- The entire digestive system section from the NCCI manual should be read.

- Surgical endoscopies include diagnostic endoscopies and should not be separated for billing or reporting purposes.

- If a lesion is biopsied but not excised, assign only the biopsy code.

- If a biopsy specimen is obtained and then the rest of the lesion excised, assign only the excision code.

- If more than one biopsy specimen is obtained, assign only the biopsy code x1.

- If a biopsy is performed on a lesion, then a different lesion is excised, assign both the biopsy and excision codes, with a modifier 59.

- Control of bleeding is not separately coded when the bleeding results from the procedure.

- Report one CPT code per polypectomy using the primary method of removal. Example: if one polyp is removed via cold biopsy *and* snare, code only the snare.

- Report one CPT code per method of removal, regardless of the number of polyps. Example: if two polyps are removed via snare, code only one snare removal, because the codes read polyp(s).

Definitions and Acronyms

ablation: Laser obliteration of a polyp or other tissue (this is not a biopsy).

achalasia: An esophageal motility disorder.

anoscopy: Examination of the anus, anal canal, and lower rectum using a speculum. The physician inserts an anoscope a few inches into the rectum. This enlarges the rectum to allow viewing of the entire anal canal.

cold biopsy: Use of a pinching or snipping instrument to obtain a biopsy.

colonoscopy: Examination of the entire lining of the large intestine from the rectum to the cecum. The procedure may or may not include examination of the terminal ileum.

dilation: Stretching or enlarging of an opening or the lumen of a hollow structure. Balloon dilation involves the insertion of a balloon catheter that is inflated at the narrowed area of the esophagus for dilation.

dysphagia: Difficulty swallowing.

endoscopic retrograde cholangiopancreatography (ERCP): Endoscopic examination through the mouth, the esophagus, the stomach, and into the duodenum. A catheter is passed into the liver and pancreatic ducts.

enteroscopy: Examination of the inside of the small intestine using an enteroscope. During the procedure, the enteroscope is threaded through the small intestine. As it travels, a tiny video camera at its tip allows the gastroenterologist to look (on a video screen) for problems in the intestine, such as bleeding or strictures.

esophagogastroduodenoscopy (EGD): Endoscopic examination of the esophagus and stomach and at least into the duodenum.

esophagoscopy: Endoscopic study of the esophagus. When the endoscope passes the diaphragm, the procedure is an esophagogastroscopy. When the pyloric channel is traversed, the procedure is described as esophagogastroduodenoscopy (EGD).

Healthcare Common Procedure Coding System (HCPCS): These are the code sets used for filing Medicare bills consisting of Level I CPT codes and Level II HCPCS codes.

hot biopsy: A unipolar or bipolar electrical instrument used to remove specimens and control bleeding.

proctosigmoidoscopy: Examination of the rectum and sigmoid colon.

sigmoidoscopy: Examination of the entire rectum and sigmoid colon. The procedure may include examination of a portion of the descending colon.

snare: A loop with an electrical current used to squeeze off a polyp.

CHAPTER EXERCISES

EXERCISE 1

Procedure: EGD endoscopy and esophageal dilation

Clinical note: The patient is a 53-year-old male with dysphagia.

Preoperative preparation: The patient received fentanyl 0.125 mg and midazolam 5 mg intravenously immediately prior to the procedure.

Endoscopic findings: A video gastroscope was passed readily into the esophagus. A hiatal hernia approximately 4 cm in diameter was noted. At the esophagogastric junction, a Schatzki's ring was clearly noted. The scope could pass readily through it. Small erosions were seen above the Schatzki's ring. Biopsies were taken from the distal esophagus. The stomach was carefully inspected throughout and appeared normal. The duodenal bulb and second portion of the duodenum appeared normal. A 20-mm TTS balloon was inflated at the Schatzki's ring and held for a minute. The scope and balloon were then removed.

Impression: 1. Erosive esophagitis, 2. Schatzki's ring, 3. Hiatal hernia

What portion(s) of this procedure can be coded and why?

EXERCISE 2

Procedure: Colonoscopy with hot biopsy destruction of sessile, 3-mm, mid-sigmoid colon polyp and multiple cold biopsies taken randomly throughout the colon.

Preoperative diagnosis: Fecal incontinence. Diarrhea. Constipation.

Anesthetic: meperidine 50 mg and midazolam 3 mg, both given intravenously.

Procedure: The digital examination revealed no masses. A pediatric variable flexion colonoscope was introduced into the rectum and advancement to the cecum was achieved. The scope was then carefully extubated. The mucosa looked normal. Random biopsies were taken from the sigmoid colon and rectum. There was a 3-mm, sessile polyp in the mid-sigmoid colon, which was destroyed by hot biopsy.

Impression: Sigmoid colon polyp destroyed by hot biopsy.

Recommendation: I have asked the patient to call my office in a week to get the results of the pathology. Cold biopsies were taken because of the history of diarrhea.

What portions of this procedure can be coded and why?

ANSWERS TO CHAPTER EXERCISES

Exercise 1

Within this operative note, there is a diagnostic endoscopy (CPT code 43235), which would be incidental to the surgical endoscopy. Also, the surgical endoscopies for the dilation (CPT code 43249) and biopsy (CPT code 43239) are both coded.

The diagnostic endoscopy is bundled into the surgical endoscopy, based on both NCCI and CPT coding guidelines. The biopsies and dilation codes do not bundle together, as they represent distinct surgical services for which there is no comprehensive code. Therefore, codes 43239 and 43249 should be reported for this operative procedure.

Exercise 2

For this procedure, the diagnostic endoscopy (CPT code 45378) is incidental to the surgical endoscopy. Also, both surgical procedures of biopsy and hot biopsy removal (CPT codes 45380 and 45384, respectively) may be coded. A modifier 59 is needed on the biopsy code (CPT code 45380).

Diagnostic endoscopies are incidental to surgical endoscopies, but the surgical endoscopies (biopsies and hot biopsy removal) are both coded, as they are on distinct polyps. Because biopsy codes bundle into excision codes, a modifier 59 is needed on the biopsy code to indicate that distinct sites are involved.

REFERENCES

1. Centers for Medicare and Medicaid Services. "Chapter VI Surgery: Digestive System." In NCCI Policy Manual for Medicare Services. www.cms.hhs.gov/NationalCorrectCodInitEd/01_overview .asp#TopOfPage. Accessed June 12, 2009.

2. Centers for Medicare and Medicaid Services. "Chapter I General Correct Coding Policies." NCCI Policy Manual for Medicare Services. www.cms.hhs.gov/NationalCorrectCodInitEd/ 01_overview.asp#TopOfPage. Accessed June 12, 2009.

3. American Medical Association. *Current Procedural Terminology (CPT®) 2009 Professional Edition*. Chicago, IL: American Medical Association; 2008.

The Urinary System

Chapter 11 provides background about the urinary system, reviews the National Correct Coding Initiative (NCCI) coding guidelines for procedures performed on the urinary system, and provides examples to reflect the logic behind the edits. As do the other chapters, this chapter provides an NCCI guideline followed by our interpretation, an example, or both.

Introduction Section of NCCI and Urinary System Guidelines

Excerpt From the Urinary System Coding Policies Section of NCCI Guidelines[1(p2)]

Introduction
The principles of correct coding discussed in Chapter I apply to the CPT codes in the range 50000-59999. Several general guidelines are repeated in this Chapter. However, those general guidelines from Chapter I not discussed in this chapter are nonetheless applicable.

Interpretation

This instruction reiterates that the overall NCCI guidelines apply to each section of the CPT codebook, and, even if they are not repeated within a chapter, they are nonetheless a guideline to be followed. The introductory guidelines were reviewed comprehensively in Chapter 2 of this book, and only those with a clear application within the urinary system are covered in the specific urinary system NCCI policies explained in this chapter.

Urinary System (50010-53899) and NCCI Guidelines

Excerpt From the Urinary System Coding Policies Section of NCCI Guidelines[1(p4)]

Insertion of a urinary bladder catheter is a component of the global surgery package. Urinary bladder catheterization (CPT codes 51701, 51702, and 51703) is not separately reportable with a surgical procedure when performed at the time of or just prior to the procedure.

Interpretation

Throughout NCCI, the guidelines state that placements of urinary catheters are not to be coded in addition to other surgery to which they are incidental or integral (see Chapter 2). Urinary catheter placements are not to be coded in addition to more major procedures for which they are a component part. When the catheter placements are purely to assist the performance of or recovery from the surgery (eg, bladder irrigation) or for postoperative drainage, the catheterization becomes a component part of the more major procedure. A case in point would be when a gastrointestinal surgeon performs a hemicolectomy and inserts a urethral catheter for the postoperative drainage, the catheter is not for treatment of an independent condition, but rather to assist in the recovery from the hemicolectomy procedure. The catheterization would not be coded.

> **Excerpt From the Urinary System Coding Policies Section of NCCI Guidelines**[1(p4)]
>
> Cystourethroscopy, with biopsy(s) (CPT code 52204) includes all biopsies during the procedure and should be reported with one unit of service.

> **Excerpt From the Urinary System Coding Policies Section of NCCI Guidelines**[1]
>
> When irrigation procedures or drainage procedures are necessary and are integral to successfully accomplish a genitourinary (or any other) procedure, only the more extensive service is reported.

Interpretation

52204 Cystourethroscopy, with biopsy(s)

The CPT codes for endoscopic biopsies include multiple biopsy sites during a single endoscopic examination. Therefore, one code for multiple biopsies obtained during a single endoscopy is used. CPT code 52204 (cystourethroscopy, with biopsy[s]) includes one or more biopsies in the description; therefore, if 1 or 10 biopsies were performed during the cystourethroscopy, this code would be billed only once.

Note: CPT code 52204 has a medically unlikely edit code of one, meaning that if more than one unit of service is billed for this code (on a single line item), it would be denied.

> **Excerpt From the Urinary System Coding Policies Section of NCCI Guidelines**[1(p4-5)]
>
> Some lesions of the genitourinary tract occur at mucocutaneous borders. The *CPT Manual*[2] contains integumentary system (CPT codes 10000-19999) and genitourinary system (CPT codes 50000-59899) codes to describe the various procedures such as biopsy, excision, or destruction. A single code from one of these two sections of the *CPT Manual* that best describes the biopsy, excision, destruction, or other procedure performed on one or multiple similar lesions at a mucocutaneous border should be reported.

Interpretation

This guideline asks that documentation is carefully read (and worded) so that it is clear whether or not the integumentary or urinary system codes should be used. Do not use codes from both systems if only one procedure at one site is involved. Use the most specific code based on the documentation.

Interpretation

This guideline reiterates that if the irrigation or drainage services are integral to the primary procedure, the irrigation and drainage should not be coded separately in addition to the major surgery. The Centers for Medicare and Medicaid Services (CMS) provides the basic principle here as to what types of services are bundled into others. See Figure 11-1.

Standard of care: The standard of care is the recognized usual treatment protocol or process providers follow for specific clinical circumstances. When the standard of care for the primary (or Column 1) procedure indicates that the component (Column 2) service is also usually performed, the component should not be separately coded.

Necessary component: A necessary component reflects when a Column 2 service is a necessary part of a Column 1 service and, therefore, should not be independently coded. If the physician had to perform the component in order to successfully accomplish the comprehensive service, it should not be separated from the comprehensive service when coding is done.

Not separately distinguishable: Services that are not separately distinguishable are those in which the component service is essentially a critical part of the comprehensive procedure, and the component should not be separately coded.

Although these all seem similar in concept, there are subtle differences.

FIGURE 11-1 *Basic Principles of Bundling Edits Categories*

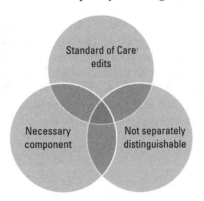

Excerpt From the Urinary System Coding Policies Section of NCCI Guidelines[1]

Unless otherwise defined by *CPT Manual* instructions, the repair and closure of surgical procedures are included in the CPT code for the more extensive procedure and are not to be separately reported. In many genitourinary services, hernia repair is included in the *CPT Manual* descriptor for the service; accordingly, a hernia repair is not separately reported. If the hernia repair performed is at a different site, this can be separately reported with modifier -59 indicating that this service occurred at a different site (i.e., via a different incision).

Interpretation

This NCCI guideline points out two principles of NCCI:

1. Surgical access and closure are included in the reimbursement for the procedure for which the approach and closure are performed. Any incidental or integral services that are performed as a part of the approach and/or closure to the primary procedure should not be coded separately. If a surgeon performs an open procedure, the code for the open procedure will include closing the surgically created wound.

2. If there is a comprehensive CPT code that includes the component parts, use the comprehensive code, rather than dividing the services into separate CPT codes. The following example shows a comprehensive procedure that includes a hernia repair as well. It would be incorrect to separately bill the hernia repair unless the herniorrhaphy was performed at a different site.

50728   Revision of urinary-cutaneous anastomosis (any type urostomy); with repair of fascial defect and hernia

However, if a hernia repair was performed, but there is no CPT code to include the hernia repair, an additional code may be used to encompass the herniorrhaphy.

Example

If a ureterocolonic conduit was created through an open incision, CPT code 50815 would be the appropriate code. The closure of the incision is incidental and integral to this service and should not be coded additionally.

50815   Ureterocolon conduit, including intestine anastomosis

Example

A urachal cyst was excised along with an umbilical hernia repair. CPT code 51500 includes both services within its description. The hernia repair would not be coded separately.

51500   Excision of urachal cyst or sinus, with or without umbilical hernia repair

Example

If a urachal cyst was excised along with an inguinal hernia repair, the hernia repair should be coded in addition to the cyst excision, because there is no CPT code that includes both services.

Excerpt From the Urinary System Coding Policies Section of NCCI Guidelines[1(p5)]

In general, multiple methods of performing a procedure (e.g., prostatectomy) cannot be performed at the same patient encounter. (See general policy on mutually exclusive services.) Therefore, only one method of accomplishing a given procedure may be reported. If an initial approach is unsuccessful and is followed by an alternative approach, only the successful or last unsuccessful approach may be reported.

Interpretation

Chapter 2 discusses NCCI edits for mutually exclusive services. Essentially, mutually exclusive edits are cases in which two codes should not be reported together because both services cannot be reasonably performed at the same anatomic site or during the same patient encounter. When planning surgical procedures, physicians want to use the least invasive and most effective approach. On occasion, the planned approach is insufficient to the overall success of the procedure, and the surgeon must convert to a different approach during the procedure. Failed approaches, or approaches that are converted to different approaches, are incidental to successful approaches, and only the successfully approached procedure should be coded.

An example of a mutually exclusive situation is the repair of an organ that can be performed by two different methods. Only one method can be chosen to repair the organ.

In normal anatomy, males have one prostate gland; therefore, if the prostate gland is resected, only one methodology could be used. If two different prostate gland resections were billed for a single patient encounter, this would create a mutually exclusive code edit.

For example, the following codes would create a mutually exclusive edit because they both represent prostate gland resections.

52601 Transurethral electrosurgical resection of prostate, including control of postoperative bleeding, complete (vasectomy, meatotomy, cystourethroscopy, urethral calibration and/or dilation, and internal urethrotomy are included)

55801 Prostatectomy, perineal, subtotal (including control of postoperative bleeding, vasectomy, meatotomy, urethral calibration and/or dilation, and internal urethrotomy)

Table 11-1 shows some of the mutually exclusive code edits for CPT code 52601. Note that the codes that are mutually exclusive include various procedures that include some level of prostate gland excision, whether a resection or destruction of tissue.

TABLE 11-1 *Mutually Exclusive Edits for Transurethral Resection of the Prostate Procedure (CPT code 52601)*

Column 1	Column 2	Modifier 0 = not allowed 1 = allowed 9 = not applicable
52601	52606	0
52601	52612	0
52601	52614	0
52601	52620	0
52601	52630	0
52601	52640	0
52601	52647	0
52601	52648	0
52601	53850	0
52601	53852	0
52601	53853	0
52601	55873	1
52606	52614	0

Excerpt From the Urinary System Coding Policies Section of NCCI Guidelines[1]

When an endoscopic procedure is performed as an integral part of an open procedure, only the open procedure is reported. If the endoscopy is confirmatory or is performed to assess the surgical field ("scout endoscopy"), the endoscopy does not represent a diagnostic or surgical endoscopy. The endoscopy represents exploration of the surgical field, and should not be separately reported under the diagnostic or surgical endoscopy codes. When an endoscopic procedure is attempted unsuccessfully and converted to an open procedure, only the open procedure is reported (see general policy on sequential procedures). If the endoscopy is performed for diagnostic purposes and a subsequent therapeutic service can be performed at the same session, the procedure is coded at the highest level of specificity. If the *CPT Manual* narrative includes endoscopy, then the diagnostic endoscopy is not separately coded. If the narrative does not include endoscopy and a separate endoscopy is necessary as a diagnostic procedure, this can be reported separately. Modifier -58 may be used to indicate that the diagnostic endoscopy and the subsequent therapeutic service are staged or planned procedures. The medical record must describe the intent and findings of the diagnostic endoscopy in these cases.

Interpretation

This guideline sums up many of the endoscopic and open procedure instructions covered throughout this book. NCCI guidelines include identification of landmarks as a part of the surgical approach (as noted in the standards of medical/surgical practice). A scout scope procedure is for landmark identification (looking at the lay of the land) and not for diagnosing or treating. It is a complementary component of the primary procedure. CMS distinguishes a scout scope procedure from a diagnostic scope procedure, which is an important principle in NCCI. If a truly diagnostic scope procedure is necessary before an open therapeutic procedure, the diagnostic scope procedure may be separately coded, as long as the scope procedure is truly diagnostic (the decision for the therapeutic open procedure is made based on the findings of the scope procedure). The physician's documentation must be very clear that the service is supported as diagnostic. The scope procedure is not separately coded if the physician:

- knows prior to the scope procedure what therapeutic open procedure is going to be performed or
- has already performed a diagnostic scope procedure or
- goes on to perform a therapeutic scope procedure.

NCCI edits state that when the diagnostic scope procedure is performed prior to an open procedure, both procedures may be coded, and modifier 58 (staged procedure) should be appended.

 CPT Coding Tip: When coding, see if the preoperative diagnosis differs from the postoperative diagnosis, as this could be an indication of whether the endoscopy is truly diagnostic. If there is a symptom or a rule-out diagnosis preoperatively, that helps support the endoscopy as diagnostic.

There should be a procedure-indications section at the beginning of the operative note. This too can help clarify whether the endoscopy is diagnostic or not.

Physicians should clearly document whether the endoscopy is diagnostic or not.

50551	Renal endoscopy through established nephrostomy or pyelostomy, with or without irrigation, instillation, or uretero-pyelography, exclusive of radiologic service;
50553	with ureteral catheterization, with or without dilation of ureter
50555	with biopsy
50557	with fulguration and/or incision, with or without biopsy
50561	with removal of foreign body or calculus
50562	with resection of tumor

Because CPT code 50551's complete description falls before the semi-colon, it is inherent in all of the codes and would never be coded in addition to any codes in this series *unless* the procedure was performed at a separate surgical session.

Excerpt From the Urinary System Coding Policies Section of NCCI Guidelines[2](p6)

When multiple endoscopic procedures are performed at the same patient encounter, the most comprehensive code accurately describing the service(s) performed should be reported. If several procedures not included in a more comprehensive code are performed at the same endoscopic session, multiple HCPCS/CPT codes may be reported with modifier -51 attached.

Excerpt From the Urinary System Coding Policies Section of NCCI Guidelines[2](p6)

CPT code 51700 (bladder irrigation, simple, lavage and/or instillation) is used to report irrigation with therapeutic agents or as an independent therapeutic procedure. It is not separately reportable if bladder irrigation is part of a more comprehensive service such as to gain access to or visualize the urinary system. Irrigation of a urinary catheter is included in the global surgical package. CPT code 51700 should not be misused to report irrigation of a urinary catheter.

Interpretation

The principles of coding in this guideline are the following:
1. Do not code component CPT codes if there is a comprehensive code that includes the components.
2. If there is no comprehensive code, the component codes may be used. Modifier 51 may be necessary on the lesser procedures.
3. Whenever billing multiple codes, remember that each service must be medically necessary in order to be billed.

NCCI offers an example:

"For example, if a renal endoscopy is performed through an established nephrostomy, a biopsy is performed, a lesion is fulgurated and a foreign body (calculus) is removed, the appropriate CPT coding would be CPT codes 50557 and 50561-51, not CPT codes 50551, 50555, 50557, and 50561."

Interpretation

Any service that is for either access or visualization should not be coded in addition to the primary procedure. The access or visualization becomes integral to the root operation and must be performed in order to carry out the primary procedure. If the urinary bladder irrigation is (1) for an independent condition, (2) unrelated to any other procedure performed, and (3) inclusive of therapeutic agents, the irrigation may potentially be coded in addition to the other procedure, but clear documentation would be necessary, illustrating the independent need for the irrigation. Note: All three requirements (1, 2, and 3) would be necessary before the irrigation could be coded separately.

Example

Diagnosis: Multiparous female desires permanent sterilization.

Operation: Laparoscopic tubal ligation with Falope ring on the right and bipolar cautery on the left.

Findings at operation: At the time of surgery, the patient was found to have a normal-sized uterus, but it was densely adherent to the posterior surface of the anterior abdominal wall in its entirety. The round ligaments were also densely adherent. The left tube was quite phimotic. The right tube appeared normal. Both ovaries appeared normal. The patient's appendix was noted to be in the cul-de-sac, but was not adherent.

Procedure: The patient was taken to the operating room, where she was laid supine on the operating table, and general endotracheal anesthesia was administered. She was then placed in the dorsal lithotomy position, and examination under anesthesia revealed her to have a normal-sized uterus. The patient's vagina, perineum, and abdomen were sterilely prepped and draped for surgery in the usual fashion. The cervix was visualized and grasped with a single-tooth tenaculum, and Kahn's cannula was placed. **The urinary bladder was drained with a Foley catheter.** A #11 blade was then used to make an infraumbilical stab incision, and a Veress needle was placed. After testing for adequate intraperitoneal placement, pneumoperitoneum was obtained with 2.5 liters of carbon dioxide gas. The Veress needle was then removed, and the 10-mm trocar and trocar sheath were placed. The trocar was removed, and the operative laparoscope was placed, and the patient's pelvic contents were visualized, with findings as noted above.

The Falope ring applicator was used to place a Falope ring at the avascular midportion of the patient's right tube without difficulty. A large knuckle of tube was performed. The patient's left tube was then located and identified by the fimbriated end, and a Falope ring was placed, but the knuckle of tube was judged to be insufficient. Therefore, the Kleppinger bipolar forceps were used to cauterize the tube in four segments until loss of ammeter resistance was found. When this was completed, the tube was basically cauterized in its entirety. No bleeding was seen.

The procedure was terminated. The instruments were removed. The pneumoperitoneum was released, and the trocar sheath was removed under direct visualization. The fascia and subcuticular tissue were closed with 3-0 Vicryl. A sterile dressing was placed. The Foley catheter and vaginal instruments were also removed, and the patient was returned to the recumbent position and taken from the operating room to the recovery room in stable condition.

Note that the urinary bladder was irrigated as a part of the procedure's access and not for an independent reason.

Excerpt From the Urinary System Coding Policies Section of NCCI Guidelines[1(p6)]

When electromyography (EMG) is performed as part of a biofeedback session, neither CPT code 51784 nor 51785 is to be reported unless a significant, separately identifiable diagnostic EMG service is provided. If either CPT code 51784 or CPT code 51785 is to be used for a diagnostic electromyogram, a separate report must be available in the medical record to indicate this service was performed for diagnostic purposes.

Interpretation

90911 Biofeedback training, perineal muscles, anorectal or urethral sphincter, including EMG and/or manometry

The CPT code description for biofeedback includes electromyography (EMG). Therefore, there would have to be sufficient support to separately report an EMG from the biofeedback. The NCCI guideline indicates that a separate report must be available in order to bill the EMG study. However, because the biofeedback does include EMG, use care in billing it separately.

51784 Electromyography studies (EMG) of anal or urethral sphincter, other than needle, any technique

51785 Needle electromyography studies (EMG) of anal or urethral sphincter, any technique

---

Excerpt From the General Correct Coding Policies Section of NCCI Guidelines[2(p6)]

When endoscopic visualization of the urinary system involves several regions (e.g., kidney, renal pelvis, calyx, and ureter), the appropriate CPT code is defined by the approach (e.g., nephrostomy, pyelostomy, ureterostomy, etc.) as indicated in the CPT descriptor. When multiple endoscopic approaches at the same patient encounter are medically reasonable and necessary (e.g., renal endoscopy through a nephrostomy and cystourethroscopy) to perform different procedures, they may be separately reported appending modifier -51 to the less extensive procedure codes. However, when multiple endoscopic approaches are utilized to attempt the same procedure, only the completed approach should be reported.

Interpretation

In normal anatomy, the urethra connects the bladder to the outside of the body. Then the bladder is connected to the kidneys through two ureters. The physician could insert an endoscope through the urethra and sequentially examine the urethra, bladder, and ureters. There is one pathway and only one endoscopy procedure coded, even if the physician commented on different anatomical parts of the examination.

However, within the urinary system, endoscopic examinations can be performed through an ostomy (artificial opening). This NCCI guideline states that if separate areas and separate approaches are used for endoscopic evaluation, then both may be coded (if medically necessary). So, if a renal endoscopy was performed through a nephrostomy and the bladder examined through a cystourethroscopy, different anatomical sites were evaluated through different endoscopic approaches, and each may be coded.

Excerpt From the General Correct Coding Policies Section of NCCI Guidelines[2(p7)]

When urethral catheterization or urethral dilation (e.g., CPT codes 51701-51703) is necessary to accomplish a more extensive procedure, the urethral catheterization/dilation is not to be separately reportable.

Interpretation

Remember, any service that is either integral or incidental to the procedure is included in the CPT code for the primary procedure. So, if the main procedure being performed requires that the urethra be catheterized or dilated, that is incidental to the procedure and should not be coded separately. For example, a cystourethroscopy (CPT code 52000) is an endoscopic examination of the urethra and bladder through an endoscope inserted through the urethra. In order to accomplish a cystourethroscopy, the physician must insert a catheter into the urethra and advance it to the bladder. Catheter placement is an integral part of the procedure and may not be separately coded. If the urethra must be dilated to insert the catheter, that procedure should not be coded separately.

On the other hand, if a cystourethroscopy was performed for a urethral stricture that had to be dilated, the patient's condition establishes that more than a diagnostic cystourethroscopy was necessary.

52281   Cystourethroscopy, with calibration and/or dilation of urethral stricture or stenosis, with or without meatotomy, with or without injection procedure for cystography, male or female

Assign code 52281 if the dilation was performed to correct a urethral stricture or stenosis. Do not assign this code if the dilation was performed to determine the size of the scope necessary to do the examination.

Last, if a surgeon performing a colectomy inserted a urethral catheter for bladder irrigation during the procedure, the catheterization should not be separately coded, as it was not a separate therapeutic service.

Excerpt From the Urinary System Coding Policies Section of NCCI Guidelines[1(p7)]

Ureteral anastomosis procedures are described by CPT codes 50740-50825, and 50860. In general, they represent mutually exclusive procedures that are not reported together. If one type of anastomosis is performed on one ureter, and a different type of anastomosis is performed on the contralateral ureter, the appropriate modifier (e.g., -LT, -RT) should be reported with the CPT code to describe the service performed on each ureter.

Interpretation

Ureteral anastomoses are procedures in which the ureter is surgically reconnected. For example, ureteroneocystostomy is the surgical reconnection of the ureter to the bladder. It would be unusual to have multiple ureter anastomoses performed during a single surgical session, which is why NCCI created mutually exclusive edits for these services. However, there are two ureters. If different procedures are performed on different ureters, lateral modifiers (LT for left, RT for right) should be appended to indicate which ureter was involved with the procedure.

Take, for example, the following CPT codes, which are unilateral. If the exact same procedure is performed on each ureter, a modifier 50 may be appended to the code to reflect that both ureters were repaired.

50780   Ureteroneocystostomy; anastomosis of single ureter to bladder

50782   anastomosis of duplicated ureter to bladder

50783   with extensive ureteral tailoring

50785   with vesico-psoas hitch or bladder flap

50800   Ureteroenterostomy, direct anastomosis of ureter to intestine

Also, if different surgeries were performed on each ureter, each procedure could be coded with the appropriate lateral (LT, RT) modifier appended. Modifier 50 would be used only when the exact same procedure was performed on both ureters. If a ureteroenterostomy with direct anastomosis of ureter to intestine was performed on the right side, and a cystourethroscopy with removal of ureteral calculus was performed on the left side, both may be coded, with an RT modifier on the ureteroenterostomy and LT modifier on the ureteral calculus.

50800-*RT*   Ureteroenterostomy, direct anastomosis of ureter to intestine

The RT modifier indicates that the procedure was performed on the right side.

52320-*LT*   Cystourethroscopy (including ureteral catheterization); with removal of ureteral calculus

The LT modifier indicates that the procedure was performed on the left side.

Excerpt From the Urinary System Coding Policies Section of NCCI Guidelines[1(p7)]

The CPT codes 53502-53515 describe urethral repair codes for urethral wounds or injuries (urethrorrhaphy). When a urethroplasty is performed, codes for urethrorrhaphy should not be reported in addition since "suture to repair wound or injury" is included in the urethroplasty service.

Interpretation

Urethroplasties are for the repair of the urethra. Because the urethroplasty service is for repairing the urethra, any incidental service (eg, suturing) is an integral part of the urethroplasty and not separately coded.

There are many CPT codes for the various types of urethroplasty procedures. Several are listed in the following:

53400   Urethroplasty; first stage, for fistula, diverticulum, or stricture (eg, Johannsen type)

53410   Urethroplasty, 1-stage reconstruction of male anterior urethra

53415   Urethroplasty, transpubic or perineal, 1-stage, for reconstruction or repair of prostatic or membranous urethra

53430   Urethroplasty, reconstruction of female urethra

Remember from earlier lessons that less extensive procedures are bundled into more extensive procedures when they are performed on the same body site during a single surgical session. The suturing of a wound of the urethra is included in the more extensive urethroplasty CPT code.

Excerpt From the Urinary System Coding Policies Section of NCCI Guidelines[1(p7-8)]

CPT code 52332 (Cystourethroscopy, with insertion of indwelling ureteral stent) describes insertion of a self-retaining indwelling stent during cystourethroscopy with ureteroscopy and/or pyeloscopy and should not be reported to describe insertion and removal of a temporary ureteral stent during diagnostic or therapeutic cystourethroscopy with ureteroscopy and/or pyeloscopy (CPT codes 52320-52355). The insertion and removal of a temporary ureteral catheter (stent) during these procedures is not separately reportable.

Interpretation

This guideline is consistent with the CPT codebook instructions that insertion of temporary stents (those left in for the duration of the surgery, then removed) are not coded as insertion of indwelling stents (left in after surgery to assist in the healing process).

A case in point would be that of a patient who presents for a cystourethroscopy with ureteroscopy and removal of a ureteral calculus. During the procedure, the physician inserted indwelling stents to ensure proper postoperative healing.

52352   Cystourethroscopy, with ureteroscopy and/or pyeloscopy; with removal or manipulation of calculus (ureteral catheterization is included)

52332   Cystourethroscopy, with insertion of indwelling ureteral stent (eg, Gibbons or double-J type)

Both of these CPT codes may be billed, as the stent was left indwelling at the conclusion of the surgery.

On the other hand, the code options for a patient who presents for a cystourethroscopy with removal of a ureteral calculus, and the physician inserted a temporary stent that was left in for the duration of the procedure, then removed are:

52320   Cystourethroscopy (including ureteral catheterization); with removal of ureteral calculus

52332   Cystourethroscopy, with insertion of indwelling ureteral stent (eg, Gibbons or double-J type)

Because the physician did not leave the stent indwelling after the procedure, only CPT code 52320 (removal of the calculus) should be coded.

Note: Prior to April 1, 2007, the NCCI edits bundled CPT code 52332 (insertion of indwelling stent) with other ureteroscopy codes. As of April 1, 2007, those edits have been deleted. However, it is still important that the services be coded correctly, and if the stent is temporary and removed at the conclusion of the procedure, do not code the stent insertion in addition to the procedure.

Excerpt From the Urinary System Coding Policies Section of NCCI Guidelines[1(p8)]

Prostatectomy procedures (CPT codes 55801-55845) include cystoplasty or cystourethroplasty as a standard of surgical practice. CPT code 51800 (cystoplasty or cystourethroplasty) should not be reported separately with prostatectomy procedures.

Interpretation

NCCI edits bundle cystoplasties into prostatectomy codes because it is a standard of practice to perform a bladder repair during a prostatectomy. The component service is an accepted standard of care when the comprehensive service is performed. This bundling edit may not be bypassed, so, regardless of the scenario, the cystoplasty would never be coded in addition to the prostatectomy.

Excerpt From the Urinary System Coding Policies Section of NCCI Guidelines[1(p8)]

CPT code 50650 (ureterectomy, with bladder cuff (separate procedure)) should not be reported with other procedures on the ipsilateral ureter. Because CPT code 50650 includes the "separate procedure" designation, CMS does not allow additional payment for the procedure when it is performed with other procedures in an anatomically related area.

Interpretation

Remember, anytime a separate procedure is performed on the same anatomic site as another more major procedure, the separate procedure code should not be coded, as it is incidental to the more major procedure. The ureterectomy is incidental to other procedures performed on the same ureter (anastomosis, ureterostomy, etc). However, if there was a procedure performed on the contralateral (opposite) ureter, both could be coded. Either lateral modifiers (LT for left, RT for right) or modifier 59 would be needed to show that different ureters were involved. If a patient underwent a right nephrectomy with ureterectomy, the separate code for ureterectomy (CPT code 50650) could not be added to the procedure if it was performed on the same ureter as the one included in the nephrectomy codes. However, if a ureterectomy was performed on the opposite ureter from the one included in the nephrectomy, it could be added to the nephrectomy code.

50220 Nephrectomy, including partial ureterectomy, any open approach including rib resection;

50650 Ureterectomy, with bladder cuff (separate procedure)

However, if a patient had an anastomosis of the right ureter to the bladder, and, during the procedure, a partial ureterectomy was performed in order to remove a diseased ureter section prior to reconnection, the ureterectomy would be incidental to the anastomosis, as it was a necessary part of the procedure.

 CMS Tip: *It is interesting that CPT code 50650 bundles into many surgeries that do not allow bypassing with a modifier. This seems odd because a contralateral ureter could be involved. Check edits prior to appending a modifier to determine whether it is appropriate. Hard copy appeals may be necessary if inappropriate denials occur.*

50900 Ureterorrhaphy, suture of ureter (separate procedure)

Note: It may seem logical that if the ureterectomy was performed on a different ureter than the ureterorrhaphy, both procedures could be coded. However, the NCCI edits do not allow bypassing the bundling edits for these codes.

Other Information and Comments About the Urinary System and NCCI Edits

Medicare Carriers Manual,[3] Chapter 12, Section 30.2: Urinary and Male Genital Systems (Codes 50010-55899)

A. Cystourethroscopy With Ureteral Catheterization (Code 52005)

Code 52005 has a zero in the bilateral field (payment adjustment for bilateral procedure does not apply) because the basic procedure is an examination of the bladder and urethra (cystourethroscopy), which are not paired organs. The work RVUs assigned take into account that it may be necessary to examine and catheterize one or both ureters. No additional payment is made when the procedure is billed with bilateral modifier "-50." Neither is any additional payment made when both ureters are examined and code 52005 is billed with multiple surgery modifier "-51." It is inappropriate to bill code 52005 twice, once by itself and once with modifier "-51," when both ureters are examined.

B. Cystourethroscopy With Fulguration and/or Resection of Tumors (Codes 52234, 52235, and 52240)

The descriptors for codes 52234 through 52240 include the language "tumor(s)."

This means that regardless of the number of tumors removed, only one unit of a single code can be billed on a given date of service. It is inconsistent to allow payment for removal of a small (code 52234) and a large (code 52240) tumor using two codes when only one code is allowed for the removal of more than one large tumor. For these three codes only one unit may be billed for any of these codes, only one of the codes may be billed, and the billed code reflects the size of the largest tumor removed.

The October 2002 issue of *CPT Assistant*[4] addressed the issue of determining the size category when multiple bladder tumors are fulgurated or resected using a cystourethroscope. The guideline was stated thus:

The tumor sizes should not be added together for a cumulative total size. Rather, each tumor should be measured individually to determine the appropriate category (eg, small, medium, large). Code 52234,

Cystourethroscopy, with fulguration (including cryosurgery or laser surgery) and/or resection of; SMALL bladder tumor(s) (0.5 to 2.0 cm), should be reported once for single or multiple tumors that individually measure 0.5-2.0 cm. Code 52235 should be reported once for medium (single or multiple) tumors that individually measure 2.0-5.0 cm. Tumors larger than 5.0 cm would be considered large tumors and would be reported using code 52235 one time.

Comment

This guideline leads one to believe that each size category of tumor removed may be coded separately. However, NCCI edits bundle the lower sized tumor removals into the larger sized tumor removals and do not allowing bypassing of the edit. Chapter 2 of this book reviews the NCCI edit guideline that CPT codebook instructions should be followed in the absence of a different guideline within NCCI. It further states that *CPT Assistant* guidelines would not be used to bypass bundling edits. Therefore, even when different-sized lesions are fulgurated or resected, only one code should be used per procedure. Use the largest tumor fulgurated to determine the code.

Cystoscopy, Urethroscopy, Cystourethroscopy

According to CPT codebook[5(p234)] instructions, the cystoscopy, urethroscopy, and cystourethroscopy codes include:
- meatotomy, urethral calibration and/or dilation, urethroscopy, and
- cystoscopy prior to a transurethral resection of the prostate gland, ureteral catheterization following extraction of a ureteral calculus, and
- internal urethrotomy and bladder neck fulguration when a cystourethroscopy is performed in the female urethral syndrome.

None of these services should be coded in addition to the endoscopic procedures. According to the NCCI edits, retrograde pyelograms are bundled into cystoscopy codes, 52320 through 52355, and cannot be unbundled under any circumstances.

Extracorporeal Shock Wave Lithotripsy

Extracorporeal shock wave lithotripsy is coded one time, regardless of how many stones are removed during the single session, unless the procedure is performed on both the right and left kidneys, and the machine must be repositioned to access the stones. Then modifier 50 may be appended to indicate bilateral procedures.

SUMMARY

- The entire urinary system section from the NCCI manual should be read.

- Urinary catheter placements are not to be coded in addition to other surgery to which they are incidental or integral.

- Any service that is either for access or visualization should not be coded in addition to the primary procedure.

- Inserting temporary stents (those left in for the duration of the surgery, then removed) are not coded as insertion of indwelling stents (left in after surgery to assist in the healing process).

Definitions and Acronyms

American Urological Association (AUA): The AUA is the national association for urological clinicians. Aside from clinical-related information and support, the AUA also offers practice management resources that include coding tips and guidance.

contralateral: On or of the opposite side.

cystourethroscopy: Endoscopic examination of the urethra and urinary bladder.

ipsilateral: On or of the same side.

transurethral resection of the prostate (TURP): During a TURP, the urethra is the point of approach to resection of a portion of the prostate gland.

urachal cyst: Fluid-filled structure occurring between the two obliterated ends of the umbilicus and urinary bladder dome.

CHAPTER EXERCISES

EXERCISE 1

When a transurethral bladder tumor resection (TUBTR) is performed during the same session as random biopsies being taken, can the biopsies be coded in addition to the TUBTR?

Comments from the operative report:
Specimens were removed from the right bladder wall.

Tumor resection was complete.

At completion of the procedure, deep biopsies were taken from the resected area.

Other biopsies were taken from the left bladder wall, anterior bladder wall, posterior bladder wall, bladder neck, and urethra.

EXERCISE 2

Operations: Cystoscopy, urethroscopy, left retrograde pyelogram, and manipulation for left ureteral calculus

Disposition: The patient tolerated the procedure well and was transported to the recovery room in stable postoperative condition.

Operative findings: At the time of cystoscopy, the urethra was found to be grossly normal in course, caliber, and length. The trigone of the bladder was visualized, and there was prominence of the left ureteral orifice, suggesting an underlying ureteral calculus. The orifice was extended into the lumen of the urinary bladder approximately 1 cm from the remaining bladder wall. The efflux noted from the left ureter seemed to be decreased. No evidence of neoplastic disease in the bladder, no active bleeding, and no intravesical calculi were noted. The bladder was not trabeculated, and no diverticula were seen.

Procedures: The patient was placed in the lithotomy position and prepped and draped in the usual fashion under suitable general anesthesia prior to beginning the procedure. At this time, cystourethroscopy was carried out using the 30-degree lens. After adequate cystoscopy was completed, a left retrograde pyelogram was performed. I was unable to catheterize the ureter with the ureteral catheter, but after advancing a wire into the deformed left ureteral orifice, I was able to follow the wire with a ureteral catheter.

At this point, a retrograde pyelogram was carried out, and this demonstrated what appeared to be a filling defect in the area of the expected ureteral calculus. This filling defect was approximately the same size as the expected calculus, which was reported at 5 mm on prior radiologic evaluation. After this was completed, it was also noted that there was evidence of hydroureter above the level of the calculus. The entire ureter was dilated, as the calculus was at the distal-most portion of the ureter.

After the retrograde pyelogram was completed, the wire was removed from the catheter. The catheter was left in the ureter. A small stone basket catheter was advanced through the ureteral catheter and placed in a position such that it was above the ureteral calculus. After the catheter was in the lower portion of the ureter, the basket was deployed, and both the stone basket catheter and ureteral catheter were closely removed from the ureter. As the basket was seen coming out of the ureteral orifice, it was apparent that the stone had been engaged. The stone was pulled through the ureteral orifice with gentle, steady traction. There was no tearing of the orifice noted on cystoscopy. The stone was recovered and sent to the laboratory for analysis. It was approximately 5 mm in size, irregularly shaped, and yellow in color. After the stone was removed, cystoscopy was again carried out. The ureteral orifice appeared to be without trauma. At that point, I again introduced contrast material into the distal portion of the left ureter, and no filling defect was present. Also, there was good drainage of the left ureter after the urethral catheter was removed.

At this point, the bladder was drained, the cystoscope was removed, and the procedure was terminated. Anesthesia was reversed, and the patient was transported to the recovery room in stable postoperative condition.

Tissue specimen to be examined: Left ureteral calculus

Macroscopic: There is an irregularly ovoid, stony hard, tan-brown, rough-surfaced calculus 0.5 cm in diameter. It was referred for chemical analysis.

Final diagnosis: Calculus consistent with ureteral calculus. What would be coded in this case and why?

ANSWERS TO CHAPTER EXERCISES

Exercise 1: As long as separate lesions other than those excised were biopsied, there is no guideline against coding both. CPT 52235 (TUBTR) is a Column 1 code to CPT code 52204; therefore, if they are separate lesions, it would be necessary to append a modifier 59 to code 52204. Note that the left bladder wall, anterior bladder, and so forth, were biopsied, whereas the resection was from the right bladder wall.

Exercise 2:

52000 Cystourethroscopy (separate procedure)

52005 Cystourethroscopy, with ureteral catheterization, with or without irrigation, instillation, or ureteropyelography, exclusive of radiologic service;

52320 Cystourethroscopy (including ureteral catheterization); with removal of ureteral calculus

---

CPT code 52000 is bundled into CPT code 52005. CPT code 52005 is bundled into CPT code 52320; therefore, the only code to be billed would be CPT code 52320. In addition, a modifier LT (on the left side) should be appended to CPT code 52320.

Code for NCCI payers = 52320-LT

REFERENCES

1. Centers for Medicare and Medicaid Services. "Chapter VII Surgery: Urinary, Male Genital, Female Genital, Maternity Care and Delivery Systems." NCCI Policy Manual for Medicare Services. www.cms.hhs.gov/NationalCorrectCodInitEd/01_overview .asp#TopOfPage. Accessed June 12, 2009.

2. Centers for Medicare & Medicaid Services. "Chapter I General Correct Coding Policies," In: NCCI Policy Manual for Medicare Services. www.cms.hhs.gov/NationalCorrectCodInitEd/01_overview.asp#TopOfPage. Accessed June 11, 2009.

3. Centers for Medicare and Medicaid Services. Physicians/Nonphysician Practitioners. In: *Medicare Claims Processing Manual*. Chapter 12, Section 30.2. www.cms.hhs.gov/manuals/downloads/clm104c12.pdf. Accessed June 13, 2009.

4. American Medical Association. *CPT Assistant*. "Coding clarification, surgery-urinary system, 52234 (Q&A)." 2002;12(10):12.

5. American Medical Association. *Current Procedural Terminology (CPT®) Professional Edition 2009*. Chicago, IL: American Medical Association; 2008.

The Male and Female Reproductive Systems

Chapter 12 provides background about both the male and female reproductive systems, reviews the National Correct Coding Initiative (NCCI) coding guidelines for procedures performed on these systems, and provides examples to reflect the logic behind the edits. As do the other chapters, this chapter provides NCCI guidelines followed by our interpretation, an example, or both.

Introduction Section of NCCI Guidelines Regarding the Male Reproductive System

Excerpt From the Male Reproductive System Coding Policies Section of NCCI[2(p2)] Guidelines

A. Introduction
The principles of correct coding discussed in Chapter I apply to the CPT codes[1] in the range 54000-55899. Several general guidelines are repeated in this chapter. However, those general guidelines from Chapter I not discussed in this chapter are nonetheless applicable.

Interpretation

The overall NCCI guidelines apply to each section of the CPT codebook, and, even if they are not repeated within a chapter, they are nonetheless a guideline to be followed. Chapter 2 of this book covers these guidelines comprehensively.

NCCI Guidelines Regarding Male Reproductive System Services

Excerpt From the Male Reproductive System Coding Policies Section of NCCI[2(p8)] Guidelines

Transurethral drainage of a prostatic abscess (e.g., CPT code 52700) is included in male transurethral prostatic procedures and should not be reported separately.

Interpretation

Transurethral drainage of a prostatic abscess involves access through the urethra (that is the transurethral part) and drainage of a pocket of infection within the prostate gland. If the physician documents a transurethral drainage of a prostatic abscess at the same surgical session as another transurethral prostatic procedure, do not code the drainage additionally. The work done for abscess drainage during another transurethral prostate gland procedure is minimal and, therefore, not separately billable. Often the drainage occurs because of the approach of the more major procedure (incidental drainage), which requires no additional work.

Excerpt From the Male Reproductive System Coding Policies Section of NCCI Guidelines[2(p8)]

The puncture aspiration of a hydrocele (e.g., CPT code 55000) is included in services involving the tunica vaginalis and proximate anatomy (scrotum, vas deferens) and in inguinal hernia repairs and should not be reported separately.

Interpretation

Whenever the aspiration (removing fluid with a needle) of a hydrocele (fluid-filled sac surrounding a testicle) is performed in conjunction with another procedure on an anatomically close (proximate) area (tunica vaginalis, scrotum, vas deferens), the hydrocele aspiration should not be coded in addition to the other procedure.

An inguinal hernia and a hydrocele share a similar etiology and pathophysiology and may coexist. Quite often a hydrocele aspiration is performed in conjunction with an inguinal hernia repair, and, according to NCCI guidelines, the work for the hernia repair includes the work for the hydrocele procedure. Do not code the aspiration additionally. However, there is no edit for these two CPT codes. Oddly, few codes have the hydrocele aspiration bundle into them.

Regardless of the edits, however, remember to follow the guideline. When an aspiration of a hydrocele is performed during an inguinal hernia repair or other procedure on the tunica vaginalis, scrotum, or vas deferens, do not add a code for the hydrocele aspiration. An exception would be if the hydrocele was on the opposite side. If that were the case, a modifier could be appended and both services coded.

The *excision* (not aspiration) of the hydrocele (CPT code 55040) has bundling edits for services performed on the scrotum as well as the inguinal hernia codes. The aspiration does not have bundling edits. Correction of a hydrocele is incidental to the more major procedure when performed at the same session as a procedure of proximate (nearby) anatomy, whether through aspiration or excision.

So, as an example, a patient has an inguinal herniorrhaphy and hydrocele aspiration within a single surgical session. There is no NCCI edit bundling CPT code 55000 (hydrocele aspiration) into the inguinal hernia repair (CPT code range of 49500). Only the hernia repair would be coded because the NCCI guidelines instruct that the hydrocele aspiration is incidental. There is no bundling edit for this code combination.

Interpretation

There is one prostate gland in normal anatomy, and when a procedure is performed to either remove or destroy the prostate tissue, all services for the removal or destruction should be coded to the most extensive procedure performed. Any other excision or destruction would be incidental to the most extensive service.

A surgeon might start out by performing a less invasive procedure, then determine that the procedure needs to be converted to a more extensive surgery. Once the more extensive procedure for prostate excision or destruction begins, the lesser procedure is not coded.

Explanation

Transurethral: In this operation, the doctor advances a cystoscope up the urethra to the prostate gland, where tiny surgical tools are used to snip away the surrounding prostate tissue. (These codes are in the urinary system section of the CPT codebook.)

Perineal: In this operation, the prostate tissue is removed through an incision between the rectum and the scrotum. Potentially cancerous lymph nodes in the area may also require removal.

Retropubic and suprapubic prostatectomy: These operations require a larger incision in the lower abdomen, through which the prostate gland and nearby lymph nodes can be removed.

As an example, if a patient has a prostatectomy following an attempted transurethral resection of the prostate gland during a single surgical encounter, the prostatectomy would be the more major procedure and should be the only code billed. The transurethral resection is incidental to the prostatectomy.

Excerpt From the Male Reproductive System Coding Policies Section of NCCI Guidelines[2(p8)]

The *CPT Manual* contains many codes (CPT codes 52601-52649, 53850-53853, 55801-55845, 55866) which describe various methods of removing or destroying prostate tissue. These procedures are mutually exclusive, and two codes from these code ranges should not be reported together.

Other Information on the Male Reproductive System

Excerpt From the Urinary System Coding Policies Section of NCCI[2(p4-5)]

Some lesions of the genitourinary tract occur at mucocutaneous borders. The *CPT Manual*[1] contains Integumentary system (CPT codes 10000-19999) and genitourinary system (CPT codes 50000-59899) codes to describe the various procedures such as biopsy, excision, or destruction. A single code from one of these two sections of the *CPT Manual* that best describes the biopsy, excision, destruction, or other procedure performed on one or multiple similar lesions at a mucocutaneous border should be reported.

Interpretation

This guideline indicates that documentation should be read carefully so that it is clear whether or not the integumentary or male reproductive system codes should be used. For instance, a physician destroys a lesion on the male genitalia. To determine whether the correct code is from the integumentary system or male reproductive system, check with the provider to determine whether the service is simply a cutaneous level of destruction (which would be coded from the integumentary system) or something more in-depth that should be coded from male reproductive system codes.

Plaque excision
Removal of penile plaque often raises questions if the code used for the procedure should be.

54110 Excision of penile plaque (Peyronie disease);

54111 with graft to 5 cm in length

54112 with graft greater than 5 cm in length

The August 1999 issue of *CPT Assistant*[3] addressed the question of whether code 54111 includes obtaining a graft. The guideline provided was this:

When procurement (harvest) of the graft is separately performed, this procedure may be reported in addition to code 54111 Excision of penile plaque (Peyronie disease); with graft to 5 cm in length. Graft procurement may occur from multiple sources (eg, fascia, tunic of testis, and cadaver sources). When the autogenous graft

is obtained through a separate incision, this procedure is separately reported; for example, code 20920 may be reported for procuring a fascia graft, or code 20926 may be reported for obtaining the tunic of testis for grafting. Placement of the autograft or allograft is an inclusive component of code 54111. Closure of the donor site is included in codes 20900-20938, and is not separately reported.

Interpretation

The code for harvesting the graft may be billed additionally if the graft is procured by making a separate incision to reach the site of the donor graft material. So, a patient has excision of a penile plaque followed at the same session by a fascia graft obtained from a cadaver donor. Only CPT code 54111 or 54112 would be coded. No additional code would be used if the graft is obtained from a cadaver. On the other hand, another patient has excision of a penile plaque followed in the same surgical session by a fascia graft obtained from the patient's left leg. CPT code 54111 or 54112 plus the harvesting code should be billed, because the graft is obtained through a separate incision from the patient undergoing the excision.

Hypospadias repair with skin graft

54332 One stage proximal penile or penoscrotal hypospadias repair requiring extensive dissection to correct chordee and urethroplasty by use of skin graft tube and/or island flap

In the September 2004 issue of *CPT Assistant*,[4] the appropriateness of reporting the flap code 15740 in conjunction with the hypospadias repair code 54332 was addressed:

From a CPT coding perspective, since the descriptor of code *54332, One stage proximal penile or penoscrotal hypospadias repair requiring extensive dissection to correct chordee and urethroplasty by use of skin graft tube and/or island flap*, states that the hypospadias repair is performed by use of skin graft tube and/or island flap, the island flap would be considered an integral component and would not be reported separately. Therefore, it would not be appropriate to report code *15740, Flap; island pedicle*, in addition to code 54332.

Interpretation

Unlike the plaque removal with skin graft, repair of hypospadias using a skin graft includes the harvesting of the skin graft. These guidelines are nuances that coders need to be very careful in understanding, researching, and applying. Reading *CPT Assistant* and understanding the NCCI edits is important to accurate and optimal coding.

NCCI Guidelines Regarding Female Reproductive System and Maternity Services

> ### Excerpt From the Female Reproductive System Coding Policies Section of NCCI Guidelines[2(p10)]
>
> When a pelvic examination is performed in conjunction with a gynecologic procedure, either as a necessary part of the procedure or as a confirmatory examination, the pelvic examination is not separately reported. A diagnostic pelvic examination may be performed for the purposes of deciding to perform a procedure. This examination is included in the evaluation and management service at the time the decision to perform the procedure is made.

Interpretation

Never code a pelvic examination in addition to any other gynecologic procedures performed during the same encounter. If the procedure is planned, the pelvic examination becomes a part of the approach (see Chapter 2 regarding surgical site exploration) and not separately reportable. If the procedure is unplanned, and the pelvic examination is part of the diagnostic process, it is most likely incidental to a more comprehensive examination and would be included in the evaluation and management (E/M) code provided on that date of service. The pelvic examination is either bundled into the procedure with which it is performed or bundled into the E/M service with which it is affiliated. To illustrate, a patient has a planned colposcopy during which the physician performs a preliminary pelvic examination before performing the colposcopy with biopsy. Do not code the pelvic examination separately from the colposcopy procedure.

> ### Excerpt From the Female Reproductive System Coding Policies Section of NCCI Guidelines[2(p10)]
>
> All surgical laparoscopic, hysteroscopic or peritoneoscopic procedures include diagnostic procedures.

Interpretation

Remember that coders must follow CPT codebook instructions, and CPT guidelines direct that all diagnostic scope procedures (endoscopies, laparoscopies, hysteroscopies, etc) are incidental to the surgical procedures when performed during the same session and in the same anatomic pathway. In the CPT codebook, most endoscopic CPT code range is preceded by this instruction: "Surgical laparoscopy always includes diagnostic laparoscopy."[1(p218,222,250)] Also, the diagnostic laparoscopy CPT code (see CPT code 49320) is designated as a separate procedure code; therefore, it would not be coded in addition to other, more major procedures performed during the same surgical session on the same anatomic pathway.

If there was a laparoscopically assisted vaginal hysterectomy, it includes the diagnostic laparoscopy as part of the approach for the procedure. The laparoscopy should not be coded separately.

> ### Excerpt From the Female Reproductive System Coding Policies Section of NCCI Guidelines[2(p10)]
>
> Pelvic examination under anesthesia (CPT code 57410) is included in all major and most minor gynecological procedures and not separately reportable. This procedure represents routine evaluation of the surgical field.

Interpretation

As mentioned in the section on the nonanesthetic pelvic examination, this service should never be coded in addition to any other gynecologic procedures performed during the same encounter. NCCI edits bundle the pelvic examination under anesthesia (CPT code 57410) into almost every other gynecologic procedure.

One basic instruction within NCCI is that the surgical approach, including identification of anatomical landmarks, incision, and *evaluation of the surgical field*, is incidental to the primary surgery and should not be coded separately.

> ### Excerpt From the Female Reproductive System Coding Policies Section of NCCI Guidelines[2(p10)]
>
> Dilation of vagina or cervix (CPT codes 57400 or 57800), when done in conjunction with vaginal approach procedures, is not reported separately unless the CPT code descriptor states "without cervical dilation."

Interpretation

The dilation of the vagina or cervix becomes an inherent part of the primary procedure. Anything performed to visualize or access a body part is inherent in the primary procedure and should not be coded separately from the primary procedure. If the dilation is necessary in order to access the specific body part during a surgery, the dilation is an inherent part of the primary procedure approach and is, therefore, not separately coded. For example, during a vaginal hysterectomy (CPT code 58260) the physician must dilate the cervix to allow access for removal of the uterus. The dilation is not for a distinct therapeutic reason, and the hysterectomy code does not exclude the dilation service.

Excerpt From the Female Reproductive System Coding Policies Section of NCCI Guidelines[2(p10)]

Colposcopy (CPT codes 56820, 57420, 57452) should not be reported separately when performed as a "scout" procedure to confirm the lesion or to assess the surgical field prior to a surgical procedure. A diagnostic colposcopy resulting in the decision to perform a non-colposcopic procedure may be reported with modifier -58. Diagnostic colposcopies (56820, 57420, 57452) are not separately reportable with other colposcopic procedures.

Interpretation

This is a reminder that coders must follow CPT codebook instructions, and CPT guidelines direct that all diagnostic endoscopies are incidental to the surgical endoscopy when performed during the same session and within the same anatomic pathway[5]. For the colposcopy, remember that NCCI includes identification of landmarks as a part of the surgical approach (as noted in the standards of medical/surgical practice). A scout scope procedure is for landmark identification (looking at the lay of the land) and not for diagnosing or treating. It is a complementary component of the primary procedure. The CMS distinguishes a scout scope procedure from a diagnostic scope procedure, which is an important principle in NCCI guidelines. If a truly diagnostic scope procedure is necessary before an open therapeutic procedure, the diagnostic scope procedure may be separately coded, as long as the scope procedure is truly diagnostic (the decision for the therapeutic open procedure is made based on the findings of the scope procedure). The physician's documentation must be very clear that the service is supported as diagnostic. The scope procedure is not separately coded if the physician:

- knows prior to the scope procedure what therapeutic open procedure is going to be performed or
- has already performed a diagnostic scope procedure or
- goes on to perform a therapeutic scope procedure.

Excerpt From the Female Reproductive System Coding Policies Section of NCCI Guidelines[2(p11)]

Laparoscopic lysis of adhesions (CPT codes 44180 or 58660) is not separately reportable with other surgical laparoscopic procedures.

Interpretation

Remember that lysis of adhesions is a standard of care and should not be separately coded unless circumstances (extensive lysis of adhesions) are met. The lysis is also not separately distinguishable from the primary procedure, because it was integral to the approach, or access to the operative site. For example, a patient presents for an abdominal hysterectomy, and during the approach (abdominal incision) to reach the uterus, the surgeon encounters significant adhesions, which were lysed, and the hysterectomy is then performed. Unless the surgeon documents the additional work (time and effort) lysing the adhesions, no additional coding or modifier is appropriate, and only the hysterectomy would be coded.

Coding for Maternity Care and Delivery Services

Excerpt From the Maternity Care and Delivery Services Coding Policies Section of NCCI[2(p11)]

The total obstetrical packages (eg, CPT codes 59400 and 59510) include antepartum care, the delivery, and postpartum care. They do not include among other services, ultrasound, amniocentesis, special screening tests for genetic conditions, visits for unrelated conditions (incidental to pregnancy) or additional and frequent visits due to high risk conditions.

Interpretation

If the pregnant patient needs more than routine care during the antepartum, delivery, or postpartum period, those nonroutine services may be coded in addition to the usual care. NCCI guidelines point out specific services not included in the antepartum/delivery/postpartum care, as mentioned earlier (eg, ultrasound, amniocentesis). It is probably a good idea to highlight in the CPT codebook those services that are separately billable.

Example

Which of the following are part of the maternity global care and which are not?

A patient who was seeing the physician for routine maternity care:

a. needed an amniocentesis.
b. fell and had vaginal bleeding.
c. was 47 years old and was diabetic.
d. came in for her monthly routine check up for the pregnancy.

Answer: All but *d* above would be billed in addition to the global maternity care, because they include care that is not part of standard care.

Excerpt From American College of Obstetricians and Gynecologists[6] (ACOG) web Site

ACOG's position is that the repair of first and second degree lacerations are not to be reported separately. However, third and fourth degree lacerations extend beyond the perineum into areas such as the rectum and anus. Since these repairs require significant additional physician work, they are separately reportable.

ACOG's Coding Committee recommends the following two options for reporting complete third and fourth degree lacerations repair:

Option 1:
Append the modifier 22 (increased procedural services) to the appropriate delivery or global package code. Documentation describing the extent of the injury should be submitted with the claim.

Option 2:
Depending on whether the repair is intermediate or complex, the physician can report a CPT-4 code from the Integumentary series, 12041–12047 (repair intermediate) or 13131–13133 (repair complex). The appropriate repair code would be reported in addition to the delivery or global package code.

Note: If the physician who performs these repairs is not the physician who delivered the baby, report CPT-4 code 59300 (Episiotomy or vaginal repair, by other than attending physician) instead.

Excerpt From the Maternity Care and Delivery System Coding Policies Section of NCCI[2(p11)]

CPT codes 59050 and 59051 (fetal monitoring during labor), 59300 (episiotomy) and 59414 (delivery of placenta) are included in CPT codes 59400 (routine obstetric care, vaginal delivery), 59409 (vaginal delivery only), 59410 (vaginal delivery and postpartum care), 59510 (routine obstetric care, cesarean delivery), 59514 (cesarean delivery only), 59515 (cesarean delivery and postpartum care), 59610 (routine obstetric care, vaginal delivery, after previous cesarean delivery), 59612 (vaginal delivery only after previous cesarean delivery), 59614 (vaginal delivery and postpartum care after previous cesarean delivery), 59618 (routine obstetric care, cesarean delivery, after previous cesarean delivery), 59620 (cesarean delivery only after previous cesarean delivery), and 59622 (cesarean delivery and postpartum care after previous cesarean delivery). They are not to be separately reportable.

Interpretation

All other procedures and services may be coded in addition to the delivery services, except for these specific procedures:

- Fetal monitoring during labor
- Episiotomy
- Delivery of placenta

Each of these services is included in the delivery codes identified in the NCCI edits.

Take, for example, a physician performing a vaginal delivery after providing all antepartum care for the mother. Additionally, the physician will continue routine postpartum care. During the vaginal delivery of the baby, an episiotomy is required to assist in the delivery, and the baby requirs fetal monitoring.

59400 Routine obstetric care including antepartum care, vaginal delivery (with or without episiotomy, and/or forceps) and postpartum care

This code would be the only one used for the entire maternity care as long as no complications were addressed. The CPT code includes in its description the episiotomy but not the fetal monitoring. However, knowing that the NCCI guidelines include the monitoring, coders should not code that service in addition to CPT code 59400.
Note: Fetal monitoring by a consulting physician may be coded with CPT code 59050 or CPT code 59051.

59050 Fetal monitoring during labor by consulting physician (ie, non-attending physician) with written report; supervision and interpretation

59051 interpretation only

SUMMARY

- The entire male/female reproductive system section from the NCCI manual should be read.

- Cystourethroscopy, with biopsy(s) (CPT code 52204) includes all biopsies during the procedure and should be reported with one unit of service.

- A pelvic examination under anesthesia is reported using code 57410. A pelvic examination performed without anesthesia is not coded separately; it is included in the evaluation and management code reported for the visit.

- Remember that lysis of adhesions is a standard of care and should not be separately coded unless circumstances (extensive lysis of adhesions) are met. The lysis is also not separately distinguishable from the primary procedure, because it was integral to the approach, or access to the operative site.

Definitions and Acronyms

dilation and curettage (D&C): This procedure is used to suction away the lining of the uterus and take tissue samples by dilating the entrance to the uterus and then scraping the uterus.

hydrocele: A fluid-filled sac that surrounds a testicle and results in swelling of the scrotum.

pelvic examination: Physical examination of the female reproductive organs. A speculum is inserted into the vagina to enable the physician to examine the vagina and cervix. The examination usually includes palpation of the ovaries as well.

CHAPTER EXERCISES

EXERCISE 1

Preoperative diagnosis: Moderate dysplasia of the cervix with human papillomavirus effect.

Postoperative diagnosis: Moderate dysplasia of the cervix with human papillomavirus effect.

Operation: Conization of the cervix.

Anesthesia: General.

History: The patient is a 29-year-old female with recurrent cervical dysplasia after colposcopy confirmed moderate dysplasia with human papillomavirus effect. A repeat Pap smear after the colposcopy remained the same; therefore, the conization of the cervix was indicated.

Procedures: Under general anesthesia, the patient was put in the dorsal lithotomy position. The skin over the abdomen, perineum, and the vagina were prepared with iodophor solution and draped in the usual fashion. The uterus was normal in size, anteverted. There was no adnexal mass. The cervix was slightly eroded on the lower portion, so a tenaculum was used to grasp the anterior lip of the cervix.

A loop electrocautery excision procedure large loop was used at 45 watt setting, and, with one sweep, a well-formed cone shape of the cervix was removed. The endocervical area also was done, and coagulation was done by cautery. There was no bleeding noted.

The patient tolerated the entire procedure well. Estimated blood loss was scanty. The patient was transferred to the recovery room in stable condition.

What would be coded in this case and why?

EXERCISE 2

Operative procedure: Circumcision

Preoperative diagnosis: Phimosis

Postoperative diagnosis: Same

Anesthesia: General

Estimated blood loss: None

Complications: None

Drains: None

Specimens: Foreskin to pathology

Indications: Eleven-year-old male with phimosis, which is symptomatic and requires circumcision.

Findings: Phimosis

Procedures: The patient was taken to the operating room. After the induction of general anesthesia, he was placed in the supine position and prepped and draped in the usual sterile fashion.

The foreskin was able to be retracted after the patient was asleep, and the glans was also prepped. After draping, the foreskin was retracted, and the frenulum was found to be tethering the glans. **We dissected out the frenulum, divided and cauterized this very carefully, straightening out the penis. We then made a circumferential incision approximately 1 cm proximal to the glans, with the foreskin retracted; we took this through the skin. We then replaced the foreskin in its normal position and made a mirror-image circumferential incision around the coronal sulcus.** We connected both incisions sharply and sharply removed the foreskin. We then achieved meticulous hemostasis with electrocautery. We took great care to avoid injury to the deep structures or the urethra.

After satisfactory hemostasis, we approximated the skin with 4-0 chromic interrupted sutures with a U-stitch ventrally.

The patient tolerated the procedure well and was transferred to the recovery area in good condition.

What would be coded in this case and why?

ANSWERS TO CHAPTER EXERCISES

Exercise 1:

57522 Conization of cervix, with or without fulguration, with or without dilation and curettage, with or without repair; loop electrode excision

Comment: There is no indication of a colposcopy during this procedure.

Exercise 2:

54161 Circumcision, surgical excision other than clamp, device, or dorsal slit; older than 28 days of age

Comment: The incision is part of the approach and not separately coded. Hemostasis and suturing are part of the procedure closure and not separately coded.

REFERENCES

1. American Medical Association. *Current Procedural Terminology (CPT®) Professional Edition 2009.* Chicago, IL: American Medical Association; 2008.

2. Centers for Medicare and Medicaid Services. "Chapter VII Surgery: Urinary, Male Genital, Female Genital, Maternity Care and Delivery Systems." In: NCCI Policy Manual for Medicare Services. www.cms.hhs.gov/NationalCorrectCodInitEd/01_overview.asp#TopOfPage. Accessed June 12, 2009.

3. American Medical Association. "Coding consultation, male genital system, 54111, (Q&A)." *CPT Assistant,* 1999;9(8):5.

4. American Medical Association. "Coding consultation, integumentary system, 15740, 54332 (Q&A)." *CPT Assistant,* 2004;14(9):12.

5. American Medical Association. "Coding communication, female genital system, endoscopy codes." *CPT Assistant,* 2003;13(2):5.

6. American College of Obstetricians and Gynecologists. *Repair of lacerations following delivery.* www.acog.org/departments/dept_notice.cfm?recno=6&bulletin=4645. Accessed June 12, 2009.

The Nervous System

Chapter 13 provides background about the nervous system, reviews the National Correct Coding Initiative (NCCI) coding guidelines for procedures performed on the nervous system, and provides examples to reflect the logic behind the edits. As with the other chapters, this chapter provides an NCCI guideline followed by our interpretation, an example, or both.

The first rule in correct coding is to understand the service or procedure being coded. Without the clinical knowledge or understanding of a service or procedure, it is difficult to correctly code the service or decide if a bundling edit should be bypassed. Coders should remember to read all the instructions within that section (eg, nervous system) of the *Current Procedural Terminology* (CPT®)[1] codebook and refer to it for additional instructions. The NCCI guidelines should also be reviewed to make sure information is being coded correctly, optimally, and compliantly.

The Nervous System and NCCI Guidelines

Excerpt From the Nervous System Section of NCCI Guidelines[2(p2)]

Introduction
The principles of correct coding discussed in Chapter I apply to the CPT codes in the range 61000-64999. Several general guidelines are repeated in this Chapter. However, those general guidelines from Chapter I not discussed in this Chapter are nonetheless applicable.

Interpretation

This instruction indicates that the overall NCCI guidelines apply to each section of the CPT codebook, and, even if they are not repeated within a chapter, they are nonetheless a guideline to be followed. The introductory guidelines were reviewed comprehensively in Chapter 2 of this book; however, those introductory guidelines that have clear application within the nervous system are reiterated in this chapter.

Excerpt From the General Correct Coding Policies Section of NCCI[3(p10)]

Exposure and exploration of the surgical field is integral to an operative procedure and is not separately reportable. If exploration of the surgical field results in additional procedures other than the primary procedure, the additional procedures may generally be reported separately. However, a procedure designated by the CPT code descriptor as a "separate procedure" is not separately reportable if performed in a region anatomically related to the other procedure(s) through the same skin incision, orifice, or surgical approach.

Interpretation

Approaches, access, and explorations for procedures are always bundled into the primary procedure and not separately coded. Because invasive procedures require the physician to reach the body part, the access (or approach) does not add to the physician's work sufficiently to warrant an additional code. Also, during the procedure the surgeon should assess the entire surgical field to decide the best route for approach, determine the extent of the condition (disease, injury), and determine whether any other procedures are needed. All of these services are usual for an invasive procedure and are not separately coded. However, if during the exploration, the surgeon determined that another procedure was needed, the additional procedure should be coded unless bundled into the primary procedure for other reasons (separate procedure, NCCI edits, etc). For example, in performing a discectomy, the physician must create a small incision to view the vertebra and disc. The incision and any exploration are included in the discectomy code. Also, in a transcranial decompression of the orbit, the approach is through a transfrontal craniotomy, which is necessary for removal of the roof of the orbit. Therefore, transcranial decompression of the orbit would include the craniotomy for access.

CPT Coding Tip: Within the nervous system section of the CPT surgery section, there is an exception to that rule. For skull-based tumors, the approach is coded separately and in addition to the root operation and the closure. Because these procedures often require the skill of different specialists (ear, nose, and throat; neurosurgery; orthopaedics; etc), the coding was established to allow the different surgeons to capture their portions of the procedure without having to code as co-surgeons or team surgeons. In coding for skull-based tumors, read the CPT codebook guidelines carefully to ensure proper coding for each surgeon involved.

Excerpt From the Nervous System Section of NCCI Guidelines[2(p4)]

A burr hole is often necessary for intracranial surgery (e.g., craniotomy, craniectomy), to access intracranial contents, to alleviate pressure, or to place an intracranial pressure monitoring device. When this service is integral to the performance of other services, CPT codes describing this service are not separately reportable if performed at the same patient encounter. A burr hole is separately reportable with another cranial procedure only if performed at a separate site unrelated to the other cranial procedure or at a separate patient encounter on the same date of service.

Interpretation

A burr hole is a small opening in the skull made with a surgical drill. If this procedure is necessary in order to perform a more major procedure of the same site on the skull, the burr hole becomes a part of the surgical approach of the more major procedure and is not separately billed. Likewise, if the burr hole is performed to either alleviate pressure as a part of the preparation for an intracranial procedure or to place a monitoring device before surgery, the burr hole creation is still an inherent part of the primary procedure.

If the burr hole is done at a separate surgical session in preparation for the later surgery, both services may be billed, and the subsequent procedure should be appended with modifier 58 (staged/related procedure). Bottom line: if

performed during the same surgical session as another, more major procedure of the same site, the burr hole is included in coding of the other procedure. If the burr hole procedure is performed at a separate session, modifier 58 may be appended to the subsequent procedure.

A burr hole is also performed for therapeutic reasons, perhaps to remove a subdural hematoma or obtain a biopsy specimen. These services are not for access but rather for treatment and may be coded separately.

For instance, a patient presents for a craniotomy for treatment of an aneurysm. During the procedure (performed under general anesthesia), the patient's head is shaved over the area of the surgical incision. An incision is made and the scalp pulled back for access to the cranium, where burr holes are made prior to opening of a flap of skull. The dura mater is then opened, an operating microscope is brought in and the brain accessed, dissecting down to the site of the aneurysm. The aneurysm is dissected and a clip placed across the neck of the aneurysm. The dura is closed, then the skull is closed (using a titanium plate), then the scalp is closed. The burr holes in this case were made simply to assist in accessing the patient's brain and would not be coded separately.

In a different situation, a burr hole is made for a subdural hematoma to remove a hemorrhage (blood clot) from the surface of the brain. The blood clot is beneath the dura mater (subdural). The head is partially shaved to expose the area of operation, and the area is then "prepped and draped" using an antibiotic solution. The surgeon makes an incision and pulls back the scalp over the area of the hematoma. Then, an air-powered drill is used to make a hole in the skull. The dura mater is opened, the hematoma is exposed, and the surgeon irrigates it out and passes a drain around the brain to provide postoperative drainage. The surgeon closes the scalp. In this case, the burr holes were the treatment and should be coded.

61108 Twist drill hole(s) for subdural, intracerebral, or ventricular puncture; for evacuation and/or drainage of subdural hematoma

---

Excerpt From the Nervous System Section of NCCI Guidelines[2(p4)]

In addition, taps, punctures or burr holes accompanied by drainage procedures (e.g., hematoma, abscess, cyst, etc.) followed by other procedures are not separately reportable unless performed as staged procedures. Modifier -58 may be used to indicate staged or planned services. Many intracranial procedures include bone grafts by CPT definition and these grafts should not be reported separately.

Interpretation

This guideline needs to be extracted a bit to make following the logic easier. If the puncture and drainage is performed in conjunction with another procedure on the same body site, the puncture/drainage is incidental to the more major procedure and should not be separately coded unless it is a staged procedure. The drainage is most likely incidental (a byproduct) of the more major procedure. Going back to an earlier example, a patient presents for a craniotomy for treatment of an aneurysm; however, there is also a suspected subdural hematoma. The surgeon can access the aneurysm site over the site of the hematoma and drain the hematoma as well as repair the aneurysm. During the procedure (performed under general anesthesia), the patient's head is shaved over the area of the surgical incision. An incision is made and the scalp pulled back for access to the cranium, where burr holes are made prior to opening a flap of skull. The hematoma is drained at that point prior to continuing down to the site of the aneurysm. The drainage of the hematoma becomes incidental to the aneurysm repair and is not separately reported.

A staged/related procedure would be coded when the puncture/drainage was performed first, and it was determined that a more extensive procedure would be done later. When the later procedure is performed, that procedure may be coded with modifier 58. So, a burr hole for drainage is done, and later that day the patient has severe head pain, and the surgeon decides to perform a craniotomy exploration. The craniotomy is a staged procedure, and both services may be coded.

Excerpt From the Nervous System Section of NCCI Guidelines[2(p4)]

Biopsies performed in the course of Central Nervous System (CNS) surgery should not be reported as separate procedures.

Interpretation

This guideline offers little leeway, but remember that if a biopsy is performed on a different and distinct site, it is separately reportable. This situation may be reported with modifier -59. In all other circumstances, the biopsy would not be coded separately from the CNS surgery as long as it is in the same course (tract, path, route, site). For instance, if a biopsy is performed during a craniectomy for excision of a bone lesion, the biopsy is incidental to the excision. If however, the biopsy was a percutaneous biopsy of the spinal cord during the same session as the craniectomy, these would obviously be separate and distinct sites, and both

the biopsy and craniectomy could be coded. No modifier should be necessary, because these are clearly distinct surgical sites, and the codes do not currently bundle together.

Excerpt From the Nervous System Section of NCCI Guidelines[2(p4)]

Craniotomies and craniectomies always include a general exploration of the accessible field. An exploratory craniectomy or craniotomy (CPT codes 61304 or 61305) should not be reported separately with another craniectomy/craniotomy procedure performed at the same anatomic site and same patient encounter.

Interpretation

NCCI general coding concepts (see complete discussion in Chapter 2 of this book) note that surgery CPT codes include the surgical approach. The approach includes identification of anatomical landmarks, incision, *evaluation of the surgical field*, debridement of traumatized tissue, and so forth. Therefore, the surgical exploration should not be separately coded from the craniotomy or craniectomy procedures. For example, a surgeon plans to implant a subdural electrode array via a craniotomy. After making the incision, the surgeon explores the surgical field to determine the best method and route to proceed.

In this case, the exploration of the surgical field is incidental to the craniotomy procedure and should not be coded separately. CPT code 61533 would be the only code necessary.

61533 Craniotomy with elevation of bone flap; for subdural implantation of an electrode array, for long-term seizure monitoring

---

Excerpt From the Nervous System Section of NCCI Guidelines[2(p5)]

A craniotomy is performed through a skull defect resulting from reflection of a skull flap. Replacing the skull flap during the same procedure is an integral component of a craniotomy procedure and should not be reported separately utilizing the cranioplasty CPT codes 62140 and 62141. A cranioplasty may be separately reportable with a craniotomy procedure if the cranioplasty is performed to replace a skull bone flap removed during a procedure at a prior patient encounter or if the cranioplasty is performed to repair a skull defect larger than that created by the bone flap.

Interpretation

Remember from our general NCCI coding edits discussion (see Chapter 2) that operative site closure and dressings are included in the global surgery reimbursement and should not be separately coded from the primary procedure. Therefore, if a bone flap that was pulled back to gain access to the main surgical site was replaced at the conclusion of the procedure, the replacement serves as part of the closure of the surgical site and should not be separately coded. If the bone flap was performed at a subsequent patient encounter, it may be coded with either a modifier 58 (staged) or 59 (separate and distinct). If the bone flap was required to repair a wound site that was more extensive than the original incision, the bone flap may be coded separately. Each of these would need to be clearly and comprehensively documented to be billed additionally.

As an example, a surgeon is performing a craniectomy for decompression of the medulla with a dural graft. During the procedure a bone flap is retracted for exposure to the skull where the incision for the craniectomy begins. At the conclusion of the surgery, the bone flap is replaced and fixed, and the scalp is closed.

The bone flap was removed for access, and the closure was the usual closure for this procedure; therefore, the bone flap closure is incidental to the primary procedure and not separately coded.

On the other hand, a patient presents with a defect in the skull remaining after a prior intracranial procedure. The surgeon repairs the site with a cranioplasty using an autogenous graft. In this scenario, the repair is not the closure of a surgical wound site immediately on conclusion of the surgery. Rather, the repair is to repair a prior (outside of the immediate surgical session) surgical wound. This repair could be coded.

Excerpt From the Nervous System Section of NCCI Guidelines[2(p5)]

The use of general intravascular access devices (e.g., intravenous lines, etc.), cardiac monitoring, oximetry, laboratory sample procurement and other routine monitoring for patient safety has been addressed in the previous policy for general anesthesia or monitored anesthesia care (MAC), or other anesthesia are included in the anesthesia service and are not separately reportable. For example, if a physician performs a spinal puncture for intrathecal injection and administers an anxiolytic agent, the vascular access and any appropriate monitoring is considered part of the spinal puncture procedure and is not separately reportable.

Interpretation

Often when providers are performing spinal injections, there is a need for monitoring the patient and perhaps having some vascular access. This policy states that any necessary components of that service are inherent in the code for the primary procedure and should not be billed separately. To recap from Chapters 2 and 4:

- When a provider codes for anesthesia, all aspects of the anesthesia are included in the anesthesia CPT code. Services inherent in performing anesthesia are not separately billable unless they are clearly unrelated to the anesthesia service. Do not code these separately.
- If the physician who performed a surgery also provided the anesthesia services for the surgery, separate CPT codes for the anesthesia may not be used. The anesthesia is included in the surgery when performed by the same physician.

Excerpt From the Nervous System Section of NCCI Guidelines[2(p6)]

When a spinal puncture is performed, the local anesthesia necessary to perform the spinal puncture is included in the procedure. The reporting of nerve block or facet block CPT codes for anesthesia for a diagnostic or therapeutic lumbar puncture is inappropriate.

Interpretation

When a physician performs a spinal puncture, there may be a need for a local anesthetic to be administered at the site of the puncture to deaden the area prior to the puncture. When the anesthetic is given solely as the anesthetic for the primary procedure (eg, puncture), the anesthesia is included in the primary procedure reimbursement and should not be separately coded. Again, if the physician who is performing a surgery also provides the anesthesia services for the surgery, separate CPT codes for the anesthesia may not be used. The anesthesia is included in the surgery when performed by the same physician.

Excerpt From the Nervous System Section of NCCI Guidelines[2(p6)]

If cerebrospinal fluid is withdrawn during a nerve block procedure, the withdrawal is not separately reportable (e.g., diagnostic lumbar puncture). It is integral to the nerve block procedure.

Interpretation

A very important principle is highlighted here. This guideline points out that coders should understand the purpose of the procedural session and code, then focus on any additional services provided and determine whether they are separately billable.

Aspiration of cerebrospinal fluid (CSF) does not support that the intention of the service was for CSF specimen collection. Rather, if the planned procedure was a facet injection that incidentally resulted in CSF aspiration, do not code the spinal puncture. The injection is the code to be billed. Basically, this tells coders to code the primary procedure and not to code those services that are incidental to the primary procedure.

> **CPT Coding Tip:** An incidental procedure is one carried out at the same time as a more complex primary procedure. An incidental procedure requires minimal additional physician resources, is clinically part of the primary procedure, and should not be billed separately.

Excerpt From the Nervous System Section of NCCI Guidelines[2(p6)]

If a dural (cerebrospinal fluid) leak occurs during a spinal procedure, repair of the dural leak is integral to the spinal procedure. CPT code 63707 or 63709 (repair of dural/cerebrospinal fluid leak) should not be reported separately for the repair.

Interpretation

If a dural (cerebrospinal fluid) leak occurs during a spinal procedure, repair of the dural leak is integral to the spinal procedure. CPT code 63707 or 63709 (repair of dural/cerebrospinal fluid leak) should not be reported separately for the repair. So, a patient presents for a spinal puncture, and a leak in the dura is created during the approach to the procedure. The leak is repaired. Only the spinal puncture should be coded. The repair of the leak is integral to the puncture and would not be coded additionally.

Excerpt From the Nervous System Section of NCCI Guidelines[2(p6)]

CPT code 29848 describes endoscopic release of the transverse carpal ligament of the wrist. CPT code 64721 describes a neuroplasty and/or transposition of the median nerve at the carpal tunnel and includes open release of the transverse carpal ligament. The procedure coded as CPT code 64721 includes the procedure coded as CPT code 29848 when performed on the same wrist at the same patient encounter. If an endoscopic procedure is converted to an open procedure, only the open procedure may be reported.

Interpretation

This guideline has several components; however, the primary point is: Never code an arthroscopic repair of a carpal tunnel with an open repair of a carpal tunnel for the same wrist during a single surgical session. If a procedure using one approach fails and is converted to a procedure using a different approach, only the successful procedure may be reported. Providers want to approach a procedure with the greatest probability of success and the least trauma to the patient. As a result, many times procedures are successfully completed using endoscopic methods, avoiding the need for a more invasive method. However, on occasion during the procedure, the provider determines that the success of the procedure will be improved by converting to an open procedure. This guideline in NCCI states that when a failed approach is followed during the same surgical session by successful approach for a single procedure, only the successful procedure may be coded. Basically, only one approach (the most successful one) will be paid for a single procedure. Therefore, if a physician attempts a carpal tunnel release through an arthroscopic approach but has to convert to an open procedure to successfully perform the repair, only the open approach should be billed. The failed procedure is incidental to the successful procedure.

Nerve repairs by suture or neurorrhaphies (CPT codes 64831-64876) include suture and anastomosis of nerves when performed to correct traumatic injury to or anastomosis of nerves which are proximally associated (e.g., facial-spinal, facial-hypoglossal, etc.). When neurorrhaphy is performed with a nerve graft (CPT codes 64885-64911), neuroplasty, transection, excision, neurectomy, excision of neuroma, etc., the neurorrhaphy is integral to the procedure and is not separately reportable.

Interpretation

Suturing a nerve is coded when suturing is the primary repair. This would occur for traumatic injuries when a nerve is being sutured closed or when a nerve is severed and being anastomosed (reconnected at two ends). When a nerve is being sutured in conjunction with other nerve procedures (neuroma excision or neuroplasty, for example), the neurorrhaphy is for closure and is an inherent part of the primary procedure. Do not code this neurorrhaphy separately.

To illustrate these points, take a patient who presents with a large, deep laceration on her arm, requiring nerve repair by suturing. This surgery would be coded as a neurorrhaphy. However, if a patient presents with a neuroma on her fourth finger. The physician excises the neuroma and creates a slight laceration in the nerve when removing the neuroma. At the conclusion of the procedure, the physician sutures the nerve for closure. This surgery would be coded as an excision of a neuroma, and the neurorrhaphy would not be coded additionally. The closure is inherent in the excision.

Implantation of neurostimulator electrodes in an area of the cerebral cortex may not be reported with two codes describing different approaches. CPT code 61860 describes implantation by craniectomy or craniotomy. CPT code 61850 describes implantation by twist drill or burr hole(s).

Interpretation

Remember from Chapter 2 of this book the NCCI guidelines stating that an excision and removal (-ectomy) includes the incision and opening (-otomy) of the organ. A Healthcare Common Procedure Coding System (HCPCS)/CPT code for an -otomy procedure should not be reported with an -ectomy code for the same organ. An excision and removal (-ectomy) includes the incision and opening (-otomy) of the organ. Also, the general coding guidelines from Chapter 2 state that multiple approaches to the same procedure are mutually exclusive of one another and should not be reported separately.

Here are a few of the neurostimulator CPT codes:

61850 Twist drill or burr hole(s) for implantation of neurostimulator electrodes, cortical

61860 Craniectomy or craniotomy for implantation of neurostimulator electrodes, cerebral, cortical

61870 Craniectomy for implantation of neurostimulator electrodes, cerebellar; cortical

The less invasive approach becomes incidental to the more invasive approach when they are performed during a single operative session. The CPT codebook often describes groups of similar codes differing in the complexity of the service. Unless services are performed at separate patient encounters or at separate anatomic sites, the less complex service is included in the more complex service and is not separately reportable. Only the most complex procedure performed during a single encounter on a single anatomic site may be coded. The lesser services are incidental to the more complex procedure.

A laminectomy includes excision of all the posterior vertebral components, and a laminotomy includes partial excision of posterior vertebral components. Since a laminectomy is a more extensive procedure than a laminotomy, a laminotomy code should not be reported with a laminectomy code for the same vertebra. CPT codes 22100-22103 (partial excision of posterior vertebral component (e.g., spinous process, lamina, or facet) for intrinsic bony lesion) are not separately reportable with laminectomy or laminotomy procedures for the same vertebra.

Interpretation

This guideline indicates that, when performed on the same spinal segment, partial excisions of vertebral components are incidental to the laminotomy/laminectomy services. Additionally, laminotomies are incidental to laminectomies when they are performed on the same lamina.

Excerpt From the Nervous System Section of NCCI Guidelines[2(p7-8)]

Some procedures (e.g., intracranial, spinal) utilize intraoperative neurophysiology testing. Intraoperative neurophysiology testing (CPT code 95920) should not be reported by the physician performing an operative procedure since it is included in the global package. The physician performing an operative procedure should report other 90000 neurophysiology testing codes for intraoperative neurophysiology testing (e.g., CPT codes 92585, 95822, 95860, 95861, 95867, 95868, 95870, 95900, 95904, 95925-95937) since they are also included in the global package. However, when performed by a different physician during the procedure, intraoperative neurophysiology testing is separately reportable by the second physician.

Interpretation

Intraoperative neurophysiologic monitoring (IONM) allows for monitoring of neurophysiologic signals during a surgical procedure whenever the neuroaxis is at risk as a consequence of either the surgical manipulation or the surgical environment. Code 95920 should not be reported by the surgeon or anesthesiologist performing an operative procedure, because it is included in the global package of the physician who serves as the IONM supervising physician. When IONM or baseline procedures are performed by a different, monitoring physician during the procedure, it is separately reportable by the monitoring supervising physician.

Excerpt From the Nervous System Section of NCCI Guidelines[2(p12)]

Medicare Global Surgery Rules prevent separate payment for postoperative pain management when provided by the physician performing an operative procedure. CPT codes 36000, 36410, 37202, 62318-62319, 64415-64417, 64450, 64470, 64475, and 90760-90775 describe some services that may be utilized for postoperative pain management. The services described by these codes may be reported by the physician performing the operative procedure only if provided for purposes unrelated to the postoperative pain management, the operative procedure, or anesthesia for the procedure.

Interpretation

Postoperative pain management performed by the surgeon would not be separately paid, as it is included in the global surgery package. See Chapter 3 of this book for additional information.

SUMMARY

- The entire nervous system section from the NCCI manual should be read.

- Approaches are bundled into primary procedures unless skull-based tumors are being removed.

Definitions and Acronyms

American Academy of Neurologists (AAN): The AAN (www.aan.com) is the national association of physicians who specialize in neurology. In addition to addressing clinical issues, the AAN also provides support for practice management, among which are resources for coding.

burr hole: A small opening in the skull made with a surgical drill.

central nervous system (CNS): The CNS is the part of the nervous system that includes the spinal cord and brain.

cerebrospinal fluid (CSF): CSF is the fluid that is contained within the CNS that helps to protect the brain and regulate pressures of the CNS. It is often sampled and used as a diagnostic tool.

craniectomy: An operation performed on the skull in which pieces of bone are removed and not replaced.

craniotomy: The surgical removal of a section of bone (bone flap) from the skull for the purpose of operating on the underlying tissues, usually the brain. The bone flap is replaced at the end of the procedure. If the bone flap is not replaced, the procedure is called a craniectomy.

discectomy: Excision of an intervertebral disk.

intraoperative neurosurgery monitoring (IONM): IONM is used during surgeries to monitor changes in the brain, spinal cord, and peripheral nerve function to catch problems before morbidity threatens. It can also be used to assist the surgeon in localizing anatomic sites.

CHAPTER EXERCISES

EXERCISE 1

For the following surgical note, determine whether the incision and closure may be coded in addition to the surgery.

Release of left carpal tunnel

Diagnosis: Bilateral carpal tunnel syndrome, left greater than right.

Operation: Release of left carpal tunnel.

After a successful axillary block was placed, the patient's left arm was prepared and draped in the usual sterile manner. A linear incision was made in the second crease in the left hand, after a local anesthetic had been injected, and this was taken down through that area, then curved slightly medially toward the hypothenar eminence, until it was approximately 1 cm proximal to the wrist crease. Once this was done, the incision was taken with a knife through the skin and subcutaneous tissue. Hemostasis was achieved with bipolar cautery. The ligament was then identified, and this was cut through with a scissors, starting proximally and working distally, until the whole ligament was freed up. The nerve was identified, and this was noted to be in

continuity all the way through. The nerve was freed up, along the bands from this ligament. Once this was done and hemostasis was achieved, a few 2-0 Dexon stitches were placed in the subcutaneous tissue, and the skin was closed with interrupted 4-0 nylon.

EXERCISE 2

A patient presented for an endoscopic hemithyroidectomy and isthmusectomy. During the procedure, the surgeon performed electromyelogram monitoring and intraoperative neurophysiology monitoring. Can the monitoring be coded in addition to the surgery?

ANSWERS TO CHAPTER EXERCISES

Exercise 1: Neither the incision nor closure is unusual or complicated. They both are inherent in the carpal tunnel release.

Exercise 2: No. Because the monitoring was performed by the surgeon, no additional coding should be given for this service. Another physician would have to be called in for the monitoring to be billed.

REFERENCES

1. American Medical Association. *Current Procedural Terminology (CPT®) Professional Edition 2009.* Chicago, IL: American Medical Association; 2008.

2. Centers for Medicare and Medicaid Services. "Chapter VIII CH13 Surgery: Endocrine, Nervous, Eye and Ocular Adnexa, and Auditory Systems." In: NCCI Policy Manual for Medicare Services. www.cms.hhs.gov/NationalCorrectCodInitEd/01_overview.asp#TopOfPage. Accessed June 10, 2009.

3. Centers for Medicare and Medicaid Services. "Chapter I General Correct Coding Policies." In: NCCI Policy Manual for Medicare Services. www.cms.hhs.gov/NationalCorrectCodInitEd/01_overview.asp#TopOfPage. Accessed June 12, 2009.

Ophthalmology Services

Chapter 14 provides background about the human body's visual system, reviews the National Correct Coding Initiative (NCCI) coding guidelines for procedures performed on the eye, and provides examples to reflect the logic behind the edits. As with the other chapters, this chapter provides an NCCI guideline followed by our interpretation, an example, or both.

The first rule in correct coding is to understand the service or procedure being coded. Without the clinical knowledge or understanding of a service or procedure, it is difficult to correctly code the service or decide whether a bundling edit should be bypassed. Coders should remember to read all the instructions within that section (eg, eye and ocular adnexa) of the *Current Procedural Terminology* (*CPT*®)[1] codebook and refer to it for additional instructions. The NCCI guidelines should also be reviewed to make sure information is being coded correctly, optimally, and compliantly.

NCCI Guidelines and the Eye and Ocular Adnexa System

Excerpt From the Ophthalmology Section of NCCI Guidelines[2(p2)]

Introduction
The principles of correct coding discussed in Chapter 1 apply to the CPT codes in the range 60000-69999. Several general guidelines are repeated in this chapter some are not. However, those general guidelines from Chapter 1 not discussed in this chapter are nonetheless applicable.

Interpretation

These instructions indicate that the overall NCCI guidelines apply to each section of the CPT codebook, and, even if they are not repeated within a chapter, they are nonetheless a guideline to be followed. The introductory guidelines were reviewed comprehensively in Chapter 2 of this book; however, those introductory guidelines that have clear application within the ophthalmology services section are reiterated in this chapter.

Excerpt From the Ophthalmology Section of NCCI Guidelines[2(p8)]

When a subconjunctival injection (e.g., CPT code 68200) with local anesthetic is performed as part of a more extensive anesthetic procedure (e.g., peribulbar or retrobulbar block), the subconjunctival injection is not separately reportable. It is part of the anesthetic procedure and does not represent a separate service.

Interpretation

When a provider codes anesthesia, the anesthesia CPT code includes all inherent services. Do not separately bill services unless they are clearly unrelated to the anesthesia service. Peribulbar and retrobulbar blocks are eye anesthetic procedures that have replaced general anesthesia for many surgeries performed on the eye. These blocks anesthetize the conjunctival sac. When a subconjunctival injection is performed as a part of the anesthesia, the injection should not be coded in addition to the blocks.

On the other hand, a therapeutic subconjunctival injection (CPT code 68200) can be coded when the documentation clearly supports the therapeutic reasons for the injection (eg, injecting antibiotics to treat an infection). For example, if a patient presents severe lid retraction (where the lid pulls away from the surface of the eye) and the physician performs a subconjunctival injection of Botox to treat the retraction, this service would be coded as CPT code 68200 (subconjunctival injection). Notice that no anesthetic procedure is being coded.

Another example in which CPT code 68200 is reported is when a patient presents for eye surgery, with a peribulbar block for anesthesia. An intravenous cannula was inserted for venous access, if needed. The conjunctival sac was injected before the peribulbar block to anesthetize with amethocaine, and two transconjunctival peribulbar injections were performed. The patient was then prepared for surgery.

Two important points:

1. The subconjunctival injection is incidental to the anesthesia.
2. The anesthesia, if performed by someone other than the surgeon, is coded. If performed by the surgeon, the anesthesia is incidental to the surgery.

CPT Coding Tip: *Remember that anesthesia (other than monitored anesthesia care for certain procedures) provided by the operating surgeon is included in the payment for the surgery and not separately coded.*

Excerpt From the Ophthalmology Section of NCCI Guidelines[2(p8)]

Iridectomy and/or anterior vitrectomy may be performed in conjunction with cataract extraction. If an iridectomy is performed in order to complete a cataract extraction, it is an integral part of the procedure and is not separately reportable. Similarly, the minimal vitreous loss occurring during routine cataract extraction does not represent a vitrectomy and is not separately reportable. If an iridectomy or vitrectomy that is separate and distinct from the cataract extraction is performed for an unrelated reason at the same patient encounter, the iridectomy and/or vitrectomy may be reported separately with an NCCI-associated modifier. The medical record must document the distinct medical necessity for each procedure.

A trabeculectomy is separately reportable with a cataract extraction if performed for a purpose unrelated to the cataract extraction. For example, if a patient with glaucoma requires a cataract extraction and a trabeculectomy is the appropriate treatment for the glaucoma, the trabeculectomy may be separately reportable. However, performance of a trabeculectomy as a preventative service for an expected transient increase in intraocular pressure postoperatively, without other evidence for glaucoma, is not separately reportable.

Interpretation

Iridectomy: The CPT codebook provides instructions that iridectomy, iridotomy, canthotomy, and capsulotomy are included in cataract extraction services and should not be coded separately. However, NCCI also states that if there is a specific diagnosis for which the iridectomy is performed (separate from the cataract diagnosis), the iridectomy may be coded with a modifier 59.

Vitrectomy: NCCI clarifies that *incidental* vitrectomies are also included in the cataract extraction codes and should not be billed separately. To determine whether a vitrectomy is incidental, look for documentation that the physician intended to perform a vitrectomy in addition to the cataract extraction. There should be verbiage describing the vitrectomy portion of the procedure as opposed to the vitreous being incidentally drained or aspirated as a part of the cataract extraction. Additionally, a diagnosis warranting a vitrectomy should be provided within the operative report as well. If vitreous fluid is aspirated as an unintended result of the cataract extraction, then the vitrectomy should not be coded. For example, if in the documentation of a cataract extraction, the surgeon notes **minimal vitreous presented into the wound**, there is no *intended* vitrectomy and the vitreous is minimal. The vitrectomy should not be coded in this instance.

Trabeculectomy: A trabeculectomy is performed to treat glaucoma by reducing the pressure on the eye. The trabeculectomy may be performed during a cataract procedure, but it would still be performed to address the glaucoma. The trabeculectomy may be coded in addition to the cataract extraction with a modifier 59; however, a diagnosis of glaucoma should be present in the documentation.

Excerpt From the Ophthalmology Section of NCCI[2(p8)]

CPT codes describing cataract extraction (66830-66984) are mutually exclusive of one another. Only one code from this CPT code range may be reported for an eye.

Interpretation

This seems to be more of a coding guideline than a bundling issue. Basically, NCCI guidelines indicate that coders should use the code that most comprehensively and specifically represents the surgery performed. Rarely does a physician have to convert from one method to a different method during this type of surgery.

Providers want to approach a procedure with the greatest probability of success and the least trauma to the patient. As a result, they carefully plan the best approach and ultimate operation. However, on occasion during the procedure, the provider determines that the success of the procedure will be improved by converting to a different procedure. This guideline in NCCI states that only one (the successful one) cataract surgery should be coded during a single operative session involving one eye.

Some of the CPT codes for cataract extraction are:

66840 Removal of lens material; aspiration technique, 1 or more stages

Aspiration technique is through a vertical capsulotomy with a needle aspiration of the cataract.

66850 phacofragmentation technique (mechanical or ultrasonic) (eg, phacoemulsification), with aspiration

Phacoemulsification is where, through a small incision, localized high-frequency waves are generated through an instrument to break the cataract into small fragments and then vacuumed out.

66852 pars plana approach, with or without vitrectomy

66920 intracapsular

Intracapsular is to remove the lens and lens capsule in one piece.

66930 intracapsular, for dislocated lens

66940 extracapsular (other than 66840, 66850, 66852)

Extracapsular is removing the lens but leaving the capsule.

Excerpt From the Ophthalmology Section of NCCI Guidelines[2(p8)]

There are numerous CPT codes describing repair of retinal detachment (e.g., 67101-67113). These procedures are mutually exclusive and should not be reported separately for the ipsilateral eye on the same date of service. Some retinal detachment repair procedures include some vitreous procedures which are not separately reportable. For example, the procedure described by CPT code 67108 includes the procedures described by CPT codes 67015, 67025, 67028, 67031, 67036, 67039, and 67040.

Interpretation

There are several CPT codes for retinal detachment repairs that include vitrectomies. See the following CPT codes for examples:

67101 Repair of retinal detachment, 1 or more sessions; cryotherapy or diathermy, with or without drainage of subretinal fluid

67105 photocoagulation, with or without drainage of subretinal fluid

67107 Repair of retinal detachment; scleral buckling (such as lamellar scleral dissection, imbrication or encircling procedure), with or without implant, with or without cryotherapy, photocoagulation, and drainage of subretinal fluid

67108 with vitrectomy, any method, with or without air or gas tamponade, focal endolaser photocoagulation, cryotherapy, drainage of subretinal fluid, scleral buckling, and/or removal of lens by same technique

67110 by injection of air or other gas (eg, pneumatic retinopexy)

67112 by scleral buckling or vitrectomy, on patient having previous ipsilateral retinal detachment repair(s) using scleral buckling or vitrectomy techniques

67113 Repair of complex retinal detachment (eg, proliferative vitreoretinopathy, stage C-1 or greater, diabetic traction retinal detachment, retinopathy of prematurity, retinal tear of greater than 90 degrees), with vitrectomy and membrane peeling, may include air, gas, or silicone oil tamponade, cryotherapy, endolaser photocoagulation, drainage of subretinal fluid, scleral buckling, and/or removal of lens

When coding this procedure in conjunction with a retinal detachment repair, choose the retinal detachment repair that includes the vitrectomy, rather than coding the vitrectomy in addition to the retinal procedure.

For example, an operative report states that the retinal tear was treated with cryopexy and the eye was then re-entered, and a vitrectomy was performed; the lens was considerably imbedded in the vitreous and was not readily moved until an extensive dissection of vitreous from the intraocular lens was made. Because both a retinal detachment repair and vitrectomy were performed during a single surgical encounter, a single CPT code (67108) for retinal detachment repair with vitrectomy should be assigned.

See Table 14-1 for a snapshot of the NCCI mutually exclusive edits for retinal detachment repairs.

TABLE 14-1 *NCCI Mutually Exclusive Edits for Retinal Detachment Repairs*

	Mutually Exclusive Edits	
Column 1	Column 2	Modifier 0 = not allowed 1 = allowed 9 = not applicable
60252	60240	1
60252	60270	1
60260	60240	1
67101	67107	1
67110	67107	1
67110	67108	1
67112	67108	1
67120	65175	1
67120	65260	1
67120	65265	1
67121	65260	1

CPT Coding Tip: *The mother of all retinal detachment repair codes; CPT code 67113 (repair of complex retinal detachment) includes, when performed, the following procedures:*

> *vitrectomy*
>
> *membrane peeling*
>
> *air, gas, or silicone oil tamponade*
>
> *cryotherapy*
>
> *endolaser photocoagulation*
>
> *drainage of subretinal fluid*
>
> *scleral buckling*
>
> *removal of lens*

Although all of these do not have to be performed to use this code (see the CPT codebook), none of these services should be billed separately when performed during a single session on a single eye.

Excerpt From the Ophthalmology Section of NCCI Guidelines[2(p9)]

The procedures described by CPT codes 68020-68200 (incision, drainage, biopsy, excision, or destruction of the conjunctiva) are included in all conjunctivoplasties (CPT codes 68320-68362). CPT codes 68020-68200 should not be reported separately with CPT codes 68320-68362 for the ipsilateral eye.

Interpretation

A conjunctivoplasty is a surgical repair of the conjunctiva. Therefore, in the repair or reconstruction of the conjunctiva, any incision into the conjunctiva is incidental to the repair and is most likely part of the approach. Any drainage would be incidental and is in all probability incidental to the access and not a distinct procedure. Additionally, any excision necessary to complete the repair is not to be coded separately as it is integral to the repair and does not add appreciably to the surgeon's work.

The general guidelines of NCCI state that the most extensive procedure is coded, and any other procedures performed as integral parts of the most extensive procedure are not coded separately. The repair is the most extensive procedure, and any incision, drainage, or excision would be integral to the repair. Only the most complex procedure performed during a single encounter on a single anatomic site may be coded. The lesser services are incidental to the more complex procedure.

For example, a physician performs a conjunctivoplasty procedure for conjunctivochalasis. The conjunctivoplasty involved a conjunctival excision to correct the disorder. Access is made via an incision. In this case, only the conjunctivoplasty would be coded, as the excision and incision are included in the repair code reimbursement. See CPT codes 68320-68362.

Again, if the procedures involved different eyes, multiple procedures may be coded.

Excerpt From the Ophthalmology Section of NCCI Guidelines[2(p9)]

CPT code 67950 (canthoplasty) is included in repair procedures such as blepharoplasties (CPT codes 67917, 67924, 67961, 67966).

Interpretation

The canthus is the corner of the eye where the upper and lower lids meet. If a blepharoplasty or other repair of the eyelids is performed, the canthoplasty is incidental to the blepharoplasty. The canthoplasty is performed to reinforce lower eyelid support by detaching the lateral canthal tendon from the orbital bone and constructing a replacement.

The terminology within this guideline is a little dated, because the term *blepharoplasty* in the CPT codebook was removed from CPT codes 67917, 67924, 67961, and 67966. Instead, the blepharoplasty codes are now found within the integumentary system in the CPT codebook. Regardless, the CPT codes referenced in the guideline are for correction to conditions (diagnoses) and not for cosmetic purposes.

Use care when coding to select the correct code from either the integumentary or eye section of the CPT codebook.

The procedures described in these CPT codes (67917, 67924, 67961, 67966) all include extensive repair of the eyelid, and because the canthus is a part of the eyelid, any service performed on the canthus during the same session as a procedure included in one of these CPT codes would be incidental to the eyelid repair. The anatomic location is too close in proximity to consider the procedures as being at a separate site.

The February 2004 issue of the *CPT Assistant*[3] addressed the question of whether code 68320 can be reported separately or is it included in the ectropion repair code when conjunctivoplasty with conjunctival graft is performed in addition to an extensive ectropion repair (code 67917). The guideline provided read:

> From a CPT coding perspective, code 68320, *Conjunctivoplasty; with conjunctival graft or extensive rearrangement*, may be reported in conjunction with code 67917, *Repair of ectropion; blepharoplasty, extensive (eg, Kuhnt- Szymanowski or tarsal strip operations)*, as it is not considered an inherent component of the ectropion repair described by code 67917.

Excerpt From the Ophthalmology Section of NCCI Guidelines[2(p9)]

Correction of lid retraction (CPT code 67911) includes a full thickness graft (e.g., CPT code 15260) as part of the procedure. A full thickness graft code such as CPT code 15260 should not be reported separately with CPT code 67911 for the ipsilateral eye.

Interpretation

There are several methods of correcting lid retraction including the following:
- Support system reinforcement (canthoplasty)
- Grafting of an internal spacer (Alloderm, ear cartilage, hard palate, dermal fat graft, etc)
- Skin grafting
- Midface lift
- Augmentation of insufficient bony support below the eye
- Augmentation of deficient orbital fat

CPT coding does not distinguish between the various types of correction surgery, so unless otherwise indicated, the repair of lid retraction would be all inclusive of the services required to repair the retracted lid. CPT guidelines

state that obtaining autogenous graft materials should be coded from CPT codes 20920, 20922, or 20926. With the exception of obtaining the autogenous graft materials, and regardless of the type of repair, CPT code 67911 should be used for correction of lid retraction. No additional codes should be added when the service is directly related to the lid retraction procedure.

Excerpt From the Ophthalmology Section of NCCI Guidelines[2(p9)]

If it is medically reasonable and necessary to inject anti-sclerosing agents at the same patient encounter as surgery to correct glaucoma, the injection is included in the glaucoma procedure. CPT codes such as 67500, 67515, and 68200 for injection of anti-sclerosing agents (e.g., 5-FU, HCPCS code J9190) should not be reported separately with other pressure-reducing or glaucoma procedures.

Interpretation

In this instance, the injection becomes an incidental part of the glaucoma surgery and is not separately distinguishable and, as a result, not separately coded.

Excerpt From the Ophthalmology Section of NCCI Guidelines[2(p9)]

Since visual field examination (CPT codes 92081-92083) would be performed prior to scheduling a patient for a blepharoplasty (CPT codes 15820-15823) or blepharoptosis (CPT codes 67901-67908) procedure, the visual field examination CPT codes should not be reported separately with the blepharoplasty or blepharoptosis procedure codes for the same date of service.

Interpretation

A visual field test measures a patient's scope of vision. The visual field test, when performed prior to a blepharoplasty or repair of blepharoptosis is incidental to that surgery when performed on the same date of service. The visual field test assists the physician in determining the patient's level of visual field loss from the drooping eyelid.

The CPT code descriptors for CPT code 67108 (repair of retinal detachment …) and 67113 (repair of complex retinal detachment …) include removal of lens if performed. CPT codes for removal of lens or cataract extraction (e.g., 66830-66984) should not be reported separately.

Interpretation

The following CPT codes illustrate that the removal of the lens is an inherent part of the code. Note, however, that the lens removal is included in this code when performed; however, if the lens is not removed, the code may still be used.

67108 Repair of retinal detachment; with vitrectomy, any method, with or without air or gas tamponade, focal endolaser photocoagulation, cryotherapy, drainage of subretinal fluid, scleral buckling, and/or removal of lens by same technique

67113 Repair of complex retinal detachment (eg, proliferative vitreoretinopathy, stage C-1 or greater, diabetic traction retinal detachment, retinopathy of prematurity, retinal tear of greater than 90 degrees), with vitrectomy and membrane peeling, may include air, gas, or silicone oil tamponade, cryotherapy, endolaser photocoagulation, drainage of subretinal fluid, scleral buckling, and/or removal of lens

Medicare Anesthesia Rules prohibit the physician performing an operative procedure from separately reporting anesthesia for that procedure except for moderate conscious sedation for some procedures. CPT codes describing ophthalmic injections (e.g., CPT codes 67500, 67515, 68200) should not be reported separately with other ophthalmic procedure codes when the injected substance is an anesthetic agent. Since Medicare Global Surgery Rules prohibit the separate reporting of postoperative pain management by the physician performing the procedure, the same CPT codes should not be reported separately by the physician performing the procedure for postoperative pain management.

Interpretation

The CPT codes referenced in this guideline are all for ophthalmic injections, and the guideline reminds coders that if the injections are local anesthetic to be used in the performance of another procedure, a code for the anesthetic injection must not be added. Remember that, as discussed in Chapter 3 of this book, anesthesia performed by the physician performing the primary procedure is already included in the primary procedure code, and is not to be coded separately.

Therefore, if a physician performs a cataract extraction and injects retrobulbar anesthetic, report CPT code 67500. CPT code 67500 represents a retrobulbar injection, but the injection would not be coded in addition to the cataract extraction service because it was anesthetic for the cataract extraction.

67500 Retrobulbar injection; medication (separate procedure, does not include supply of medication)

Medical Unlikely Edits

Because, in normal anatomy, there are two eyes, the medically unlikely edits (MUEs) for most procedures coded within the eye and ocular adnexa section of CPT codebook are limited to a unit of service of two. See Table 14-2 for an example of the MUEs for eye surgeries.

TABLE 14-2 *Mutually Exclusive Edits (MUEs) for Eye Procedures*

HCPCS\CPT Code	Practitioner DME Supplier MUE
66940	2
66982	2
66983	2
66984	2
66985	2
66986	2
66990	2
67005	2
67010	2
67015	2
67025	2
67027	2
67028	2
67030	2
67031	2
67036	2
67039	2

SUMMARY

- The entire ophthalmology section of the NCCI manual should be read.

- Incidental procedures (eg, vitrectomies) are not separately coded from the primary surgery being performed (eg, cataract extractions).

- Incidental procedures are those not intended by the surgeon and that are not associated with a specific, documented condition being treated.

- Review all the instructions within the CPT codebook for eye and ocular adnexa system procedures. They are often consistent with the NCCI guidelines.

Definitions and Acronyms

American Academy of Ophthalmology (AAO) (www.aao.org)

conjunctivochalasis: Excessive conjunctiva visibly overlapping the lid margin and punctum of the inferior lid.

glaucoma: Dangerous buildup of intraocular pressure.

CHAPTER EXERCISES

EXERCISE 1

The procedure performed was a bilateral pterygium removal with placement of autologous, free-floating, conjunctival grafts (nasal and temporal).

Would the graft be coded in addition to the pterygium removal?

EXERCISE 2

Procedures: Pars plana vitrectomy for complex retinal detachment, membrane peeling, scleral buckle, endolaser, and gas-fluid exchange

Which of the following represents correct coding for these procedures? (Descriptions of codes follow.)

A. CPT codes 67108 and 67036

B. CPT code 67113

67108   Repair of retinal detachment; with vitrectomy, any method, with or without air or gas tamponade, focal endolaser photocoagulation, cryotherapy, drainage of subretinal fluid, scleral buckling, and/or removal of lens by same technique

67036   Vitrectomy, mechanical, pars plana approach;

67113   Repair of complex retinal detachment (eg, proliferative vitreoretinopathy, stage C-1 or greater, diabetic traction retinal detachment, retinopathy of prematurity, retinal tear of greater than 90 degrees), with vitrectomy and membrane peeling, may include air, gas, or silicone oil tamponade, cryotherapy, endolaser photocoagulation, drainage of subretinal fluid, scleral buckling, and/or removal of lens

EXERCISE 3

A patient has complex phacoemulsification cataract extraction with insertion of an intraocular lens, a pars plana vitrectomy with epiretinal membrane peeling, panretinal endolaser photocoagulation, and peripheral cryopexy with air-fluid exchange.

Would the following CPT codes include all procedures performed, or would additional codes be needed?

66982   Extracapsular cataract removal with insertion of intraocular lens prosthesis (one stage procedure), manual or mechanical technique (eg, irrigation and aspiration or phacoemulsification), complex, requiring devices or techniques not generally used in routine cataract surgery (eg, iris expansion device, suture support for intraocular lens, or primary posterior capsulorrhexis) or performed on patients in the amblyogenic developmental stage

67040   Vitrectomy, mechanical, pars plana approach; with endolaser panretinal photocoagulation

ANSWERS TO CHAPTER EXERCISES

Exercise 1: Because there is a CPT code that includes the graft (CPT code 65426), no additional code would be billed.

65420   Excision or transposition of pterygium; without graft

65426   with graft

LESSON: *Never separately code components of a surgery when there is a comprehensive code.*

Exercise 2: CPT code 67113 is the correct code because it comprehensively covers the procedure (with the information provided). It would be incorrect to use CPT codes 67108 and 67036 with modifier 59.

Exercise 3: These two codes support the entire surgery and should both be reported.

REFERENCES

1. American Medical Association. *Current Procedural Terminology (CPT®) Professional Edition 2009.* Chicago, IL: American Medical Association; 2008.

2. Centers for Medicare and Medicaid Services. "Chapter VIII Surgery: Endocrine, Nervous, Eye and Ocular Adnexa, and Auditory Systems." In: NCCI Policy Manual for Medicare Services. www.cms.hhs.gov/NationalCorrectCodInitEd/01_overview.asp#TopOfPage. Accessed June 10, 2009.

3. American Medical Association. "Coding communication: eye and ocular adnexa, 67917 (Q&A)." *CPT Assistant,* 2004;14(2):11.

The Auditory System

Chapter 15 provides background about the auditory system, reviews the National Correct Coding Initiative (NCCI) coding guidelines for procedures performed on the ear, and provides examples to reflect the logic behind the edits. As do the other chapters, this chapter provides an NCCI guideline followed by our interpretation, an example, or both.

The first rule in correct coding is to understand the service or procedure being coded. Without the clinical knowledge or understanding of a service or procedure, it is difficult to correctly code the service or decide whether a bundling edit should be bypassed. Coders should remember to read all the instructions within that section (eg, auditory) of the *Current Procedural Terminology (CPT®)*[1] codebook and refer to it for additional instructions. The NCCI guidelines should also be reviewed to make sure information is being coded correctly, optimally, and compliantly.

The Auditory System and NCCI Guidelines

The auditory section of NCCI is very brief.

> **Excerpt From the Auditory System Section of NCCI Guidelines**[2(p2)]
>
> **Introduction**
> The principles of correct coding discussed in Chapter I apply to the CPT codes in the range 60000-69999. Several general guidelines are repeated in this Chapter. However, those general guidelines from Chapter I not discussed in this Chapter are nonetheless applicable.

Interpretation

This instruction indicates that the overall NCCI guidelines apply to each section of the CPT codebook, and, even if they are not repeated within a chapter, they are nonetheless a guideline to be followed. The introductory guidelines were reviewed comprehensively in Chapter 2 of this book; however, those introductory guidelines that have clear application within the auditory system section are reiterated in this chapter.

> **Excerpt From the Auditory System Section of NCCI Guidelines**[2(p10)]
>
> If the code descriptor for a procedure of the auditory system includes a mastoidectomy (e.g. CPT codes 69530, 69802, 69910), an additional code describing a mastoidectomy (e.g., 69502-69511) is not separately reportable for the ipsilateral mastoid.

Interpretation

This guideline reiterates that if a CPT code description includes a procedure, do not separately code that procedure if performed on the same ear. The following CPT code illustrates that the mastoidectomy is included in the petrous apecectomy and, therefore, it would be erroneous to add a mastoidectomy code when performed on the same ear.

69530 Petrous apicectomy including radical mastoidectomy

Be careful with the coding to ensure that the most specific and descriptive code is being used. If the physician was performing a revision mastoidectomy and also included an apicectomy during the surgery, CPT 69530 would not be the correct code—rather, CPT code 69605, which specifies revision would be more appropriate.

69601 Revision mastoidectomy; resulting in complete mastoidectomy

69605   with apicectomy

On the other hand, if the apicectomy was performed as the primary planned procedure, and a mastoidectomy was also provided, CPT code 69530 would be more appropriate than the mastoidectomy codes.

CPT Coding Tip: There are several different types of mastoidectomy.

Simple (closed): The operation is performed through the ear or through an incision behind the ear. The surgeon opens the mastoid bone and removes the infected air cells. The eardrum is incised to drain the middle ear. Topical antibiotics are then placed in the ear.

Radical mastoidectomy: The eardrum and most middle ear structures are removed, but the innermost small bone (the stapes) is left behind so that a hearing aid can be used later to offset the hearing loss.

Modified radical mastoidectomy: The eardrum and the middle ear structures are saved, which allows for better hearing than is possible after a radical operation.

Excerpt From the Auditory System Section of NCCI Guidelines[2(p10)]

A myringotomy (e.g., CPT codes 69420, 69421) is included in a tympanoplasty or tympanostomy procedure and is not separately reportable.

Interpretation

A myringotomy is a small surgical incision in the eardrum (the tympanic membrane). When tubes are placed during the same surgical encounter, this becomes a tympanostomy. An opening is created in the eardrum (tympanostomy) for insertion of the ventilating tubes. A tympanoplasty is the surgical repair of an eardrum. Because a myringotomy is an incision into the eardrum, it becomes incidental (for coding purposes) to any other surgical procedure performed on the eardrum. For the tympanostomy and tympanoplasty, an incision is required in order to complete the procedure—the incision is integral to the approach and not separately coded.

For example, a child has chronic otitis media with effusion that does not respond to drug treatment, and the physician decides to place ear tubes after a course of antibiotics. The physician begins the procedure by washing the ear, then creates a small incision in the eardrum (myringotomy). The fluid is removed through the incision

(part of the myringotomy), a tube is inserted (tympanostomy), and the ear is then packed with cotton.

In this case, the myringotomy is the surgical approach, and surgical approaches are not coded separately from the primary procedure; therefore, only the tympanostomy would be coded.

CPT Coding Tip: If different procedures were performed on different ears or during different encounters, each could be coded separately. If, for example, a myringotomy for drainage was performed on the left ear and a tympanostomy on the right, each could be coded, with the lateral (LT - left, RT - right) modifiers appended.

Medical Unlikely Edits

Because, in normal anatomy, there are two ears, one would think the medically unlikely edits (MUEs) for most procedures coded within the auditory section of the CPT codebook would be limited to a unit of service of two. However, there are quite a few procedures that have a limitation of one. This is because the type of service would not likely be needed on both ears at the same time. See Table 15-1 for an example of the MUEs for ear surgeries.

TABLE 15-1 *Medically Unlikely Edits (MUEs) for Ear Procedures*

HCPCS\CPT Code	Practitioner DME Supplier MUE
69530	1
69535	1
69540	2
69550	1
69552	1
69554	1
69601	1
69602	1
69603	1
69604	1
69605	1
69610	2
69620	2
69631	2
69632	1
69633	1
69635	1

Other General Information from the Auditory System Section of NCCI Guidelines

Removal of impacted cerumen: In myringotomies, the general NCCI guidelines (see Chapter 2) point out that in order to perform the myringotomy, the provider must reach the tympanic membrane. For a patient who has impacted cerumen, the removal of the cerumen becomes a part of the myringotomy approach and would not be separately reported when performed on the same ear during the same operative session. The cerumen removal is a necessary component of the myringotomy.

Likewise, this guideline can be taken a step further and applied to any inner ear procedure. If removal of impacted cerumen is necessary for any middle or inner ear procedure, do not add the code for the removal of the cerumen—it is part of the access or approach.

The CMS created another code for removal of impacted cerumen (Healthcare Common Procedure Coding System [HCPCS] G0268) when performed on the same date of service as audiologic function testing. This code should be billed only in those situations in which a physician's expertise was needed to remove impacted cerumen on the same day as audiologic function testing performed by an employed audiologist. The audiologist and physician must share the same billing number. The G0268 code cannot be billed by independent audiologists. Routine removal of cerumen, as defined by CMS, is the use of softening drops, cotton swabs, and/or a cerumen spoon to remove ear wax and is not paid separately. It is considered incidental to the office visit and cannot be reimbursed on the same day as the evaluation and management (E/M) service.

According to AAO[3] CMS only makes payment for the removal of cerumen only when *all* of the following criteria are met:

1. The service is the sole reason for the patient encounter.
2. Service is personally performed by a physician or non-physician, (ie, nurse practitioner, physician assistant, clinical nurse specialist).
3. Service is provided to a patient who is symptomatic.
4. The documentation shows significant time and effort spent in performing the service.

E/M and cerumen removal: In addition, CMS will consider payment for both an E/M visit and the cerumen removal only when *all* of the following criteria are met:

1. The nature of the E/M visit is for anything other than the removal of cerumen.
2. During an unrelated patient encounter, the physician observed impacted cerumen, or the patient complains about an ear problem during the encounter.

3. Otoscopic examination of the tympanic membrane is not possible because of the impacted cerumen.
4. Removal of the impacted cerumen requires the expertise of the physician or nonphysician practitioner and is personally performed by the practitioner.
5. The procedure requires a significant amount of time and effort, and all of the stated criteria are clearly documented in the patient's medical record.

Excerpt from the American Academy of Otolaryngology web Site[3]

Tips for Billing an E/M, Cerumen Removal and Audiometric Evaluations: When all of the above conditions have been met, report the E/M, G0268, and audiometric function tests (CPT Codes 92553 through 92598, except for non-covered codes 92559 and 92560) appending a 25 modifier to the E/M visit. When this service is reported in addition to the E/M, the medical record must clearly reflect that this procedure was separate from the reason for the E/M visit. Also, remember that G0268 is a bilateral procedure and should be reported with one unit of service even if both ears were cleaned. The HCPCS/CPT code(s) may be subject to CCI edits. Please refer to CCI for correct coding guidelines and specific applicable code pairs prior to billing Medicare.

For example: A patient is seen for a scheduled audiometric function test in your office. On examination, impacted cerumen is noted in both ears. You remove the impacted cerumen and send them down the hall to your audiologist for audiometric testing.

In this circumstance, report the proper level E/M service, appending the 25 modifier, bill the G0268 and the appropriate audiometric testing code(s). Remember, the reporting of G0268 designated that the physician remove the impacted cerumen at a separate encounter from the audiometric function testing. If code 69210 were reported, payment for the impacted cerumen would be denied.

In addition, the removal of impacted cerumen is designated as a separate procedure code. If a HCPCS/CPT code descriptor includes the term *separate procedure*, the HCPCS/CPT code may not be reported separately with a related procedure. CMS interprets this designation to prohibit the separate reporting of a separate procedure when performed with another procedure in an anatomically related region, often through the same skin incision, orifice, or surgical approach. A HCPCS/CPT code with the *separate procedure* designation may be reported with another procedure if it is performed at a separate patient encounter on the same date of service or at the same patient encounter in an anatomically unrelated area, often through a separate skin incision, orifice, or surgical approach. Modifier -59 may be appended to the separate procedure HCPCS/CPT code to indicate that it qualifies as a separately reportable service.

Whenever a CPT code description includes the term *separate procedure*, that service is usually incidental to other services provided during the same encounter on the same anatomic site. Do not code the separate procedure service in addition to another service when performed in the same anatomic region. However, if the separate procedure service is performed in a different anatomic site than that for any other code also being used, or during a separate encounter, both services may be coded.

Note: There are no current NCCI edits bundling the audiometric tests, G0268 and E/M services.

CPT Coding Tip: *A coder might well ask, "If a therapeutic procedure is performed on one ear after bilateral removal of cerumen, could removal of impacted cerumen from the other ear be coded with a modifier 59? After all the code states 'one or both ears'."*

The answer is no—consider the entire code bundled into the major procedure on that date. It is splitting hairs and too risky to code separately for the other ear unless there is strong documentation supporting the therapeutic rationale.

SUMMARY

- Read the entire auditory system section from the NCCI manual (very brief section).

- Review all the instructions within the CPT codebook for the auditory system procedures.

Definitions and Acronyms

American Academy of Otolaryngology (AAO): The AAO (www.entnet.org) is the national association devoted to physicians who specialize in otolaryngology. The Academy focuses on clinical and practice management support for their members.

CHAPTER EXERCISES

Yes or No. Ear wax removal should be coded when the cerumen:

1. is impacted, and the removal is performed without any other therapeutic procedure on the same day.
2. must be removed in order to visualize the eardrum for diagnosing the condition.
3. must be removed in order to gain access for a mastoidectomy.

ANSWERS TO CHAPTER EXERCISES

1. **Yes.** This should be coded as long as the removal is for treatment of the condition and not for gaining access or visualizing.

2. **No.** When the removal is solely to visualize the middle or inner ear, the removal is not coded. It becomes incidental to other procedures.

3. **No.** When the removal is solely for access for another procedure, the removal of cerumen is not separately coded.

REFERENCES

1. American Medical Association. *Current Procedural Terminology (CPT®) Professional Edition 2009*. Chicago, IL: American Medical Association; 2008.

2. Centers for Medicare and Medicaid Services. "Chapter VIII Surgery: Endocrine, Nervous, Eye and Ocular Adnexa, and Auditory Systems." In: NCCI Policy Manual for Medicare Services. www.cms.hhs.gov/NationalCorrectCodInitEd/ 01_overview .asp#TopOfPage. Accessed June 10, 2009.

3. American Academy of Otolaryngology. *Cerumen Removal Codes*. 2006; August. www.entnet.org/Practice/upload/Cerumen-Removal. pdf. Accessed June 13, 2009.

Radiology Services

Chapter 16 provides background about services in the radiology section of the *Current Procedural Terminology* (*CPT*®)[1] codebook, reviews the National Correct Coding Initiative (NCCI) coding guidelines for radiology services, and provides examples to reflect the logic behind the edits. As do the other chapters, this chapter provides an NCCI guideline followed by our interpretation, an example, or both.

Introduction Section of NCCI Radiology Services Guidelines

Excerpt From the Radiology Section of NCCI Guidelines[2(p2)]

Introduction
The principles of correct coding discussed in Chapter I apply to the CPT codes in the range 70000-79999. Several general guidelines are repeated in this Chapter. However, those general guidelines from Chapter I not discussed in this chapter are nonetheless applicable.

Interpretation

These instructions indicate that the overall NCCI guidelines apply to each section of the CPT codebook, and, even if they are not repeated within a chapter, they are nonetheless a guideline to be followed. The introductory guidelines were covered comprehensively in Chapter 2 of this book; those introductory guidelines that have clear application within radiology services will be reiterated in this chapter.

Excerpt From the General Coding Policies Section of NCCI Guidelines[3(p2)]

CPT and HCPCS Level II code descriptors usually do not define all services included in a procedure. There are often services inherent in a procedure or group of procedures.

Interpretation

Even though the CPT codes should reflect the service provided, every element of the service cannot be included in the CPT code description. It would make the descriptors too long to be practical. Therefore, this NCCI concept is to remind coders that inherent and integral components to the service represented by a specific CPT code should not be separately coded.

For example, a patient presents for a CT scan of the chest with contrast media, and the contrast media is given intravascularly. The CPT code does *not* reflect an intravascular instillation of contrast medium; however, the CPT codebook introductory guidelines do indicate the methods of contrast media administration that are inherent in the codes. Because the inherent contrast media administrations are not included in every code description, it demonstrates the importance of reading all appropriate instructions within the CPT codebook. Read all the guidelines carefully to ensure proper coding for the services.

Excerpt From the CPT Codebook[1](p304) Radiology Guidelines

Administration of Contrast Material(s)

The phrase "with contrast" used in the codes for procedures performed using contrast for imaging enhancement represents contrast material administered intravascularly, intra-articularly, or intrathecally.

For intra-articular injection, use the appropriate joint injection code. If radiographic arthrography is performed, also use the arthrography supervision and interpretation code for the appropriate joint (which includes fluoroscopy). If computed tomography (CT) or magnetic resonance (MR) arthrography are performed without radiographic arthrography, use the appropriate joint injection code, the appropriate CT or MR code ("with contrast" or "without followed by contrast"), and the appropriate imaging guidance code for needle placement for contrast injection.

For spine examinations using computed tomography, magnetic resonance imaging, magnetic resonance angiography, "with contrast" includes intrathecal or intravascular injection. For intrathecal injection, use also 61055 or 62284.

Injection of intravascular contrast material is part of the "with contrast" CT, computed tomographic angiography (CTA), magnetic resonance imaging (MRI), and magnetic resonance angiography (MRA) procedures.

Oral and/or rectal contrast administration alone does not qualify as a study "with contrast."

TABLE 16-1 *Contrast Media Administration and Coding for Radiology*

Contrast Media Administration Worksheet

Mode of Administration	Contrast Radiology Code Used	Administration Code Added
intravascularly	Yes, use 'with contrast' radiology code	No
intra-articularly	Yes, use 'with contrast' radiology code	Yes
intra-thecal	Yes, use 'with contrast' radiology code	Yes
oral	No, do not use the 'with contrast' or 'without followed by with contrast' code	No
rectal	No, do not use the 'with contrast' or 'without followed by with contrast' code	No

Comments:

Interpretation

Here the CPT codebook instructs coders that intravascular administration is included in the CPT code for the procedure. Also, note that it is important to have the method of administration documented, because intra-articular administration can be coded additionally, but oral or rectal contrast medium administration does not qualify for using the "with contrast" procedure code. See Table 16-1.

71250 Computed tomography, thorax; without contrast material

(This code would be used if no contrast medium was administered or if the medium was administered orally or rectally.)

71260 with contrast material(s)

(This code would be used if contrast medium was administered intravascularly.)

Excerpt From the Radiology Section of NCCI Guidelines[2](p2)

Physicians should report the HCPCS/CPT code that describes the procedure performed to the greatest specificity possible. A HCPCS/CPT code should be reported only if all services described by the code are performed. A physician should not report multiple HCPCS/CPT codes if a single HCPCS/CPT code exists that describes the services. This type of unbundling is incorrect coding.

Interpretation

If one code includes all the services provided, choose that code over splitting the service into individual CPT codes for the components. For instance, if a patient presents for an MRI of the chest and has imaging provided without contrast medium, and then contrast medium is administered and additional imaging performed, the code should be CPT code 71552, as this code includes imaging without administration of contrast medium followed by administration of contrast medium and additional imaging.

71550 Magnetic resonance (eg, proton) imaging, chest (eg, for evaluation of hilar and mediastinal lymphadenopathy); without contrast material(s)

71551 with contrast material(s)

71552 without contrast material(s), followed by contrast material(s) and further sequences

If both CPT codes 71550 and 71551 were billed instead of the comprehensive code, that would be unbundling and erroneous.

Excerpt From the Radiology Section of NCCI Guidelines[2(p2)]

Medicare Global Surgery Rules define the rules for reporting evaluation and management (E&M) services with procedures covered by these rules.

Interpretation

There are a few of different instructions covered within this guideline.

1. NCCI edits incorporate the CMS guidelines surrounding global codes for surgeries. The radiology services are designated as "XXX" procedures, and therefore, the global period does not apply.

2. The "XXX" procedures can have some preprocedure/intraprocedure/postprocedure work performed each time the procedure is provided. If so, do not code that usual work in addition to the "XXX" procedure (the radiology service).

3. If the provider does indeed provide a medically necessary and well-documented evaluation and management (E/M) service on the same date as the "XXX" procedure, it may be coded separately. A modifier 25 may be appended to the E/M service, but most radiology procedures do not bundle with the E/M service, so the modifier should not be necessary. If the E/M service is billed separately from the radiology service, any time or work spent directly related to the radiology service cannot be used to support the level of E/M service billed.

Excerpt From the Radiology Section of NCCI Guidelines[2(p4)]

When physician interaction with a patient is necessary to accomplish a radiographic procedure, typically occurring in invasive or interventional radiology, the interaction generally involves limited pertinent historical inquiry about reasons for the examination, the presence of allergies, acquisition of informed consent, discussion of follow-up, and the review of the medical record. In this setting, a separate evaluation and management service is not reported. As a rule, if the medical decision making that evolves from the procurement of the information from the patient is limited to whether or not the procedure should be performed, whether comorbidity may impact the procedure, or involves discussion and education with the patient, an evaluation/management code is not reported separately. If a significant, separately identifiable service is rendered, involving taking a history, performing an exam, and making medical decisions distinct from the procedure, the appropriate evaluation and management service may be reported.

Interpretation
Noninvasive Radiology

Radiologists who are performing and interpreting plain film X-rays rarely must evaluate the patient as separate from the radiology service. They are usually working from an order by the patient's treating provider and, therefore, not making any clinical determinations as to the efficacy of the ordered service. In this case, because no E/M service is determined, only the radiology procedures would be billed.

However, if the physician is the one who is medically evaluating the patient and determining a need for a radiology service, and the radiology procedure is performed within that provider's office, both the radiology and E/M service should be billed, as the E/M service determined the need for the radiology service. This would occur in a practice that has its own radiologic equipment. The E/M service must be documented as separate from the radiology service, significant, and medically necessary.

Invasive Radiology

On the other hand, it is standard medical practice for a radiologist who performs invasive procedures to perform a minimal patient examination and evaluation prior to the procedure to ensure that the patient can safely undergo the procedure and that the correct procedure was ordered.

This is considered part of the invasive radiology service and is included in the code for the invasive service.

Here again, if the radiologist performing the invasive procedure is the physician who is evaluating the patient, and that provider determines a need for a radiology procedure, which is performed within that provider's office, both services should be coded, because the E/M service determined the need for the radiology service and should be documented as separate and significant. The documentation must support a level of E/M beyond that typical for the radiology service, and the service must be medically necessary as demonstrated by the documentation.

To illustrate the points here, consider these three scenarios:

1. A patient's primary care physician orders a chest X-ray. The radiology technician at the imaging center takes the X-ray, and the radiologist at the imaging center interprets the film and provides the requesting physician with the formal interpretation. In this case, the radiologist never sees or evaluates the patient and cannot bill a medical visit.

2. A patient's primary care physician refers the patient to a neurointerventionalist for evaluation and consult regarding the patient's headaches. The neurointerventionalist performs a complete work-up on the patient prior to deciding to perform a cerebral carotid angiography. The angiography is completed.

    In this case, the neurointerventionalist may bill both the E/M service, with a modifier 25 appended, and the angiography, as the E/M service was necessary to determine the need for the angiography.

3. A patient with shortness of breath presents to a cardiologist. The cardiologist completes a full work-up on the patient (history, examination, and medical decision making) and determines that a chest X-ray should be performed. The X-ray is taken and reviewed by the cardiologist while the patient is still in the office.

    In this scenario, the cardiologist is the treating provider and the radiologist and can bill for both the E/M service with a modifier 25 appended and the chest X-ray, assuming both were appropriately documented.

CPT Coding Tip: Physicians billing for an E/M service and a radiology interpretation during the same encounter should not consider the interpretation of the X-ray when determining their level of medical decision making for the E/M service, because they are billing for the interpretation separately. Likewise, if the physician merely reviews an X-ray film but does not perform a formal interpretation (report), the provider should not bill for the radiology interpretation but use the film review as a part of their medical decision making for the E/M service billed.

Noninterventional Diagnostic Radiology Services and NCCI Guidelines

Excerpt From the Radiology Section of NCCI Guidelines[2(p5)]

If radiographs have to be repeated in the course of a radiographic encounter due to substandard quality, only one unit of service for the code can be reported.... When limited comparative radiographic studies are performed (e.g., post-reduction radiographs, post-intubation, post-catheter placement, etc.), the CPT code for the radiographic series should be reported with modifier -52, indicating that a reduced level of interpretive service was provided. This requirement does not apply to OPPS services reported by hospitals.

Interpretation

Medicare will pay only for medically necessary imaging. If the original image was unsuccessful and must be repeated, only the successful image should be billed. However, if a second image is necessary and must be repeated to determine the patient's current condition, both images may be coded. The second image, if identical to the first, should be billed as a repeat procedure (modifiers 76 or 77). If the second imaging differs in some way (different number of views, for example), a modifier 59 would be appended to the second procedure.

Often, a second image is necessary to see if the treatment provided was successful. For example, for fractures, often a postreduction film would be made to determine whether proper alignment was obtained through the manipulation. For these limited comparative studies, a modifier 52 should be appended, indicating that a reduced level of interpretation was provided.

For example, a patient presents for a chest X-ray because of chest pain. The physician performs an X-ray but cannot read the film because of poor quality of the X-ray machinery. A second study is successfully performed using different equipment. Only the second X-ray should be coded, as the first was unsuccessful because of equipment failure, and only one film is supported as being medically necessary.

On the other hand, if another patient presents with what was expected to be a broken hand and has a two-view hand X-ray performed. The interpreting physician confirms the fracture, and the patient has fracture reduction with casting. Once the procedure is completed, a second, one-view hand X-ray is performed to confirm the alignment and success of the treatment.

Both the prereduction and postreduction films may be coded, with the postreduction service appended with modifier 59.

Note: There is no code for a one-view hand X-ray, therefore, a reduced-service modifier (52) would also be necessary for the second film.

Excerpt From the Radiology Section of NCCI Guidelines[2(p5)]

If the radiologist elects to obtain additional views after reviewing initial films in order to render an interpretation, the Medicare policy on the ordering of diagnostic tests must be followed. The CPT code describing the total service should be reported, even if the patient was released from the radiology suite and had to return for additional services.

Interpretation

According to the *Medicare Benefit Policy Manual*,[4] Chapter 15, Section 80.6 (see in the following), there are fairly strict but clear guidelines on when an interpreting physician may or may not perform additional studies. This NCCI instruction is a reminder that those guidelines must be followed. Additionally, and this is important, if the radiologist appropriately follows the guidelines and performs additional views, the CPT code used must be for the total number of views, rather than for the services as two separate films. This is true regardless of whether the additional films are obtained during the same encounter or not. For example, a patient's physician orders a one-view plain film of the cervical spine, but the rendering radiologist believes a three-view film to be more appropriate based on the interpretation of the one-view film. Therefore, in order to perform a three-view study, the radiologist has to obtain a new order for the expanded test. The radiologist releases the patient for lunch after performing the one-view film, and asks that the patient return later after the new order is received. The new order arrives, and the radiologist completes the additional two views later that same day.

72020	Radiologic examination, spine, single view, specify level
72040	Radiologic examination, spine, cervical; 2 or 3 views
72050	minimum of 4 views
72052	complete, including oblique and flexion and/or extension studies

In this case, CPT code 72050 for three views would be the only code billed. The two visits for the complete test (three views) are combined for coding purposes.

Figure 16-1 shows the decision tree for determining when an additional study may be performed.

Excerpt From the *Medicare Benefit Policy Manual*,[4] Chapter 15, Section 80.6

80.6.2 - Interpreting Physician Determines a Different Diagnostic Test is Appropriate
When an interpreting physician… at a testing facility determines that an ordered diagnostic radiology test is clinically inappropriate or suboptimal, and that a different diagnostic test should be performed… the interpreting physician/testing facility may not perform the unordered test until a new order from the treating physician/practitioner has been received. Similarly, if the result of an ordered diagnostic test is normal and the interpreting physician believes that another diagnostic test should be performed… an order from the treating physician must be received prior to performing the unordered diagnostic test.

80.6.3 - Rules for Testing Facility to Furnish Additional Tests
If the testing facility cannot reach the treating physician/practitioner to change the order or obtain a new order and documents this in the medical record, then the testing facility may furnish the additional diagnostic test if all of the following criteria apply:
- The testing center performs the diagnostic test ordered by the treating physician/practitioner;
- The interpreting physician at the testing facility determines and documents that, because of the abnormal result of the diagnostic test performed, an additional diagnostic test is medically necessary;
- Delaying the performance of the additional diagnostic test would have an adverse effect on the care of the beneficiary;
- The result of the test is communicated to and is used by the treating physician/practitioner in the treatment of the beneficiary; and
- The interpreting physician at the testing facility documents in his/her report why additional testing was done.

80.6.4 - Rules for Testing Facility Interpreting Physician to Furnish Different or Additional Tests
The following applies to an interpreting physician of a testing facility who furnishes a diagnostic test to

(continued)

FIGURE 16-1 *Decision Tree for Radiologists Performing Additional Studies Outside of Original Orders*

1. Treating Physician is defined as radiologist performing a therapeutic interventional procedure, and is therefore, considered a treating physician. A radiologist performing a diagnostic interventional or diagnostic procedure is not considered a treating physician.
2. An "order" is a communication from the treating physician/practitioner requesting that a diagnostic test be performed for a beneficiary. The order may conditionally request an additional diagnostic test for a particular beneficiary if the result of the initial diagnostic test ordered yields to a certain value determined by the treating physician/practitioner.
3. An order may be delivered via the following forms of communication:
   - A written document signed by the treating physician/practitioner, which is hand-delivered, mailed, or faxed to the testing facility;
   - A telephone call by the treating physician/practitioner or his/her office to the testing facility; and
   - An electronic mail by the treating physician/practitioner or his/her office to the testing facility.

If the order is communicated via telephone, both the treating physician/practitioner or his/her office and the testing facility must document the telephone call in their respective copies of the beneficiary's medical records. While a physician order is not required to be signed, the physician must clearly document, in the medical record, his or her intent that the test be performed.

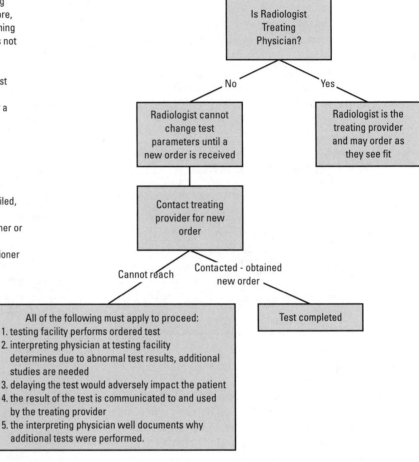

Excerpt From the *Medicare Benefit Policy Manual*[4], Chapter 15, Section 80.6 *(continued)*

a beneficiary who is not a hospital inpatient or outpatient. The interpreting physician must document accordingly in his/her report to the treating physician/practitioner. **Test Design** Unless specified in the order, the interpreting physician may determine, without notifying the treating physician/practitioner, the parameters of the diagnostic test... **Clear Error** The interpreting physician may modify, without notifying the treating physician/practitioner, an order with clear and obvious errors that would be apparent to a reasonable layperson, such as the patient receiving the test.... **Patient Condition** The interpreting physician may cancel, without notifying the treating physician/practitioner, an order because the beneficiary's physical condition at the time of diagnostic testing will not permit performance of the test.... When an ordered diagnostic test is cancelled, any medically necessary preliminary or scout testing performed is payable.

Excerpt From the Radiology Section of NCCI Guidelines[2(p5)]

The CPT descriptor for many of these services refers to a "minimum" number of views. If more than the minimum number specified is necessary and no other more specific CPT code is available, only that service should be reported.

Example

73600 Radiologic examination, ankle; 2 views

73610   complete, minimum of 3 views

If four-view imaging of the ankle is performed, CPT code 73610 would be the only code needed. This code description reads "minimum of 3 views," meaning that there must be at least three views before this code may be used, but it does not limit the maximum number of views included in this code. So, if three, four, five, six, or more views were taken of one ankle, CPT code 73610 would be the only coded needed.

Interpretation

Remember the discussion from earlier on repeated films. If images have to be repeated in the course of a radiographic encounter because of a change or suspected change in the patient's condition, each imaging procedure may be coded. The second, medically necessary image procedure should be appended with either a modifier to indicate repeat service (76 or 77) or a modifier to indicate a separate session (59).

Reminder: Do not code a separate, repeat film because of substandard quality of the first film.

Interpretation

70450 Computed tomography, head or brain; without contrast material

70460 with contrast material(s)

70470 without contrast material, followed by contrast material(s) and further sections

In looking at the CPT codes for studies with contrast material, note that there is no number of views specified. Therefore, the code is based on type of study (eg, CT, MRI), body site, and whether or not contrast material was used. The number of radiographs does not impact the coding.

Interpretation

The CPT codebook offers some combination codes in which the primary radiology service and the scout film are coded with a single CPT code. When documentation supports a combined service, the combination code should be used. If, however, the primary radiology service does not have a combination code option, the primary radiology code would be the only code used, as the scout film would be an inherent part of the primary radiology service CPT code. To illustrate, a scout film is an image that is taken of a body part before a contrast medium is given. For example, an abdominal X-ray (kidneys, ureters, bladder [KUB]) is taken before a barium enema to determine whether the bowel is cleaned out enough to perform the examination. The following CPT codes indicate when the scout film is included in the procedure:

74240 Radiologic examination, gastrointestinal tract, upper; with or without delayed films, without KUB

74241 with or without delayed films, with KUB

The KUB would be the scout film, and, when documented, CPT code 74241 would be used to include the scout film in the procedure. If the scout KUB was not documented, then CPT 74240 would be the appropriate code.

Many services utilizing contrast are composed of a procedural component (CPT codes outside the 70000 section) and a radiologic supervision and interpretation component (CPT code in the 70000 section). If a single physician performs both components of the service, the physician may report both codes. However, if different physicians perform the different components, each physician reports the CPT code corresponding to that component.

Interpretation

In catheter angiographies, catheters are inserted into an artery through a small incision (percutaneously) in the skin. Once the catheter is guided to the area being examined, a contrast material is injected through the tube, and images are captured using a small dose of ionizing radiation (X-rays). These services have both an invasive component (inserting the catheter, stent, or other device into the vessel) and a radiologic component (X-ray imaging of the vessel). These two components are coded from different sections of the CPT codebook. The invasive portion is coded from the appropriate surgical section (cardiovascular, for example), and the radiologic component is coded from the radiology code range.

This method of coding was created so that when different providers were rendering each component, the services could be easily separated within the code structure without providers having to share the same CPT code. This NCCI edit guideline supports the coding structure as it is, without bundling edits to conflict with the CPT code structure.

Diagnostic angiography (arteriogram/venogram) performed on the same date of service by the same provider as a percutaneous intravascular interventional procedure should be reported with modifier -59. If a diagnostic angiogram (fluoroscopic or computed tomographic) was performed prior to the date of the percutaneous intravascular interventional procedure, a second diagnostic angiogram cannot be reported on the date of the percutaneous intravascular interventional procedure unless it is medically reasonable and necessary to repeat the study to further define the anatomy and pathology. Report the repeat angiogram with modifier -59.

Interpretation

An interventional radiology diagnostic study involves placement of a catheter and performing angiography. A diagnostic angiography is an X-ray of arteries and veins achieved by the injection of radiopaque contrast medium to evaluate vessel structure and function. Diagnostic codes should *not* be used with interventional procedures for the following:
- Roadmapping and/or fluoroscopic guidance
- Vessel measurements
- Postangioplasty/stent angiography
  (This work is captured in the interventional procedure codes)

Diagnostic codes *are* reported with interventional procedures if:
- no prior catheter-based angiographic study is available, and a full diagnostic study is performed, and the decision to intervene is based on the diagnostic study, or a prior study is available, however:
  - the patient's condition has changed, or
  - there is inadequate visualization of the anatomy and/or pathology, or
  - there is a clinical change during the procedure that requires new evaluation.

If there is a medically necessary diagnostic angiography on the same date as a therapeutic angiography, both may be coded, with a modifier 59 added to the code for the diagnostic study.

For instance, a patient who was status post radiation therapy to the neck because of a malignancy presents with a *diagnosed* right internal carotid lesion. The interventional radiologist has planned to perform a percutaneous transluminal angioplasty (PTA) with stent placement and is performing an angiography for roadmapping the site. In this case, the angiography does not appear to be diagnostic and, therefore, would not be coded in addition to the stent placement.

However, a patient who was status post radiation therapy to the neck because of a malignancy presents with a *suspected* right internal carotid lesion. The interventional radiologist performs selective cervical, carotid, and vertebral angiographies, establishing the need for a PTA with adjunctive stent angioplasty. In this case, the angiography appears to be diagnostic and, therefore, would be coded in addition to the stent placement.

Notice that in the first example, the procedure and diagnosis were known, whereas in the second example, they were not known, and the angiographies were used to establish what type of treatment was needed.

If it is medically reasonable and necessary to repeat only a portion of the diagnostic angiogram, append modifier -52 to the angiogram CPT code.

Interpretation

Even if the entire study was repeated, if only a portion was medically necessary, the modifier 52 (reduced services) should be appended. Only medically necessary studies are to be coded for Medicare patients.

Consider again the patient whose status post-radiation therapy to the neck because of a malignancy and presents with a *diagnosed* right internal carotid lesion, in which the interventional radiologist planned to perform a PTA with stent placement. Let us say that the patient presents at the time of the stent placement with acute migraine headaches with sudden onset, and the provider feels the need to perform an additional selective internal carotid angiography as well as an external angiography for roadmapping the site.

Because the patient's condition has changed, the internal carotid angiography was diagnostic and should be coded in addition to the stent placement. The external angiography was not diagnostic and should not be coded. There is a code for the internal angiography, so there would be no need for a reduced service modifier in this instance.

If an intravenous line is inserted (e.g., CPT code 36000) for access in the event of a problem with the procedure or for administration of contrast, it is integral to the procedure and is not separately reportable. CPT code 36005 describes the injection procedure for contrast venography of an extremity and includes the introduction of a needle or an intracatheter (e.g., CPT code 36000). CPT code 36005 should not be reported for injections for arteriography or venography of sites other than an extremity.

Interpretation

There is a separate CPT code for administering contrast medium for a venography, which includes the introduction of the needle or catheter.

36005   Injection procedure for extremity venography (including introduction of needle or intracatheter)

The CPT code description even indicates that the needle/catheter insertion is included, and is not to be coded separately.

When urologic radiologic procedures require insertion of a urethral catheter (e.g., CPT code 51701-51703), this insertion is integral to the procedure and is not separately reportable.

Interpretation

Although it seems a bit odd to discuss urologic procedures and surgeries within the radiology section of NCCI, remember that there are many invasive urologic radiology services. Chapter 2 of this book noted that NCCI principles under the Standards of Medical/Surgical Practice offered some examples of the services that are integral to large numbers of procedures, including insertion of a urinary catheter. For procedures that usually require urinary catheters, the catheter placements should not be coded additionally. For example, a voiding urethrocystography is an X-ray of the urinary bladder and the urethra. A catheter is placed in the bladder, and the bladder is filled with fluid, after which the catheter is removed and X-rays are taken of the bladder and as the person passes the urine. Because the catheter is an inherent and integral component of the urethrocystography, the catheter placement would not be separately coded.

74455   Urethrocystography, voiding, radiological supervision and interpretation

Nuclear Medicine Services and NCCI Guidelines

Note: Although the NCCI guidelines include CPT codes 90760-90776, please note that these codes were deleted and replaced with CPT codes 96360-96375.

Interpretation

As discussed in prior sections of this chapter, whenever a primary procedure (in this case nuclear medicine using instilled radiopharmaceuticals) *requires* (meaning it is an integral, necessary component) administration of a substance, the administration (injection) and/or vascular access (insertion of a catheter) may not be coded in addition to the primary service. The nuclear medicine code includes the administration of the radiopharmaceutical. See Table 16-2.

TABLE 16-2 *NCCI Edits for Radionuclide Administration and Intravenous Administration*

Column 1/Column 2 Edits		
Column 1	Column 2	Modifier 0 = not allowed 1 = allowed 9 = not applicable
70010	G0351	1
70010	G0353	1
70010	G0354	1
79403	96372	1
79403	96374	1
79403	96375	1
79403	96408	1
79403	96409	1
79403	96410	1
79403	96413	1
79403	96414	1

Interpretation

In planar imaging, the gamma camera remains stationary. The resulting images are two-dimensional images of the part or organ being studied. Single photon emission computed tomography, or SPECT, produces three-dimensional images because the gamma camera rotates around the patient.

The CPT codebook often describes groups of similar codes differing in the complexity of the service. Unless services are performed at separate patient encounters or at separate anatomic sites, the less complex service is mutually exclusive to the more complex service and is not separately reportable. In this case, the SPECT study is the more complex procedure, and, therefore, the less complex procedure should not be coded additionally.

Take, as an example, if liver imaging is performed as standard planar and SPECT imaging, there would be no medical necessity for two different studies, and only the most complex study (the SPECT) should be coded. Within the NCCI edits, these services are mutually exclusive to one another, and the edit cannot be bypassed with any modifier.

78201	Liver imaging; static only
78202	with vascular flow
78205	Liver imaging (SPECT);
78206	with vascular flow

 CPT Coding Tip: *It is very important to code these correctly because if both of these services were billed together, the lower reimbursed service would be paid (the static code). For mutually exclusive services, usually the least complex service is paid because it is expected that the two procedures could not be performed during a single encounter.*

Excerpt From the Radiology Section of NCCI Guidelines[2(p8)]

Myocardial perfusion imaging (CPT codes 78460-78465) is not reportable with cardiac blood pool imaging by gated equilibrium (CPT codes 78472-78473) because the two types of tests utilize different radiopharmaceuticals.

Interpretation

In reading the guideline, one would think that these services are mutually exclusive, rather than bundled services, because different radiopharmaceuticals are used. However, they are Column 1/Column 2 codes, not mutually exclusive.

Excerpt From the Radiology Section of NCCI Guidelines[2(p8)]

CPT codes 76376 and 76377 (3-D rendering) are not separately reportable for nuclear medicine procedures (CPT codes 78000-78999). However, CPT code 76376 or 76377 may be separately reported with modifier -59 on the same date of service as a nuclear medicine procedure if the 3D rendering procedure is performed in association with a third procedure (other than nuclear medicine) for which 3D rendering is appropriately reported.

Interpretation

The CPT codebook instructs that CPT code 76376 is not to be added to the nuclear medicine codes. See the following excerpt from the CPT codebook.[1(p321)]

76376 3D rendering with interpretation and reporting of computed tomography, magnetic resonance imaging, ultrasound, or other tomographic modality; not requiring image postprocessing on an independent workstation

(Do not report 76376 in conjunction with 70496, 70498, 70544-70549, 71275, 71555, 72159, 72191, 72198, 73206, 73225, 73706, 73725, 74175, 74185, 75635, 75557-75564, 76377, 78000-78999, 0066T, 0067T, 0144T-0151T, 0159T)

Note: The CPT parenthetical coding guideline specifically states that code 76376 is not to be coded when the procedure is performed for nuclear medicine services. It would be incorrect coding to add code 76376 to nuclear medicine services.

Radiation Oncology Services and NCCI Guidelines

The October 1997 issue of *CPT Assistant*[5] is a great outline and explains radiation oncology in wonderful detail.

Excerpt From the Radiology Section of NCCI Guidelines[2(p8-9)]

Continuing medical physics consultation (CPT code 77336) is reported "per week of therapy." It may be reported after every five radiation treatments. (It may also be reported if the total number of radiation treatments in a course of radiation therapy is less than five.) Since radiation planning procedures (CPT codes 77261-77334) are generally performed before radiation treatment commences, the NCCI contains edits preventing payment of CPT code 77336 with CPT codes 77261-77295, 77301-77328, and 77332-77334. Because radiation planning procedures may occasionally be repeated during a course of radiation treatment, the edits allow modifier -59 to be appended to CPT code 77336 when the radiation planning procedure and continuing medical physics consultation are reported on the same date of service.

Interpretation

77336 Continuing medical physics consultation, including assessment of treatment parameters, quality assurance of dose delivery, and review of patient treatment documentation in support of the radiation oncologist, reported per week of therapy

(a) reported after every five radiation treatments. (It may also be reported if the total number of radiation treatments in a course of radiation therapy is less than five.)

This CPT code is designated as *per week*, which would be reported one time for every five fractions per treatment week. Additionally, if the final week of treatment has fewer than five fractions, CPT code 77336 may still be billed. CPT code 77336 includes the overall quality control, machine calibration, and other physics related to the radiation treatment. This code represents the oversight by the medical physicist in the care of the patient. This is to ensure that the physician's plan of treatment for the patient is being carried out appropriately.

(b) NCCI contains edits preventing payment of CPT code 77336 with CPT codes 77261 through 77295, 77301 through 77328, and 77332 through 77334.

CPT code 77336 is to ensure that the radiation oncologist's plan is being effectively followed; therefore, the physics consultation (CPT code 77336) cannot be performed before treatment starts. NCCI edits the physics consultations into the treatment planning.

(c) The edits allow modifier 59 to be appended to CPT code 77336 when the radiation planning procedure and continuing medical physics consultation occur on the same date of service.

NCCI does allow the edit between the physics consultation and treatment planning to be overridden when they occur on the same day if the physicist is following a prior treatment plan and, on the same day, the physician is performing a subsequent treatment planning session.

To illustrate, a physicist monitoring a radiation therapy patient performs a continuing physics consultation five times the first week, five times the second week, and three times the last week. This should be billed as CPT code 77336 × 3 (three different weeks with at least five fractions each week except the last). Because three is the total for the last week, the weekly code is still used.

Another example would be for a physicist monitoring a radiation therapy patient, and the service date was billed on the same date as the radiation treatment planning (CPT code 77261). Both may be billed, with a modifier 59 appended to code 77336 only if:

1. the physicist was monitoring a plan from prior dates of service.
2. the treatment planning was truly to monitor and potentially update the prior plan.

Other Information on Intensity Modulated Radiation Therapy

The current Medicare policy is that CPT code 77336 (Continuing medical physics consultation) may not be reported when the service is part of the IMRT planning process (CPT code 77301). Remember, CPT code 77336 is for the *weekly* continuing medical physics process and reports the work and oversight of the medical physicist in the care of the patient.

Some patients start with an initial IMRT plan (CPT code 77301) and then need another IMRT plan several weeks later. This is sometimes called a *boost plan*.

CPT Changes 2002: An Insider's View[6] states the following, "Only one intensity modulated radiotherapy plan may be reported for a given course of therapy to a specific treatment area. However, if there is a clinical indication to change the treatment plan, because of either changes in clinical condition or the need to change the parameters of treatment, such as would be encountered in 'boost' situation, then the additional plan would be reported."

Excerpt From the Radiology Section of NCCI Guidelines[2(p9)]

The *Internet-Only Manuals (IOM), Medicare Claims Processing Manual*, Publication 100-04, Chapter 13, Section 70.2 (Services Bundled Into Treatment Management Codes)(4) defines services that may not be reported separately with radiation oncology procedures. Based on these requirements, the NCCI contains edits bundling the following CPT codes into all radiation therapy services:

11920-11921 (Tattooing)

16000-16030 (Treatment of burns)

36000, 36410, 36425 (Venipuncture or introduction of catheter)

51701-51703 (Urinary bladder catheterization)

90760, 90768 (Intravenous infusion)

90804-90822 (Psychotherapy)

90846 (Psychotherapy)

90847 (Psychotherapy)

90862, M0064 (Pharmacologic management)

97802-97804 (Medical nutrition therapy)

99143-99144 (Anesthesia – Moderate conscious sedation)

99185 (Regional hypothermia)

99201-99215 (Evaluation & Management)

99217-99239 (Evaluation & Management)

99281-99456 (Evaluation & Management)

TABLE 16-3 *Excerpt From NCCI Edit Table for Radiation Oncology Evaluation and Management Bundled Services*

Column 1/Column 2 Edits		
Column 1	Column 2	Modifier 0 = not allowed 1 = allowed 9 = not applicable
70010	G0351	1
70010	G0353	1
70010	G0354	1
77261	99201	0
77261	99202	0
77261	99203	0
77261	99204	0
77261	99205	0
77261	99211	0
77261	99212	0
77261	99213	0
77261	99214	0
77261	99215	0

Cannot bypass this edit.

Note: Although the NCCI guidelines include CPT codes 90760 through 90775, please note that these codes were deleted and replaced with CPT codes 96360 through 96375.

Interpretation

NCCI edits bundle the E/M services into the treatments, much as global surgeries CPT codes include related E/M encounters. The radiation oncology provider may bill a consult E/M service for the initial visit to evaluate the patient and determine how to proceed with the treatment.

This initial visit may be billed as a consultation as long as it is appropriately documented. Consultation E/M services do not bundle into radiation oncology services, whereas the nonconsultation E/M services do bundle into the radiation

oncology services. Procedures that bundle may not be bypassed with a modifier. See Table 16-3 for an excerpt from the NCCI Column 1/Column 2 edits for radiation oncology.

The Medicare Claims Processing Manual Chapter 13 - Radiology Services and Other Diagnostic Procedures[7] lists services included in the radiation treatment management procedures. This manual should be reviewed by anyone billing for radiology-related services.

Example

A patient is sent to a radiation oncologist for determination of the best treatment for the patient's cancer. The radiation oncologist evaluates the patient and determines that radiation is the best mode of treatment and notifies the requesting physician of the evaluation and determination. During this same encounter, the radiation oncologist begins the treatment planning. Both the consultation and treatment planning could be billed.

Example

A patient currently undergoing radiation therapy presented for treatment (CPT codes 77401-77421), and the radiation oncologist performs an updated evaluation. The treatment would be the only service billed for this encounter, as the E/M service would be bundled into the treatment code.

Excerpt From the Radiology Section of NCCI Guidelines[2(p10)]

Based on CPT coding instructions xeroradiography (e.g., CPT code 76150) is not separately reportable with mammography studies.

Interpretation

As a reminder (refer to Chapter 2 of this book), NCCI edits advise that CPT codebook instructions should be followed when services are being coded. Within the CPT codebook, the xeroradiography code (CPT code 76150) is followed by a parenthetic instruction:

(76150 is to be used for non-mammographic studies only)[1(p321)]

As NCCI edits follow CPT guidelines, providers must use CPT-4 codes 77055 for unilateral diagnostic mammography and 77056 for bilateral diagnostic mammography whether or not xeroradiography was used in the examination. CPT-4 code 76150 should be billed when xeroradiography is used for nonmammographic studies. If providers use code 76150 with either 77055 or 77056, the claim will be denied, and the bundling edit may not be bypassed.

Tip: Xeroradiography is an X-ray that records the image on paper rather than on film. It requires more radiation exposure.

Excerpt From the Radiology Section of NCCI Guidelines[2(p10-11)]

Guidance for placement of radiation fields by computerized tomography or ultrasound (CPT code 77014 or 76950) for the same anatomical area are mutually exclusive of one another.

Interpretation

The CMS will pay one CPT code to capture a single objective. If two methods are used to reach a single purpose for one anatomical site during a single encounter, only the successful method should be coded. Therefore, if both a CT method and an ultrasonic guidance method are used for the same end result, only the successful procedure (usually the later performed) should be coded.

For instance, a patient presents for a needle biopsy, and the physician uses a CT guidance method. The CT method is unsuccessful, so the physician used ultrasonic radiologic guidance for the needle placement, which is successful. Only the successful guidance method (ultrasound) may be coded.

77012 Computed tomography guidance for needle placement (eg, biopsy, aspiration, injection, localization device), radiological supervision and interpretation

76942 Ultrasonic guidance for needle placement (eg, biopsy, aspiration, injection, localization device), imaging supervision and interpretation

These codes bundle as Column 1/Column 2 codes. Because the ultrasonic guidance was successful, CPT code 76942 would be the only code billed.

Excerpt From the Radiology Section of NCCI Guidelines[2(p11)]

Ultrasound guidance and diagnostic ultrasound (echography) procedures may be reported separately only if each service is separate and distinct.

Excerpt From the Radiology Section of NCCI Guidelines[2(p11)]

CPT code 77790 (supervision, handling, loading of radiation source) is not separately reportable with any of the remote afterloading brachytherapy codes (e.g., CPT codes 77781-77784) since these procedures include the supervision, handling, and loading of the radioelement.

Interpretation

CPT codes 77781 through 77784 have been replaced with 77785 through 77787; however, the edit and guidelines still apply. The new CPT codes 77785 through 77787, still include supervision of the radioelement. Also, *CPT Assistant*[8] (September 2005) states that CPT code 77790 is for low dose rate brachytherapy, and CPT codes 77785 through 77787 are for high dose rate brachytherapy, because guidelines based on the American College of Radiology (ACR) indicate that during low dose brachytherapy procedures, the provider may need to handle and supervise the radiation source. However, during high-dose brachytherapy, the higher dose of radiation is already encased in the catheter. Therefore, the handling and supervision of the radiation source is not required.

Excerpt From the Radiology Section of NCCI Guidelines[2(p11)]

Bone studies such as CPT codes 77072-77076 require a series of radiographs. Separate reporting of a bone study and individual radiographs obtained in the course of the bone study is inappropriate.

Interpretation

Bone studies coded with CPT codes 77072 through 77076 require a series of radiographs. Separate reporting of a bone study and individual radiographs obtained in the course of the bone study is inappropriate. So, if a physician performs a complete osseous survey (CPT code 77075) and a separate, one-view cervical spine X-ray, the one-view spine procedure (CPT code 72020) should not be coded separately.

77075 Radiologic examination, osseous survey; complete (axial and appendicular skeleton)

Note that these two codes do not bundle together, and, therefore, no modifier would be required for coding; however, it would be incorrect to bill both together, unless there was a medically necessary separate and distinct cervical spine X-ray. The documentation would have to clearly support the medical necessity and the separate and distinct performance of the one-view X-ray.

Excerpt From the Radiology Section of NCCI Guidelines[2(p11)]

Radiologic supervision and interpretation codes include all radiological services necessary to complete the service procedure. CPT codes for fluoroscopy/fluoroscopic guidance (e.g., CPT codes 76000, 76001, 77002, 77003) or ultrasound/ultrasound guidance (e.g., CPT codes 76942, 76998) should not be reported separately.

Interpretation

The CPT codebook states that radiological supervision and interpretation (S&I) codes, additional codes should not be added for fluoroscopic guidance, because the guidance is captured in the radiological S&I code(s). NCCI further clarifies that the S&I codes also include the ultrasonic guidance. If, however, a second procedure was performed on the same date as the S&I procedure, and the second procedure was performed using fluoroscopic guidance, the guidance could be billed for that procedure as long as:
- the documentation clearly distinguished the two procedures, and
- the procedure with which the fluoroscopy was billed is not one that includes the work for the fluoroscopic guidance.

The following *CPT Assistant* discusses when fluoroscopic guidance may be reported in addition to procedures. The February 2007 issue of *CPT Assistant*[9] considered the issue of whether certain procedures require fluoroscopic guidance and when additional reporting is warranted.

Fluoroscopic guidance can be used independently or in combination with other imaging methods; therefore, it is important to refer to the code descriptors, parenthetical instructions, and introductory notes for specific reporting instruction. For example, fluoroscopic guidance (77002) is inclusive of all radiographic arthrography with the exception of supervision and interpretation for computed tomography and magnetic resonance arthrography. Therefore, it is not appropriate to report 77002 in addition to codes 70332, 73040, 73085, 73115, 73525, 73580, and 73615.

Fluoroscopic guidance is inclusive of organ or anatomic specific radiological supervision and interpretation procedure codes 74320, 74350, 74355, 74445, 74470, 74475, 75809, 75810, 75885, 75887, 75980, 75982, and 75989.

If the physician is not present in the operating room during a procedure that uses fluoroscopy or fluoroscopic guidance, that physician should not submit a code for fluoroscopy because fluoroscopic imaging requires personal supervision. However, the appropriate radiographic code to report the anatomy evaluated should be submitted in the event that (1) the radiologist's contract with the hospital requires that a radiologist issue a formal interpretation or (2) the physician performing the study requests that a radiologist produce a formal report of the procedure from permanent images recorded.

To illustrate, take the example of a patient who presents for a needle biopsy of the liver. The physician performing the biopsy asks a radiologist to provide fluoroscopic guidance for the procedure. In this case, the surgeon would bill 47000 (Biopsy of liver, needle; percutaneous), and the radiologist would bill 77002 (Fluoroscopic guidance for needle placement [eg, biopsy, aspiration, injection, localization device]). If the only imaging provided is fluoroscopy for needle placement guidance, code 77002 is reported. Code 77002 is not reported in addition to a radiological S&I code because those codes include the fluoroscopic guidance for the needle placement.

Another example would be for a patient who presents for a shoulder arthrography. The provider performs a fluoroscopically guided arthrography. The radiologist would bill 73040 (Radiologic examination, shoulder, arthrography, radiological supervision and interpretation) and 23350 (Injection procedure for shoulder arthrography or enhanced CT/MRI shoulder arthrography). The S&I includes any fluoroscopy element of the procedure.

> ### Excerpt From the Radiology Section of NCCI Guidelines[2(p12)]
>
> Abdominal ultrasound examinations (CPT codes 76700-76775) and abdominal duplex examinations (CPT codes 93975, 93976) are generally performed for different clinical scenarios, although there are some instances where both types of procedures are medically reasonable and necessary. In the latter case, the abdominal ultrasound procedure CPT code should be reported with an NCCI-associated modifier.

Interpretation

An abdominal ultrasound is a sonography to capture the structure and movement of the abdomen's internal organs. A duplex scan combines an abdominal ultrasound and a Doppler (where a special technique is used to evaluate the blood as it flows through a blood vessel).

76700	Ultrasound, abdominal, real time with image documentation; complete
76705	limited (eg, single organ, quadrant, follow-up)
76770	Ultrasound, retroperitoneal (eg, renal, aorta, nodes), real time with image documentation; complete
76775	limited
93975	Duplex scan of arterial inflow and venous outflow of abdominal, pelvic, scrotal contents and/or retroperitoneal organs; complete study
93976	limited study

The NCCI guideline indicates that in order to bill for both an abdominal ultrasound (sonography of an organ) and an abdominal duplex scan (vascular study), the documentation must support that different clinical issues (medical necessity for both) are being explored and that separate and distinct studies were also performed. Do not code a duplex scan if color is turned on to determine whether a structure is vascular. The duplex is for vascular analysis of blood flow.

> ### Excerpt From the Radiology Section of NCCI Guidelines[2(p12)]
>
> Tumor imaging by positron emission tomography (PET) may be reported with CPT codes 78811-78816. If a concurrent computed tomography (CT) scan is performed for attenuation correction and anatomical localization, CPT codes 78814-78816 should be reported rather than CPT codes 78811-78813. A CT scan for localization should not be reported separately with CPT codes 78811-78816. However, a medically reasonable and necessary diagnostic CT scan may be separately reported with an NCCI-associated modifier.

Interpretation

78811	Positron emission tomography (PET) imaging; limited area (eg, chest, head/neck)
78812	skull base to mid-thigh
78813	whole body
78814	Positron emission tomography (PET) with concurrently acquired computed tomography (CT) for attenuation correction and anatomical localization imaging; limited area (eg, chest, head/neck)
78815	skull base to mid-thigh
78816	whole body

PET scans produce digital pictures that can help identify many forms of cancer, damaged heart tissue, and brain disorders (eg, Alzheimer's disease). The PET scan images the biology of disorders at the molecular level before anatomical changes are visible. A PET scan differs from other imaging techniques (eg, X-ray, MRI, CT), which detect changes in the body structure or anatomy. A PET scan can distinguish between benign and malignant disorders (or between alive and dead tissue).

When a PET scan with CT is performed, the physician overlays the PET and CT images in a computer to create images of anatomic correlation. The physician reviews images at three different points (PET scan, CT data, and a combined set of data). So, PET and CT images acquired on a single machine (CT data is first and separate from the PET data) are coded with the PET with concurrent CT CPT codes (78814-78816).

If a CT procedure is performed for other than attenuation correction and anatomical localization, then a diagnostic CT of that site may be reported in addition to the PET study by appending a modifier 59 to the diagnostic CT study code.

Take the case of a patient with a history of squamous cell carcinoma of the neck who presented for a CT study of the chest to determine whether there was progression of the cancer. The CT study was performed, with findings of potential progression. Therefore, a subsequent PET-CT scan of the head/neck and chest was done to evaluate the extent of the metastasis and document precise anatomic distribution prior to consideration for surgery and/or radiation therapy.

In this scenario, both the CT study and the PET-CT should be coded, with a modifier appended to the CT study. They are both medically appropriate and should be separately documented.

Excerpt From the Radiology Section of NCCI Guidelines[2(p12)]

Axial bone density studies may be reported with CPT codes 77078 or 77080. Peripheral site bone density studies may be reported with CPT codes 77079, 77081, 76977, or G0130. Although it may be medically reasonable and necessary to report both axial and peripheral bone density studies on the same date of service, NCCI edits prevent the reporting of multiple CPT codes for the axial bone density study or multiple CPT codes for the peripheral site bone density study on the same date of service.

Interpretation

Here are some comments about bone density studies:

The CPT/Healthcare Common Procedure Coding System (HCPCS) codes are as follows:

G0130 Single-energy X-ray absorptiometry (SEXA) bone density study, one or more sites; appendicular skeleton (peripheral) (eg, radius, wrist, heel)

76977 Ultrasound bone density measurement and interpretation, peripheral site(s), any method

77078 Computed tomography, bone mineral density study, 1 or more sites; axial skeleton (eg, hips, pelvis, spine)

77079 appendicular skeleton (peripheral) (eg, radius, wrist, heel)

77080 Dual-energy X-Ray absorptiometry (DXA), bone density study, 1 or more sites; axial skeleton (eg, hips, pelvis, spine)

77081 appendicular skeleton (peripheral) (eg, radius, wrist, heel)

77082 vertebral fracture assessment

The *axial* skeleton forms the central axis of the body. It consists of the skull, the vertebral column, the ribs, and the sternum or breastbone. The *appendicular* (peripheral) skeleton consists of the girdles and the skeleton of the limbs. The upper (anterior) limbs are attached to the pectoral (shoulder) girdle, and the lower (posterior) limbs are attached to the pelvic (hip) girdle.

There are several different methods of performing a bone density study (OCT, DXA, SEXA, ultrasound), and there are different codes for each method as shown in the previously listed codes.

This NCCI guideline states that different body areas could be surveyed during a single encounter. However, it would not be medically necessary to perform different types (eg, CT and DXA) on the same body part during the same encounter, and they are deemed mutually exclusive.

So, if both a DXA appendicular survey and a CT appendicular survey are billed for a patient during a single encounter, they would be considered mutually exclusive and only one reimbursed. This edit may not be bypassed. However, if both a DXA appendicular and DXA axial study are performed on a patient during a single encounter, they could both be billed if the documentation supported both services being performed and if the services are medically necessary. There is an edit that bundles these as mutually exclusive, but the edit may be bypassed with a modifier 59.

Excerpt From the Radiology Section of NCCI Guidelines[2(p12)]

When existing vascular access lines or selectively placed catheters are used to procure arterial or venous samples, billing for the sample collection separately is inappropriate. CPT codes 36500 (venous catheterization for selective organ blood sampling) or 75893 (venous sampling through catheter with or without angiography...) may be reported for venous blood sampling through a catheter placed for the sole purpose of venous blood sampling with or without venography. CPT code 75893 includes concomitant venography. If a catheter is placed for a purpose other than venous blood sampling with or without venography (CPT code 75893), it is a misuse of CPT codes 36500 or 75893 to report them in addition to CPT codes for the other venous procedure(s). CPT codes 36500 or 75893 should not be reported for blood sampling during an arterial procedure.

Interpretation

Billing for venous access via catheterization is appropriate only when the catheter is placed solely for the specimen collection and is independent of any other procedures. If a catheter is placed for other primary reasons (eg, diagnostic imaging or therapeutic procedures), it would include any specimen collection through the same catheter.

Excerpt From the Radiology Section of NCCI Guidelines[2(p12-13)]

Radiologic studies with contrast (eg, CT, CTA, MRI, MRA, angiography) utilize subtraction techniques as a standard of practice. CPT code 76350 (subtraction in conjunction with contrast studies) should not be reported with procedures that typically utilize contrast.

Interpretation

Subtraction radiography and digital subtraction angiography (DSA) are image enhancing methods. Report procedure code 76350, subtraction, only in conjunction with contrast studies—when image subtraction radiography or DSA with a contrasted radiographic study is performed. Medicare will not pay for radiographic imaging techniques, such as image subtraction, used with contrasted radiographic studies. See Table 16-4 for an excerpt from NCCI edits for CPT code 76350. Note all the contrasted radiology services that include the subtraction angiography.

Subtraction radiography (or DSA) eliminates overlying bone images that may obscure the vascular pattern in an angiogram. Subtraction allows for visualization of blood vessels without interference from surrounding structures. In DSA, a computer subtracts a radiographic image taken prior to the administration of an intravascular contrast material from an image obtained with the contrast present. This technique produces an image in which only the contrast-filled vessels are visible.

Excerpt From the Radiology Section of NCCI Guidelines[2(p13)]

CPT codes 70540-70543 are utilized to report magnetic resonance imaging of the orbit, face, and/or neck. Only one code may be reported for an imaging session regardless of whether one, two, or three areas are evaluated in the imaging session.

TABLE 16-4 *NCCI Edits for Subtraction With Contrast*

(No codes listed)

During 01 2009, Code 76350 is considered a Column 2 Code to:

70450°	70460°	70470°	70480°	70481°	70482°
70486°	70487°	70488°	70490°	70491°	70492°
70496°	70498°	70540°	70542°	70543°	70544°
70545°	70546°	70547°	70548°	70549°	70551°
70552°	70553°	70557°	70558°	70559°	71250°
71260°	71270°	71275°	71550°	71551°	71552°
71555°	72125°	72126°	72127°	72128°	72129°
72130°	72131°	72132°	72133°	72141°	72142°
72146°	72147°	72148°	72149°	72156°	72157°
72158°	72191°	72192°	72193°	72194°	72195°
72196°	72197°	72198°	73200°	73201°	73202°
73206°	73218°	73219°	73220°	73221°	73222°
73223°	73700°	73701°	73702°	73706°	73718°
73719°	73720°	73721°	73722°	73723°	73725°
74150°	74160°	74170°	74175°	74181°	74182°
74183°	74185°	75561°	75563°	75600°	75605°
75625°	75630°	75635°	75650°	75658°	75660°
75662°	75665°	75671°	75676°	75680°	75685°
75705°	75710°	75716°	75722°	75724°	75726°
75731°	75733°	75736°	75741°	75743°	75746°
75756°	75774°	75790°	75801°	75803°	75805°
75807°	75809°	75810°	75820°	75822°	75825°
75827°	75831°	75833°	75840°	75842°	75860°
75870°	75872°	75880°	75885°	75887°	75889°
75891°	76376°	76377°	77058°	77059°	C8900°
C8901°	C8902°	C8903°	C8904°	C8905°	C8906°
C8907°	C8908°	C8909°	C8910°	C8911°	C8912°
C8913°	C8914°	C8918°	C8919°	C8920°	

During 01 2009, Code 76350 is considered Mutually Exclusive with:

Interpretation

The CPT codes for these MRI studies read *and/or*; therefore, regardless of the combination of sites imaged, only one code would be used.

70540   Magnetic resonance (eg, proton) imaging, orbit, face, and/or neck; without contrast material(s)

70542   with contrast material(s)

70543   without contrast material(s), followed by contrast material(s) and further sequences

Therefore, CPT code 70540 should be reported for the MRI studies of orbit without contrast, face without contrast, face and/or neck without contrast.

Excerpt From the Radiology Section of NCCI Guidelines[2(p13)]

An MRI study of the brain (CPT codes 70551-70553) and MRI study of the orbit (CPT codes 70540-70543) are separately reportable only if they are both medically reasonable and necessary and are performed as distinct studies. An MRI of the orbit is not separately reportable with an MRI of the brain if an incidental abnormality of the orbit is identified during an MRI of the brain since only one MRI study is performed.

Interpretation

Remember, only medically necessary and separately distinguishable services are coded and billed. If two different anatomic sites are viewed within a single imaging series, only one study should be billed. However, if there are separate studies and both are medically necessary, both may be coded.

SUMMARY

- The entire radiology section from the NCCI manual should be read.

- Careful reading (and rereading) of the CPT codebook guidelines for radiology services is important.

- Repeated procedures performed on the same date should be medically necessary in order to be billed. If procedures are repeated because of poor image quality or other reasons that are not related to reassessing the patient's condition, only the successfully performed procedure should be coded.

- Diagnostic angiography services prior to therapeutic services should be coded only if they are truly diagnostic, and a prior diagnostic study has not been performed or if a prior diagnostic study was performed, but the patient's condition had changed.

Definitions and Acronyms

computed tomography (CT)

intra-arterial: Into an artery.

intrathecal: Into the spine.

intravascular: Into a blood vessel.

intravenous (IV): Into a vein.

parenteral: Administered other than by the alimentary tract.

CHAPTER EXERCISES

EXERCISE 1
Is it appropriate to bill for a diagnostic ultrasound study in addition to the guidance and procedure? Example: Ultrasound-guided needle biopsy of a muscle.

EXERCISE 2
What would be coded for a CT scan of the upper extremity with orally administered contrast material?

EXERCISE 3
What would be coded for a three-view hand X-ray done before fracture treatment and a one-view hand X-ray done after fracture reduction, performed on the same date for the same patient?

ANSWERS TO CHAPTER EXERCISES

Exercise 1: The correct coding for this service would be CPT codes 76942 and 20206:

76942 Ultrasonic guidance for needle placement (eg, biopsy, aspiration, injection, localization device), imaging supervision and interpretation

20206 Biopsy, muscle, percutaneous needle

The diagnostic ultrasound of a muscle would not be additionally reported unless there was a distinct and separate diagnostic study.

Exercise 2:

73200 Computed tomography, upper extremity; without contrast material

Oral and/or rectal contrast material administration alone does not qualify as a study with contrast.

Exercise 3: CPT 73130 would be coded for the three-view X-Ray, and CPT 73120-59-52 would be coded for the postreduction one-view X-ray. The postreduction X-ray would normally be bundled into the three-view procedure and should be appended with a modifier 59 to bypass the coding edit. Additionally, there is no code for a one-view hand X-ray; therefore, modifier 52 (reduced service) should also be appended.

73120 Radiologic examination, hand; 2 views

73130 minimum of 3 views

REFERENCES

1. American Medical Association. *Current Procedural Terminology (CPT®) Professional Edition 2009*. Chicago, IL: American Medical Association; 2008.

2. Centers for Medicare and Medicaid Services. "Chapter IX Radiology Services." In: NCCI Policy Manual for Medicare Services. www.cms.hhs.gov/NationalCorrectCodInitEd/01_overview.asp#TopOfPage. Accessed June 14, 2009.

3. Centers for Medicare and Medicaid Services. "Chapter I General Correct Coding Policies." In: NCCI Policy Manual for Medicare Services. www.cms.hhs.gov/NationalCorrectCodInitEd/01_overview.asp#TopOfPage. Accessed June 14, 2009.

4. Centers for Medicare and Medicaid Services. *Medicare Benefit Policy Manual*. Chapter 15; Section 80.6. www.cms.hhs.gov/manuals/Downloads/bp102c15.pdf. Accessed June 14, 2009.

5. American Medical Association. "Coding clarification, radiation oncology." *CPT Assistant*, 1997;7(10):1.

6. American Medical Association. "*CPT Changes 2002: An Insider's View.*" Chicago, IL: American Medical Association; 2001.

7. Centers for Medicare and Medicaid Services. *Medicare Claims Processing Manual*. Chapter 13. www.cms.hhs.gov/manuals/downloads/clm104c13.pdf. Accessed June 14, 2009.

8. American Medical Association. "Clinical Brachytherapy." *CPT Assistant*, 2005;(9):1.

9. American Medical Association. "Coding communication: radiology: radiologic guidance." *CPT Assistant*, 2007;17(2):11.

Pathology and Laboratory Services

Chapter 17 provides background about services in the pathology/laboratory section of the *Current Procedural Terminology (CPT®)*[1] codebook, reviews the National Correct Coding Initiative (NCCI) coding guidelines for laboratory/pathology services, and provides examples to reflect the logic behind the edits. As do the other chapters, this chapter provides an NCCI guideline followed by our interpretation, an example, or both.

Background About the Services in the Pathology/Laboratory Guidelines in the CPT Codebook

Excerpt From the Pathology/Laboratory Section of NCCI Guidelines[2(p2)]

Pathology and laboratory CPT coding includes services primarily reported to evaluate specimens obtained from patients (body fluids, cytological specimens, or tissue specimens obtained by invasive/surgical procedures) in order to provide information to the treating physician. This information, coupled with information obtained from history and examination findings and other data, provides the physician with the background upon which medical decision making is established.

Introduction Section of NCCI Guidelines for Laboratory/Pathology Services

Excerpt From the Pathology/Laboratory Section of NCCI Guidelines[2(p2)]

Introduction
The principles of correct coding discussed in Chapter I apply to the CPT codes in the range 80000-89999. Several general guidelines are repeated in this Chapter. However, those general guidelines from Chapter I not discussed in this chapter are nonetheless applicable.

Interpretation

This instruction indicates that the overall NCCI guidelines apply to each section of the CPT codebook, and, even if they are not repeated within a chapter, they are nonetheless a guideline to be followed. The introductory guidelines were covered comprehensively in Chapter 2 of this book; those introductory guidelines that have clear application to laboratory/pathology services are reiterated in this chapter.

Excerpt From the Pathology/Laboratory Section of NCCI Guidelines[2(p2-3)]

Certain types of specimens and tests are reviewed personally by the pathologist. CPT coding for this section includes few codes requiring patient contact or evaluation and management services rendered directly by the pathologist. On the occasion that a pathologist provides evaluation and management services…appropriate coding should be rendered from the evaluation and management section of the *CPT Manual*.

Interpretation

The CPT codes within the pathology and laboratory section do not require the billing provider to interact personally with the patient, as a specimen is sent for remote examining. However, should a pathologist meet personally (or face-to-face) with a patient to provide additional information regarding the results of the testing, an evaluation and management (E/M) CPT code might very well be billable. The guidelines for coding E/M would be followed as with other providers. For example, a patient asks for more details regarding her test results reflecting cancer, and her primary care provider asks the pathologist to meet with the patient. The pathologist meets with the patient to review, in detail, the test results and what the results meant. In this case, the encounter is going to mostly involve counseling time. If the encounter is medically necessary and documented, the pathologist may bill for an E/M service, probably based on the time element.

 CPT Coding Tip: *Counseling and coordinating care services may be billed based on the total face-to-face time the provider spends with the patient, if the time spent in counseling and coordinating care exceeds more than half the total visit time. In order to use time as the driving element, the following must be documented:*

1. *Total face-to-face time between the physician and patient*
2. *Total time spent counseling and coordinating care. Time spent counseling and coordinating care may be indicated by specific time (in minutes, for example) or by the provider attesting that more than half of the total face-to-face time was spent counseling and coordinating care.*
3. *Some information as to what was discussed during the time spent counseling and coordinating care*

If the total time spent counseling and coordinating care exceeded 50% of the total visit time, the total visit time could be used to drive the level of E/M service coded.

Excerpt From the Pathology/Laboratory Section of NCCI Guidelines[2(p3)]

If, after a test was ordered and performed, additional related procedures are necessary to provide or verify the result, these would be considered part of the ordered test. For example, if a patient with leukemia had thrombocytopenia, and a manual platelet count (CPT code 85032) was performed in addition to an automated hemogram with automated platelet count (CPT code 85027), it would be inappropriate to report CPT codes 85032 and 85027, because the former provides verification for the automated hemogram and platelet count (CPT code 85027). As another example, if a patient had an abnormal test result, and repeat performance of the test was done to verify the result, the test is reported as one unit of service rather than two.

Interpretation

Remember, as discussed in prior chapters, Medicare will pay for only those services that are medically necessary. To repeat a test solely to validate or verify the original test result does not support a medically necessary service. If the original test was medically necessary, any later verification test would not be, as it represents an internal quality control on the test, not a test of the patient's condition. Therefore, positive results from drug testing are often rerun to make certain the positive test results are accurate. Although this is a good practice for ensuring accuracy of a patient's medical history (positive drug results can have far-reaching and damaging ramifications for a patient), the second result does not provide new clinical data, or at least it should not. Even when the results differ (a false positive), that merely means one of the results was inaccurate, and Medicare chooses not to pay for the unsuccessful or inaccurate testing.

If a treating physician orders an automated complete blood count with automated differential WBC count (CPT code 85025) or without automated differential WBC count (CPT code 85027), the laboratory sometimes examines a blood smear in order to complete the ordered test based on laboratory selected criteria flagging the results for additional verification. The laboratory should NOT report CPT code 85007 (microscopic blood smear examination with manual WBC differential count) or CPT code 85008 (microscopic blood smear examination without manual WBC differential count) for the examination of a blood smear to complete the ordered automated hemogram test (CPT codes 85025 or 85027). The same principle applies if the treating physician orders any type of blood count and the laboratory's practice is to perform an automated complete blood count with or without automated differential WBC count.

Interpretation

This guideline is, in part, the same as the last, in that any tests that are performed to verify *or complete* the ordered service are not separately coded. Additional testing performed as a part of the laboratory policy for quality control cannot be billed.

Tip: Examination of a blood smear is primarily ordered to evaluate blood cell populations when a complete blood count (CBC) with differential count, performed with an automated blood cell counter, indicates the presence of abnormal or immature cells. Historically, a blood smear was performed for just about anyone having a CBC performed. Now, with the automated instruments currently used, an automated differential count is also provided. If the automated results reflect the presence of abnormal white blood cells (WBC), red blood cells (RBC), or platelets, many laboratories perform the additional test of a blood smear.

This NCCI guideline indicates that the laboratory cannot code the blood smear to complete an ordered test. It would be bundled into the ordered service, rather than being coded separately. To illustrate this point, consider that a physician orders a CBC. The laboratory runs the CBC on automated equipment. The printout of the CBC result generates a flag that a manual blood smear examina-tion should be performed because of aberrant results. A manual blood smear examination is performed.

85025 Blood count; complete (CBC), automated (Hgb, Hct, RBC, WBC and platelet count) and automated differential WBC count

85008 Blood count; blood smear, microscopic examination without manual differential WBC count

Only the CBC (CPT code 85025) should be billed in this scenario.

If a treating physician orders an automated hemogram (CPT code 85027) and a manual differential WBC count (CPT code 85007), both codes may be reported. However, a provider may not report an automated hemogram with automated differential WBC count (CPT code 85025) with a manual differential WBC count (CPT code 85007) because this combination of codes results in duplicate payment for the differential WBC count. CMS does not pay twice for the same laboratory test result even if performed by two different methods unless the two methods are medically reasonable and necessary.

Interpretation

Tests of specific measures (differential WBC counts, for example) may be performed through different methodologies (automated vs manual); however, they provide basically the same measurement (percentages of each type of WBC). Because only one result (or measure) should be medically necessary, only one differential count should be coded. Frankly, the manual differential count is often performed for verification, because it is felt by some to be superior testing over the automated method.

There are many different forms of blood count services, and the physician may request the tests he or she believes to be best for a specific patient's clinical indications. If a physician orders tests for which there is a single CPT code that includes the entire testing by the specified methodology, only that code may be used. If, however, a physician orders a test for which there is no single CPT code to include the entire service, multiple codes may be billed. So, if a physician orders an automated CBC with automated differential count, and the laboratory performs an additional manual differential count for verification, only the ordered test should be coded. The manual differential count duplicates the measurement from the automated differential count. In addition, the manual differential count was not ordered. However, if a physician orders an automated CBC with a manual differential WBC count, there is no single code that incorporates both a manual differential count with an automated CBC. Therefore, both may be coded with CPT codes 85027 (CBC) and 85007 (manual differential WBC count). On the other hand, if the physician ordered an automated CBC with automated differential WBC count, there is a single code that encompasses the CBC and differential count using automated testing methodology (CPT code 85025).

Documentation Tip: *If the differential count is repeated at a later time on the same date to determine whether the patient's condition has changed, it would be acceptable to code the second procedure, because it was truly distinct and separate from the first service. The documentation should clearly reflect when and why the second, later service was ordered.*

Excerpt From the Pathology/Laboratory Section of NCCI Guidelines[2(p4)]

By contrast some laboratory tests if positive require additional separate follow-up testing which is implicit in the physician's order. For example, if an RBC antibody screen (CPT code 86850) is positive, the laboratory routinely proceeds to identify the RBC antibody. The latter testing is separately reportable. Similarly, if a urine culture is positive, the laboratory proceeds to organism identification testing which is separately reportable. In these cases, the initial positive results have limited clinical value without the additional testing. The additional testing is separately reportable because it is not performed to complete the ordered test. Furthermore, the ordered test if positive requires the additional testing in order to have clinical value.

Interpretation

This guideline differs from the others discussed so far, in that the subsequent tests are based on a finding (or positive result) from the first test and are performed through different measures or testing methodologies. If the subsequent test was performed as a result of positive test results, and the subsequent test added clinical specificity, relevancy, and detail, it should be coded in addition to the initial test, even without a physician's order for the subsequent test. There should be protocols in place in the laboratory

that indicate when additional different (eg, methodology) testing is appropriate after an initial positive result. This subsequent reflex testing is called automatic laboratory-initiated testing.

Tip: *Subsequent reflex testing benefits the patient, physician, and payer. Because the laboratory is the first to receive the results of an initial laboratory test, subsequent reflex testing can often be automatically performed. This helps expedite patient care, saves physician visits, and leads to more timely diagnosis and appropriate treatment.*

NCCI Guidelines Regarding Organ or Disease Oriented Panels

Excerpt From the Pathology/Laboratory Section of NCCI Guidelines[2(p6)]

The *CPT Manual* assigns CPT codes to organ or disease oriented panels consisting of a group of specified tests. If all tests of a CPT defined panel are performed, the provider may bill the panel code or the individual component test codes. The panel codes may be used when the tests are ordered as that panel or if the individual component tests of a panel are ordered separately. For example, if the individually ordered tests are cholesterol (CPT code 82465), triglycerides (CPT code 84478), and HDL cholesterol (CPT code 83718), the service could be billed as a lipid panel (CPT code 80061).

Interpretation

This element of the CPT and NCCI coding guidelines is often misunderstood, but if read carefully, the guidelines state that *either* the individual tests or the panel may be coded *if* all the tests within a panel are performed. Coding either way is acceptable. The payers are challenged to make sure that one method of coding does not pay differently from the other. In other words, if the individual tests were all billed on a single date of service, they should not generate more pay than the panel of tests that includes all the individual components. For example, an electrolyte panel (CPT code 80051) includes measurement of carbon dioxide (82374), chloride (82435), potassium (84132), and sodium (84295). If all these tests are performed, the provider could bill the individual test CPT codes (82374, 82435, 84132, 84295) or the panel CPT code (80051). The payment should be the same, regardless of which coding method was used. However, if carbon dioxide, chloride, and potassium tests are performed, only the individual test CPT codes could be billed, because all tests in the electrolyte panel are not performed. The sodium test is not done.

Tip: *The term profile or panel means a grouping of laboratory tests, which is usually performed automatically on a single piece of testing equipment.*

Excerpt From the Laboratory/Pathology Section of NCCI Guidelines[2(p6)]

NCCI contains edits pairing each panel CPT code (column one code) with each CPT code corresponding to an individual laboratory test that is included in the panel (column two code). These edits allow use of NCCI-associated modifiers to bypass them if one or more of the individual laboratory tests are reported on the same date of service. The repeat testing must be medically reasonable and necessary. Modifier -91 may be utilized to report this repeat testing. Based on the *Internet-Only Manuals (IOM), Medicare Claims Processing Manual*, Publication 100-04, Chapter 16, Section 100.5.1,(2) the repeat testing cannot be performed to "confirm initial results; due to testing problems with specimens and equipment or for any other reason when a normal, one-time, reportable result is all that is required."

Interpretation

Because panel CPT codes include multiple laboratory tests, NCCI edits bundle the individual tests into the panel test. In other words, the individual tests should not be billed in addition to the panel to which they belong. If, on occasion, one or more of the individual tests needs to be performed a second time on the same date of service, it may be coded when certain criteria are met:

1. The second, separate, and subsequent test was indeed performed. Otherwise, the test is included in the panel.

2. The subsequently performed test was medically necessary. If the second test serves to confirm initial results, do not code it. If the second test was performed due to equipment or other problems with the first test, do not code it. The second test must be performed to compare to the initial results.

3. A modifier 91 should be appended to the subsequent test code to indicate that it should be paid separately from the panel.

Take the example of an electrolyte panel being performed (CPT code 80051) because a patient presents with a symptom of confusion, and it is determined that the patient's potassium and sodium levels are out of the normal range. The physician provides infusions or medications to improve the electrolyte levels. Once the treatment is completed, the physician orders that only the potassium and sodium tests be performed again.

In this scenario, because the electrolyte panel includes four tests (carbon dioxide, chloride, potassium, and sodium), the NCCI edits bundle each of these tests into the panel. If, however, it is medically necessary to perform the sodium and potassium tests a second time, they may be billed in addition to the initial panel by appending a modifier 91 to each of the subsequent CPT codes. They are as follows:

80051	Electrolyte panel
	This panel must include the following:
	Carbon dioxide (82374)
	Chloride (82435)
	Potassium (84132)
	Sodium (84295)
84132-91	Potas
84132-91	Potassium; serum, plasma or whole blood
	Modifier 91 represents a repeated procedure
84295-91	Sodium; serum, plasma or whole blood
	Modifier 91 represents a repeated procedure

CPT code 80051 would be coded for the original panel, CPT code 84132-91 would be coded for the subsequently performed potassium test, and CPT code 84295-91 would be coded for the subsequently performed sodium test.

NCCI Guidelines Regarding Evocative/Suppression Testing Services

Excerpt From the Pathology/Laboratory Section of NCCI Guidelines[2(p7)]

Evocative/suppression testing involves administration of agents to determine a patient's response to those agents (CPT codes 80400-80440 are to be used for reporting the laboratory components of the testing). When the test requires physician administration of the evocative/suppression agent … these codes can be separately reported. However, when physician attendance is not required, and the agent is administered by ancillary personnel, these codes are not to be separately reported. In the inpatient setting, these codes are only reported if the physician performs the service personally. In the office setting, the service can be reported when performed by office personnel if the physician is directly supervising the service.

Interpretation

This NCCI principle makes sense, but it is a bit complicated. Because evocative/suppression testing is for the measurement of the impact of evocative/suppressive agents on patients, the agents must be administered prior to the testing. The laboratory codes (CPT codes 80400-80440) are for the measurement tests and do not include the administration of the agents. This administration is separately coded (using CPT codes 96360-96361, 96372-96375) if the testing is done in the:

- physician's office and is administered by the physician or a nonphysician provider under direct supervision.
- hospital setting and is administered by the physician.

Medically Unlikely Edits

Excerpt From the Pathology/Laboratory Section of NCCI Guidelines[2(p8)]

CMS payment policy allows only one unit of service for CPT codes 88321, 88323, and 88325 per beneficiary per provider on a single date of service. Providers should not report these codes on separate lines of a claim utilizing CPT modifiers to bypass the MUEs for these codes.

Interpretation

88321 Consultation and report on referred slides prepared elsewhere

88323 Consultation and report on referred material requiring preparation of slides

88325 Consultation, comprehensive, with review of records and specimens, with report on referred material

These codes represent consultations on slides, other referred material, potentially medical records, and actual specimens. The codes are to be billed as one unit per surgical case, which can include multiple specimens.

To code CPT code 88321, slides that were prepared elsewhere must be received and reviewed. To code CPT code 88323, the referred unprepared material (specimen, tissue block) must be received and the slides then prepared. To code CPT code 88325, the laboratory must not only review the material received but also the patient's medical records (more than just pathology reports). Because the unit of service is *per surgical case*, CMS created medically unlikely edits (MUEs) to limit the services to one.

Additionally, remember from Chapter 1 of this book that the less complex service is included in the more complex service and is not separately reportable. Only the most complex procedure performed during a single encounter may be coded. The lesser services are incidental to the more complex procedure.

General Policy Statements for Pathology/Laboratory Services and NCCI Guidelines

Excerpt From the Pathology/Laboratory Section of NCCI Guidelines[2(p8-9)]

Multiple CPT codes are descriptive of services performed for bone and bone marrow evaluation. When a biopsy is performed for evaluation of bone matrix structure, the appropriate code to bill is CPT code 20220 for the biopsy and CPT code 88307 for the surgical pathology evaluation.

When a bone marrow aspiration is performed alone, the appropriate coding is CPT code 38220. Appropriate coding for the interpretation is CPT code 85097 when the only service provided is the interpretation of the bone marrow smear. When both are performed by the same provider, both CPT codes may be reported.

Interpretation

The difference between CPT codes 20220 and 38220 is that CPT code 20220 is for the bone matrix (actual bone) biopsy, and CPT code 38220 is for the bone marrow (substance in the hollow of the bone) biopsy. The documentation should clearly indicate whether bone marrow or bone is the biopsied material. If bone is the biopsied material, the surgical pathology examination code would be CPT code 88307 (level V gross and microscopic examination). If bone marrow is the biopsied material, the interpretation code would be CPT code 85097 (bone marrow, smear interpretation). If the physician obtained the specimen and performed the pathology analysis, both the surgery and pathology codes should be billed. If a physician takes a specimen of bone marrow from a patient and performs a smear interpretation, both the biopsy (CPT code 38220) and interpretation (CPT code 85097) may be coded.

 CPT Coding Tip: If a bone biopsy was taken and includes some bone marrow in the specimen, only a bone biopsy should be coded, because a single procedure was performed. Obtaining the marrow becomes incidental to the bone biopsy when both procedures are performed on the same anatomic site.

Excerpt From the Pathology/Laboratory Section of NCCI Guidelines[2(p9)]

The pathological interpretations (CPT code 88300-88309) are not reported in addition to CPT code 85097 unless separate specimens are processed.

Interpretation

The bone marrow aspirate that is used for a smear preparation is coded with CPT code 85097. If the aspirate was allowed to clot for the cell block, the most appropriate code would be CPT code 88305 (most extensive procedure). Two different specimens would be required to bill for both codes; therefore, a different aspirate would be required for additional coding.

Excerpt From the Pathology/Laboratory Section of NCCI Guidelines[2(p9)]

When it is medically necessary to evaluate both bone structure and bone marrow, and both services can be provided with one biopsy, only one code (CPT code 38221 or CPT code 20220) can be reported. If two separate biopsies are necessary, then both can be reported using modifier -59 on one of the codes. Pathological interpretation codes 88300-88309 may be separately reported for multiple separately submitted specimens. If only one specimen is submitted, only one code can be reported regardless of whether the report includes evaluation of both bone structure and bone marrow morphology or not.

Interpretation

Throughout the NCCI bone and bone marrow guidelines, the message is clear that before additional codes may be used, different specimens must be obtained. If coding is for the acquisition of the specimen, either CPT code 38221 or 20220 would be used but not both. If bone and bone marrow were obtained through a single biopsy, code the most extensive procedure only. A distinctly separate biopsy (not through the same needle) would be necessary before both codes could be billed. The same guidelines apply for the pathology coding. Two distinct specimens would be necessary before both services could be coded. If bone and bone marrow were within the same specimen, only one code could be used. Consider when a physician obtains a bone marrow biopsy, and some bone matrix is also incidentally retrieved through the trocar. The sample is sent for pathology interpretation. The physician and the pathologist would each bill only a single code as follows:

- The physician obtaining the specimen would report CPT code 38221 (bone marrow biopsy).
- The pathologist performing the gross and microscopic examination would report CPT code 88305 (bone marrow tissue examination).

The bone biopsy and pathology are incidental services and not coded in addition to the bone marrow procedures.

Excerpt From the Pathology/Laboratory Section of NCCI[2(p9)]

The family of CPT codes 87040-87158 refers to microbial culture studies. The type of culture is coded to the highest level of specificity regarding source, type, etc. When a culture is processed by a commercial kit, report the code that describes the test to its highest level of specificity. A screening culture and culture for definitive identification are not performed on the same day on the same specimen and therefore are not reported together.

Interpretation

The culture codes are designated by the following:
- Specimen (blood, fungus, bacteria, etc.)
- Type of culture (presumptive, screening, aerobic)

The codes assigned should capture the specimen type and culture type specifically. If multiple specimens are being cultured, a modifier 59 may be appended to the second culture to avoid bundling edits.

To illustrate this point, if bacterial cultures on both stool and blood are performed on the same patient on the same date of service, both codes could be billed, based on the different specimens obtained.

87040 Culture, bacterial; blood, aerobic, with isolation and presumptive identification of isolates (includes anaerobic culture, if appropriate)

87045 stool, aerobic, with isolation and preliminary examination (eg, KIA, LIA), Salmonella and Shigella species

---

Excerpt From the Pathology/Laboratory Section of NCCI Guidelines[2(p9-10)]

When cytopathology codes are reported, the appropriate CPT code to bill is that which describes, to the highest level of specificity, what services were rendered.

Interpretation

88104 Cytopathology, fluids, washings or brushings, except cervical or vaginal; smears with interpretation

88106 simple filter method with interpretation

88107 smears and simple filter preparation with interpretation

88108 Cytopathology, concentration technique, smears and interpretation (eg, Saccomanno technique)

88112 Cytopathology, selective cellular enhancement technique with interpretation (eg, liquid based slide preparation method), except cervical or vaginal

These CPT codes represent examples for some of the cytopathology services. Note that the codes include different techniques (selective cellular enhancement vs concentration). NCCI guidelines indicate that only one code from a group of cytopathology codes may be reported per specimen. If distinct and separate specimens are obtained, the cytopathology study for each specimen may be coded separately, with modifier 59 appended.

Excerpt From the Pathology/Laboratory Section of NCCI[2(p10)]

The CPT codes 80500 and 80502 are used to indicate that a pathologist has reviewed and interpreted, with a subsequent written report, a clinical pathology test. These codes additionally are not to be used with any other pathology service that includes a physician interpretation (e.g., surgical pathology). If an evaluation and management service (face-to-face contact with the patient) takes place by the pathologist, then the appropriate E&M code is reported, rather than the clinical pathology consultation codes.

Interpretation

Clinical pathology involves a pathologist assisting in diagnosing diseases based on the analysis of bodily fluids such as blood and urine. Clinical pathology is one area of pathology; the other is anatomic pathology.

Clinical pathology consultations are not unlike the E/M consultation guidelines in that there must be:

1. a request (in this case, a written order) for the consultation,
2. a written report from the pathologist as to the findings, and
3. a demonstrated need for the additional medical interpretation (why does the physician need a consultation on the particular specimen?).

As stated in the CPT codebook,[1(p345)] "reporting of a test result(s) without *medical interpretive judgment* is not considered a clinical pathology consultation." That is why a written report of interpretation is a requirement for billing this code. Only one pathology interpretation should be coded on a single date. Therefore, if a pathologist performed a tissue examination and clinical pathology consultation for a single patient, only the tissue examination would be billed. There is also an MUE code limiting these services to one per day. The specialty societies are lobbying to remove this NCCI edit, because this policy would not allow for proper patient management in cases in which a patient is seen for multiple conditions on a single day.

80500 Clinical pathology consultation; limited, without review of patient's history and medical records

80502 comprehensive, for a complex diagnostic problem, with review of patient's history and medical records

If the consultation required the physician to personally examine the patient, the service would be coded from the E/M section, rather than the pathology/laboratory section of codes.

Physicians at teaching facilities often receive a request from a local physician asking for an interpretation on a patient's clinical pathology. If the pathologist reviews the patient's history, records, and test results, he or she may bill CPT code 80502. If, however, the consulting physician performed a physical examination of the patient in addition to rendering an interpretation for clinical pathology, the consultation codes from the E/M section of the CPT codebook should be used.

Excerpt From the Pathology/Laboratory Section of NCCI Guidelines[2(p10)]

The CPT codes 88321-88325 are to be used to review slides, tissues, or other material obtained and prepared at a different location and referred to a pathologist for a second opinion. (These codes should not be reported by pathologists reporting a second opinion on slides, tissue, or material also examined and reported by another pathologist in the same provider group.) Medicare generally does not pay twice for an interpretation of a given technical service (e.g., EKGs, radiographs, etc.).

Interpretation

If a physician requested a second opinion by a pathologist, CPT codes 88321 through 88325 may be billed. If the second opinion was driven by an initial opinion from another pathologist within the same provider group, these codes could not be used. These codes may be used only on slides or materials coming from outside the pathologist group. See the earlier discussion of these codes in this chapter. Therefore, if two pathologists from the same group practice each perform an interpretation on the same specimen, only one should bill for the service. The second interpretation would be deemed medically unnecessary.

Excerpt From the Pathology/Laboratory Section of NCCI Guidelines[2(p11)]

Multiple tests to identify the same analyte, marker, or infectious agent should not be reported separately. For example, it would not be appropriate to report both direct probe and amplified probe technique tests for the same infectious agent.

Interpretation

Whenever multiple services are performed to achieve a single goal, only the more extensive service is to be coded. Medicare will reimburse only for those services deemed medically necessary. If the results from the less extensive service did not yield the desired information, and a second, more extensive test was performed, only the successful service is to be coded.

87490 Infectious agent detection by nucleic acid (DNA or RNA); Chlamydia trachomatis, direct probe technique

87491 Chlamydia trachomatis, amplified probe technique

If two probe techniques are employed to identify *Chlamydia*, only one should be billed. The successful method should be the one billed.

Excerpt From the Pathology/Laboratory Section of NCCI Guidelines[2(p11)]

Medicare does not pay for duplicate testing. CPT codes 88342 (immunocytochemistry, each antibody) and 88184, 88187, 88188, 88189 (flow cytometry) should not in general be reported for the same or similar specimens. The diagnosis should be established using one of these methods. The provider may report both CPT codes if both methods are required because the initial method is nondiagnostic or does not explain all the light microscopic findings. The provider can report both methods utilizing modifier -59 and document the need for both methods in the medical record.

Interpretation

This is where laboratory bundling issues get very tricky. One would have to understand that these different methods yield duplicative results. This is where the coder must rely on the NCCI bundling edits and information from the providers to work through whether or not a modifier should be appended.

The safest way is to not bypass the edit for any of the tests that bundle together, unless the documentation is clear that distinct and dissimilar specimens (not the same or similar) were involved. If the initial method was nondiagnostic, both methods may be billed, but remember that other NCCI guidelines indicate that payers will pay for only successful testing, so a word of caution is needed here.

Within the NCCI guideline, there are examples of specimens considered similar. If immunocytochemistry was performed on one lymph node, and cytometry was performed on a different lymph node, the lymph nodes are considered similar, and only one service may be billed. However, if immunocytochemistry was performed on a lymph node, and cytometry was performed on blood, both services could be billed because the specimens are not considered similar.

Excerpt From the Pathology/Laboratory Section of NCCI Guidelines[2(p12)]

CPT code 83721 (lipoprotein, direct measurement; direct measurement, LDL cholesterol) is used to report direct measurement of the LDL cholesterol. It should not be used to report a calculated LDL cholesterol. Direct measurement of LDL cholesterol in addition to total cholesterol (CPT code 82465) or lipid panel (CPT code 80061) may be reasonable and necessary if the triglyceride level is too high (greater than or equal to 400 mg/dl) to permit calculation of the LDL cholesterol. In such situations, CPT code 83721 should be reported with modifier -59.

Interpretation

Calculations are just that, mathematically calculated results of other tests. The calculations do not represent actual tests themselves. Because there is no test being performed for a calculated result, there is no code to be billed for the calculation. Sometimes, the calculated result is insufficient to properly assess the patient's condition. When the results from a cholesterol or lipid panel drive the need for a direct measurement, low-density lipoprotein (LDL) test, the direct measurement LDL may be performed and billed. When it is medically necessary and documented as performed, it may be coded with a modifier 59 appended.

Excerpt From the Pathology/Laboratory Section of NCCI Guidelines[2(p12)]

...quantitative or semi-quantitative *in situ* hybridization (tissue or cellular) performed by manual methods should be reported as CPT code 88368 when performed by a physician (limited to M.D./D.O.). Do not report CPT code 88365 with CPT codes 88367 or 88368 for the same probe. Only one unit of service may be reported for CPT code 88365, 88367 or 88368 for each reportable probe.

Interpretation

In order for these codes to be used, the services must be performed by a physician. A notation in the CPT codebook next to these services might be warranted as a reminder.

The principle also states that the qualitative service code (CPT code 88365) would not be added to the quantitative service code (CPT code 88367 or 88368). Either the qualitative or quantitative service would be billed. Also, each of these services is limited to one per probe. The documentation would have to support multiple probes before multiple units of service could be billed for any of these services.

Excerpt From the Pathology/Laboratory Section of NCCI[2(p12-13)]

When *in situ* hybridization is performed on tissue or cytology specimens by a non-physician (provider other than M.D./D.O.), it should be reported using appropriate CPT codes in the range 88271-88275. For each reportable probe, a provider should not report CPT codes both from the range 88365-88368 and the range 88271-88275. *In situ* hybridization reported as CPT codes 88365-88368 includes both physician (limited to M.D./D.O.) and non-physician (non-M.D./D.O.) services to obtain a reportable probe result. The physician (limited to M.D./D.O.) work component of 88365-88368 requires that a physician (limited to M.D./D.O.) rather than laboratory scientist or technician read, quantitate (88367,88368), and interpret the tissues/cells stained with the probe(s). If this work is performed by a laboratory scientist or technician, CPT codes 88271-88275 should be reported.

Interpretation

If the service was performed by a nonphysician, the CPT code differs. Physician services would be coded with CPT codes 88365, 88367, or 88368. If nonphysicians performed the tests, the CPT codes would be 88271 through 88275. Again, this would be a good note to make in the CPT codebook.

Additionally, only one of the codes (physician or non-physician) may be used for any single probe. If both the physician and nonphysician were involved in the testing, the nonphysician's work is included in the CPT code for the physician's work. Therefore, if a technician performs a fluorescence in situ hybridization study, and the physician performs the interpretive and quantitative portion, only the physician-related CPT code (88365) would be billed, as this code includes any of the nonphysician's work as well.

Excerpt From the Pathology/Laboratory Section of NCCI Guidelines[2(p13)]

… flow cytometry interpretation should be reported using CPT codes 88187-88189. Only one code should be reported for all flow cytometry performed on a specimen. Since Medicare does not pay for duplicate testing, do not report flow cytometry on multiple specimens on the same date of service unless the morphology or other clinical factors suggest differing results on the different specimens. There is no CPT code for interpretation of one marker. The provider should not bill for interpretation of a single marker using another CPT code. Quantitative cell counts performed by flow cytometry (CPT codes 86064, 86359-86361, and 86379, and 86587) should not be reported with the flow cytometry interpretation CPT codes 88187-88189 since there is no interpretative service for these quantitative cell counts.

Interpretation

As shown in the CPT code descriptions, the flow cytometry codes include a minimum of two markers. The interpretation of a single marker is not billed in addition to the technical component.

CPT codes for technical component:

88184 Flow cytometry, cell surface, cytoplasmic, or nuclear marker, technical component only; first marker

+88185 each additional marker (List separately in addition to code for first marker)

Interpretation CPT codes:

88187 Flow cytometry, interpretation; 2 to 8 markers

88188 9 to 15 markers

88189 16 or more markers

The total number of markers (in flow cytometry experiments, fluorescence is often achieved by the deliberate labeling of a cellular component using a fluorescent marker, usually a type of dye) should be used to determine which code to bill. If multiple specimens are used for testing, they are not separately reported unless clear documentation supports that the separate specimens are expected to have different morphology or different results from the testing.

Infectious agent molecular diagnostic testing utilizing nucleic acid probes is reported with CPT codes 87470-87801, 87901-87904. These CPT codes include all the molecular diagnostic processes, and CPT codes 83890-83913 should not be additionally reported with these CPT codes. If the provider performs infectious agent molecular diagnostic testing utilizing nucleic acid probes (87470-87801, 87901-87904) on the same date of service as non-infectious agent molecular diagnostic testing or infectious agent molecular diagnostic testing utilizing methodology that does not incorporate nucleic acid probes, the molecular diagnostic testing CPT codes 83890-83913 may be reported separately with an NCCI-associated modifier.

Interpretation

Basically, the difference between these two code sets is that one is for infectious agents, and the other is for non-infectious agents. In coding, the most appropriate code (infectious or noninfectious agent) should be used, based on the tests performed. Both the infectious and noninfectious agent services would not be billed together unless a separate test was performed using the different methodology.

Infectious agent molecular diagnostic testing is by infectious agent (eg, *Bartonella henselae, Chlamydia*) and by technique (eg, direct probe, amplified probe), whereas the molecular diagnostic testing is by technique (eg, molecular isolation or extraction) and type (eg, nucleic acid, enzyme) and is billed per procedure.

CPT code 83912 describes a medically reasonable and necessary "interpretation and report" associated with molecular diagnostic testing described with CPT codes 83890-83906. CPT code 83912 should not be reported as an "interpretation and report" with CPT codes 87470-87801, 87901-87904 or 88271-88275.

Interpretation

CPT code 83912 is for the interpretation and reporting of molecular diagnostic testing for analysis of nucleic acids only (CPT codes 83890-83906) and should not be used for billing any other testing procedures. Code for each procedure used in an analysis. Take, as an example, a 20-year-old woman with a strong family history of ovarian and breast carcinomas who presents for genetic testing. The clinician requests analysis for BRCA1 because the patient's mother had recently tested positive for the mutation. The laboratory performs known mutation, single-site DNA analysis for BRCA1. The following CPT codes should be reported:

83891   Molecular diagnostics; isolation or extraction of highly purified nucleic acid, each nucleic acid type (ie, DNA or RNA)

83894   separation by gel electrophoresis (eg, agarose, polyacrylamide), each nucleic acid preparation

83898   amplification, target, each nucleic acid sequence

83904   mutation identification by sequencing, single segment, each segment

83912   interpretation and report

Rationale: In this example, the extraction, amplification, and interpretation steps are being used exclusively for the BRCA1 mutation analysis. All the codes are appropriately reported.

Free thyroxine (CPT code 84439) is generally considered to be a better measure of the hypothyroid or hyperthyroid state than total thyroxine (CPT code 84436). If free thyroxine is measured, it is not considered appropriate to measure total thyroxine with or without thyroid hormone binding ratio (CPT code 84479). NCCI does not permit payment of CPT codes 84436 or 84479 with CPT code 84439.

Interpretation

This is a fairly simple principle—do not code the free thyroxine and the total thyroxine, because the free thyroxine is considered the better measurement of the thyroid state. This edit may not be bypassed with a modifier if a patient who is undergoing hypothyroidism treatment (thyroxine medication) presents for thyroid function tests, and both the free and total thyroxine tests are performed to assess the adequacy of treatment.

84436 Thyroxine; total

84439 free

Only the free thyroxine test (CPT code 84439) would be covered for this service, because there is no additional benefit in performing the total thyroxine test. This edit may not be bypassed with a modifier.

Excerpt From the Pathology/Laboratory Section of NCCI Guidelines[2(p14)]

If array-based evaluation of multiple molecular probes is performed by a laboratory scientist or technician rather than a physician, it should not be reported with global CPT code 88385 or 88386 since these codes include physician work. Rather, it should be reported as 88385-TC or 88386-TC which includes the non-physician work including interpretation.

Interpretation

This is not a bundling issue. It's an NCCI guidelines coding instruction to clarify that the reimbursement for CPT codes 88385 through 88386, include physician work and can be coded if a technician performs the service (including interpretation). For billing of the technician work, a modifier TC (technical component) should be appended. Therefore, an oncologist orders a comparative genomic hybridization array on a patient's bone marrow and the marrow is sent to the laboratory for analysis. The analysis is performed for 350 different loci. A pathologist reviews the smear and determines that the findings were sufficient to recommend further testing. The technician performs the gene dosage test, and then the pathologist assesses the assay performance and reviews all the data (including other clinical information). The pathologist documents a clinical interpretation. CPT code 88386 would be the correct code.

88386 Array-based evaluation of multiple molecular probes; 251 through 500 probes

However, if the pathologist had no involvement in the testing and interpretation, NCCI guidelines advise that a modifier TC should be appended to the CPT code.

SUMMARY

- The entire laboratory/pathology section from the NCCI manual should be read.

- CMS has a Medicare manual for laboratory services.[2] Read through this manual for complete understanding of the Medicare guidelines related to laboratory services.

Definitions and Acronyms Important to Chapter 17

complete blood count (CBC): A CBC is a blood test to measure various types of cells in the blood (red blood cells, white blood cells, platelets).

direct supervision: Direct supervision means that a physician must be immediately available to provide assistance and direction, whereas a nonphysician provider provides services that the physician plans to bill as incidental-to. Although the physician does not have to be in the same room as the nonphysician provider, the physician must be in the same office suite.

reflex testing: Secondary testing usually performed after a positive initial test.

white blood cell (WBC): A WBC count is a blood test to measure the number of white blood cells.

CHAPTER EXERCISES

EXERCISE 1

If the following tests are performed together, could each individual code be billed? Why?

Complete blood count, automated with an automated differential WBC count (85025)

Thyroid stimulating hormone (84443)

Albumin (82040)

Bilirubin, total (82247)

Calcium, total (82310)

Carbon dioxide (bicarbonate) (82374)

Chloride (82435)

Creatinine (82565)

Glucose (82947)

Phosphatase, alkaline (84075)

Potassium (84132)

Protein, total (84155)

Sodium (84295)

Transferase, alanine amino (ALT) (SGPT) (84460)

Transferase, aspartate amino (AST) (SGOT) (84450)

Urea Nitrogen (BUN) (84520)

EXERCISE 2

A physician orders a CBC. The automated results of the test flag that a manual differential count be performed. The laboratory provides a manual differential count, documents the results, and notifies the physician. What code or codes should be used?

ANSWERS TO CHAPTER EXERCISES

Exercise 1: Yes. Each test could be coded individually, or the panel code (CPT 80050) could be billed. Either is acceptable. However, if one of the above tests was not performed, the panel could not be coded.

Exercise 2:

85025   Blood count; Blood count; complete (CBC), automated (Hgb, Hct, RBC, WBC and platelet count) and automated differential WBC count

Only this code is needed in this scenario.

REFERENCES

1. American Medical Association. *Current Procedural Terminology (CPT®) Professional Edition 2009*. Chicago, IL: American Medical Association; 2008.

2. Centers for Medicare and Medicaid Services. "Chapter X Pathology/Laboratory Services." In: NCCI Policy Manual for Medicare Services. www.cms.hhs.gov/NationalCorrectCodInitEd/01_overview.asp#TopOfPage. Accessed June 14, 2009.

Medicine Services

Chapter 18 provides background about services in the medicine section of the *Current Procedural Terminology* (*CPT*®)[1] codebook, reviews the National Correct Coding Initiative (NCCI) coding guidelines for medicine services, and provides examples to reflect the logic behind the edits. As do the other chapters, this chapter provides an NCCI guideline followed by our interpretation, an example, or both.

The medicine section of the CPT codebook runs the gamut of services from eye examinations to psychiatric care. Rather than discuss within this section all the different elements of the medicine section, this chapter will directly focus on the NCCI edits within each subsection of the medicine services contained in the CPT codebook.

Introduction Section of NCCI Medicine Section Guidelines

Excerpt From the Medicine Section of NCCI Guidelines[2(p2)]

Introduction
The principles of correct coding discussed in Chapter I apply to the CPT codes in the range 90000-99999. Several general guidelines are repeated in this Chapter. However, those general guidelines from Chapter I not discussed in this chapter are nonetheless applicable.

Interpretation

This instruction indicates that the overall NCCI guidelines apply to each section of the CPT codebook, and, even if they are not repeated within a chapter, they are nonetheless a guideline to be followed. The introductory guidelines were covered comprehensively in Chapter 2 of this book; those introductory guidelines that have clear application within the medicine section are reiterated in this chapter.

Therapeutic or Diagnostic Infusions/Injections and Immunizations and Chemotherapy Administration and NCCI Guidelines

Excerpt From the Medicine Section of NCCI Guidelines[2(p2)]

The CPT codes 90760, 90765, 90774, 96409, and 96413 represent "initial" service codes. For a patient encounter only one "initial" service code may be reported unless it is medically reasonable and necessary that the drug or substance administrations occur at separate vascular access sites. To report two different "initial" service codes use NCCI-associated modifiers.

Note: Although the NCCI guidelines reference codes 90760, 90765, and 90774, these codes have been deleted for 2009, and have been replaced with CPT codes 96360, 96365, and 96734.

Interpretation

In 2009, CPT codes were updated to move the therapeutic infusions and injections to a section that includes hydration, therapeutic, prophylactic, diagnostic injections and infusions, chemotherapy, and other highly complex drug or highly complex biologic agent administration services. This way, services with similar coding guidelines and structures are together.

Regardless of the changes, the guideline remains the same:

Only one initial drug administration code may be billed per patient encounter unless separate vascular access sites were employed. If different sites were used, each site may have one initial drug administration code with an appropriate NCCI-guideline-associated modifier. Use the initial code that best reflects the primary reason for the encounter. Take a patient who presents for chemotherapy and has hydration performed before the chemotherapy infusion. In this case, even though the hydration is the first administered substance, the patient presents for chemotherapy, and chemotherapy would be the primary reason for the visit. The chemotherapy code would be the one used for the *initial* administration.

Excerpt From the Medicine Section of NCCI Guidelines[2(p3)]

Because the placement of peripheral vascular access devices is integral to vascular (intravenous, intra-arterial) infusions and injections, the CPT codes for placement of these devices are not to be separately reported. Accordingly, insertion of an intravenous catheter (e.g., CPT codes 36000, 36410) for intravenous infusion, injection or chemotherapy administration … should not be reported separately.

Interpretation

Remember from Chapter 2 of this book, services that are integral to the procedure are included in the procedure's CPT code. In order to perform infusions and intravenous (IV) injections, an IV catheter must be inserted. The infusion cannot be performed without the IV catheter. Therefore, the peripheral catheter placement is included in the infusion services and should not be billed separately. An example would be for a patient who presents for a chemotherapy infusion, and the provider places an IV catheter to use for the infusion. The catheter placement is included in the chemotherapy administration code and should not be billed separately.

Excerpt From the Medicine Section of NCCI Guidelines[2(p3)]

Because insertion of central venous access is not routinely necessary to perform infusions/injections, these services may be reported separately. Because intra-arterial infusion often involves selective catheterization of an arterial supply to a specific organ, there is no routine arterial catheterization common to all arterial infusions. Selective arterial catheterization codes may be reported separately.

Interpretation

A central line is different from a peripheral line. The peripheral line is the usual access point for infusions, and the placement of the peripheral line would be incidental to the chemotherapy. However, placement of a central line is not included in the chemotherapy administration CPT code and may be coded additionally. Selective arterial catheterization may also be reported separately.

To illustrate, take the patient who presents for chemotherapy to be administered through a peripheral line. A catheter is inserted in her right arm and chemotherapy administered. Peripheral lines are usual for chemotherapy administration, and no additional code is used for insertion of the catheter.

However, if a patient presents for chemotherapy, but she has peripheral venous insufficiency, a central line is inserted for administration of the chemotherapy. In this case, the central line insertion may be coded in addition to the chemotherapy administration.

Excerpt From the Medicine Section of NCCI Guidelines[2(p3)]

If the sole purpose of fluid administration (e.g., saline, D5W, etc.) is to maintain patency of an access device, the infusion is neither diagnostic nor therapeutic and should not be reported separately. Similarly, the fluid utilized to administer drug(s)/substance(s) is incidental hydration and should not be reported separately.

Interpretation

Any drugs administered to facilitate infusions or to maintain the patency (natural opening) of a vessel are not separately coded because they do not serve a diagnostic or therapeutic purpose separate from the primary infusion. Each administration of a drug must serve its own diagnostic or therapeutic purpose to be coded. Otherwise, the administration is integral to the primary substance infusion.

Often, between the administration of one chemotherapy agent and another, normal saline is infused to flush the line for patency. In this case, the saline does not serve a diagnostic or therapeutic service outside of the chemotherapy administration and, therefore, is not separately coded.

Excerpt From the Medicine Section of NCCI Guidelines[2(p3)]

If therapeutic fluid administration is medically necessary (e.g., correction of dehydration, prevention of nephrotoxicity) before or after transfusion or chemotherapy, it may be reported separately.

Interpretation

A patient presents for chemotherapy administration, and prior to the beginning of chemotherapy, normal saline is infused to treat dehydration. In this scenario, the normal saline serves a therapeutic purpose (to correct dehydration) and may be coded separately from the chemotherapy.

Excerpt From the Medicine Section of NCCI Guidelines[2(p3-4)]

…drug administration services should not be reported by physicians for services provided in a facility setting such as a hospital outpatient department or emergency department. Drug administration services performed in an Ambulatory Surgical Center (ASC) related to a Medicare approved ASC payable procedure are not separately reportable by physicians. Hospital outpatient facilities may separately report drug administration services when appropriate.

Interpretation

Usually, the administration of drugs is not personally performed by the physician. Rather, the physician supervises the administration. Because the physician's staff performs the service when the physician is in the office, these services may be billed, even though the physician did not personally perform the service. However, in the hospital setting, hospital staff often perform the administration, and, therefore, the physician should not bill for hospital staff work.

An additional note to this NCCI principle is that for ambulatory surgical centers, if the administration is provided as part of a surgical procedure, the administration is incidental to the surgery and is not separately coded.

If a patient receives chemotherapy in the office setting, and a registered nurse performs the administration under direct physician supervision, the physician may bill for the chemotherapy, as long as the individual performing the service is qualified to administer the drug and the physician provides direct supervision.

Excerpt From the Medicine Section of NCCI Guidelines[2(p4)]

The drug and chemotherapy administration CPT codes…have been valued to include the work and practice expenses of CPT code 99211 (evaluation and management service, office or other outpatient visit, established patient, level I). Although CPT code 99211 is not reportable with chemotherapy and non-chemotherapy drug/substance administration HCPCS/CPT codes, other non-facility based evaluation and management CPT codes (e.g., 99201-99205, 99212-99215) are separately reportable with modifier -25 if the physician provides a significant and separately identifiable E&M service.

Interpretation

The low level established patient evaluation and management (E/M) visit code 99211 may not be added to the drug administration services. These codes are reimbursed to include the work of the low level visit. However, if the documentation supports a higher level of E/M service that is separate and distinct from the drug administration care, both may be coded. A modifier 25 should be appended to the E/M service code. Take a patient who, on chemotherapy, develops excessive fatigue. The physician evaluates the patient to determine her current status and see if there are any new problems in her health. To determine the cause of the fatigue, the physician orders laboratory tests, inquires about the patient's success with the treatment thus far, asks about any signs or symptoms resulting from the treatment, and performs a detailed examination. Severe anemia is discovered, and the physician treats the patient with an infusion of erythropoietin. In this case, both the visit and the infusion would be appropriately coded.

Excerpt From the Medicine Section of NCCI Guidelines[2(p4)]

Since physicians should not report drug administration services in a facility setting, a facility based evaluation and management CPT code (e.g., 99281-99285) should not be reported by a physician with a drug administration CPT code unless the drug administration service is performed at a separate patient encounter in a non-facility setting on the same date of service.

Interpretation

Remember from the prior guideline that a physician may not bill for the drug administration in a hospital setting. Even if the physician performed an E/M service in the outpatient hospital setting, the drug administration service may not be billed unless performed in the physician's office (or other nonfacility setting).

Excerpt From the Medicine Section of NCCI Guidelines[2(p4)]

Flushing or irrigation of an implanted vascular access port or device of a drug delivery system prior to or subsequent to the administration of chemotherapeutic or non-chemotherapeutic drugs is integral to the drug administration service and is not separately reportable. Do not report CPT code 96523.

Interpretation

Any flushing of a line, be it a port or peripheral catheter, is incidental to the drug administration if performed during the same session.

Excerpt From the Medicine Section of NCCI Guidelines[2(p5)]

CPT codes 96522 and 96523 (irrigation of implanted venous access device for drug delivery system) should NOT be reported for accessing or flushing an indwelling peripherally-placed intravenous catheter port (external to skin), subcutaneous port, or non-programmable subcutaneous pump. Accessing and flushing these devices is an inherent service facilitating these infusion(s) and is not reported separately.

Interpretation

Again, any flushing of a line, be it a port or peripheral catheter, is incidental to the drug administration if performed during the same session.

Excerpt From the Medicine Section of NCCI Guidelines[2(p5)]

CPT code 96522 (refilling and maintenance of implantable pump or reservoir for systemic drug delivery) and CPT code 96521 (refilling and maintenance of portable pump) should not be reported with CPT code 96416 (initiation of prolonged intravenous chemotherapy infusion (more than eight hours), requiring use of a portable or implantable pump) or CPT code 96425 (chemotherapy administration, intra-arterial; infusion technique, initiation of prolonged infusion (more than eight hours) requiring the use of a portable or implantable pump). CPT codes 96416 and 96425 include the initial filling and maintenance of a portable or implantable pump. CPT codes 96521 and 96522 are used to report subsequent refilling of the pump.

Interpretation

This clarifies that the initiation services for prolonged infusion include the initial filling and maintenance of the pump. Coding the refilling and maintenance (CPT codes 96522 or 96521) additionally would be double billing for the refilling and maintenance portion.

Excerpt From the Medicine Section of NCCI Guidelines[2(p6)]

Similar to drug and chemotherapy administration CPT codes, CPT code 99211 (evaluation and management service, office or other outpatient visit, established patient, level I) is not reportable with vaccine administration HCPCS/CPT codes 90465-90474, G0008-G0010.

Interpretation

The vaccine administration codes include the work of the low level visit CPT code 99211. The low level visit is not separately reported. However, if the documentation supports a higher level of E/M service that is separate and distinct from the drug administration care, both may be coded. A modifier 25 should be appended to the E/M service code. For example, a patient presents to a clinic after a fall. There are multiple lacerations, and the physician performs an expanded, problem-focused history and examination and decides to bandage the lacerations without sutures but does provide a tetanus vaccine. In this case, both the visit (because it exceeds the complexity of a low level visit), with modifier 25, and vaccine administration may be coded.

Excerpt From the Medicine Section of NCCI Guidelines[2(p6)]

CPT codes 90761 and 90766 are utilized to report each additional hour of intravenous hydration and intravenous infusion for therapy, prophylaxis, or diagnosis respectively. These codes may be reported only if the infusion is medically reasonable and necessary for the patient's treatment or diagnosis. They should not be reported for "keep open" infusions as often occur in the emergency department or observation unit.

Note: Although the NCCI guidelines reference CPT codes 90760 and 90766, those codes are deleted and replaced with CPT codes 96360 and 96366.

Interpretation

A keep-open IV is used as a maintenance IV that is established to have prophylactic (in case of need) access. Because the keep-open IV is not for treatment, it should not be coded. Very clear documentation should support how long infusion is ordered and for what purpose. For example, a patient in the emergency department undergoes infusion therapy. At the conclusion of the therapeutic infusion, the hospital nursing staff infuses 5% dextrose and water through the IV line so that the medication does not remain in the line, and the line will remain available for later access if needed. The time spent in running the solution through the IV line would not be used in billing for the infusion, as it was not for treatment, but rather for maintenance of the line.

Psychiatric Services and NCCI Guidelines

Excerpt From the Medicine Section of NCCI Guidelines[2(p7)]

CPT codes for psychiatric services include general and special diagnostic services as well as a variety of therapeutic services. By *CPT Manual* definition, therapeutic services (e.g., HCPCS/CPT codes 90804-90829) include psychotherapy and continuing medical diagnostic evaluation; therefore, CPT codes 90801 and 90802 are not reported with these services.

Interpretation

The diagnostic interview services (CPT codes 90801 and 90802) should not be separately coded from actual psychotherapy services. Most often the initial interview is provided on a day other than that of the psychotherapy, as the interview is usually used to determine the best treatment plan for the patient. Any adjustments in treatment planning are included in the psychotherapy codes and are not to be billed separately.

For instance, a patient presents for the first time and is interviewed by the psychiatrist. The psychiatrist determines the best treatment plan for the patient and schedules follow-up psychotherapy sessions. In this scenario, the CPT code for the psychotherapy interview (90801 Psychiatric diagnostic interview examination) would be used. However, if during a follow-up psychotherapy session, the provider changes the plan of treatment based on the patient's success with the current treatment plan, the change of treatment is included in the psychotherapy, and should not be coded separately using the psychiatric interview codes.

Excerpt From the Medicine Section of NCCI Guidelines[2(p7)]

Interactive services (diagnostic or therapeutic) are distinct forms of services for patients who have "lost, or have not yet developed either the expressive language communication skills to explain his/her symptoms and response to treatment...." Accordingly, non-interactive services would not be possible at the same session as interactive services and are not to be reported together with interactive services.

Interpretation

Because interactive and noninteractive psychotherapy are used for patients with different types of conditions, both services should not be used for a single patient. A patient requiring interactive psychotherapy does not have the communication skills to benefit from noninteractive psychotherapy. If a patient requires interactive psychotherapy because he or she cannot use traditional communication skills, noninteractive psychotherapy is ineffective. Likewise, if a patient can use traditional communication skills in working with the therapist, interactive therapy is not required.

Excerpt From the Medicine Section of NCCI Guidelines[2(p7)]

Drug management is included in some therapeutic services (e.g., HCPCS/CPT codes 90801-90829, 90845, 90847-90853, 90865-90870) and therefore CPT code 90862 (pharmacologic management) is not to be reported with these codes.

Interpretation

Pharmacologic management services should be billed when no other psychotherapy service is provided on the same date. Pharmacologic management is used in the following scenarios:

- A patient's psychotherapy is being managed by another health professional, and the billing physician is managing the psychotropic medication.
- A patient's psychotherapy involves psychotropic medication, and the visit is solely focused on prescribing medication, monitoring the effect of the medication and its side effects, and adjusting the dosage. For example, a psychiatric patient being treated with antianxiety pharmaceuticals sees the psychiatrist every other week for psychotherapy sessions. Once a month, during the psychotherapy, the physician also reviews the patient's antianxiety medications. During this visit, in-depth psychotherapy is provided, and the physician determines, based on the counseling session and the patient's current condition, whether adjustments are needed in the medication therapy. The medication management piece of the encounter is included in the psychotherapy and is not separately coded.

Dialysis and NCCI Guidelines

Excerpt From the Medicine Section of NCCI Guidelines[2(p8)]

Renal dialysis procedures coded as CPT codes 90935, 90937, 90945, and 90947 include evaluation and management (E&M) services related to the dialysis procedure. If the physician additionally performs on the same date of service medically reasonable and necessary E&M services that are significant and separately identifiable, these services may be separately reportable.

Interpretation

Within the CPT codebook,[1(p393)] we are instructed that CPT codes 90935, 90937, 90945, and 90947 include all the E/M services related to the hemodialysis provided on the same day as the hemodialysis. If the physician provided an unrelated E/M service on the same day as the hemodialysis (but not during the hemodialysis), the E/M with modifier 25 may be billed in addition to the hemodialysis. The documentation must clearly indicate that the E/M was unrelated and was not provided during the hemodialysis for the service to be billed separately.

If a patient presents for hemodialysis and the physician evaluates the patient at the beginning of the treatment and then again midway through the treatment, the E/M services are related to the hemodialysis and not separately reported. However, take the patient who is scheduled for hemodialysis and is involved in a minor motor vehicle accident on the same day, but before the hemodialysis appointment. The patient presents to the provider well before the dialysis appointment to be evaluated for her injuries. The provider evaluates the patient to ensure that the patient's injuries are minor and does not require further evaluation by an orthopedist or in the emergency department. The physician concludes that the patient does not need further evaluation and is able to undergo the hemodialysis. In this scenario, both the hemodialysis and separate E/M service should be billed. A modifier 25 should be appended to the E/M service.

Gastroenterology and NCCI Guidelines

Excerpt From the Medicine Section of NCCI Guidelines[2(p8)]

Gastroenterological tests included in CPT codes 91000-91299 are frequently complementary to endoscopic procedures. Esophageal and gastric washings for cytology are described as part of upper endoscopy (e.g., CPT code 43235); therefore, CPT codes 91000 (esophageal intubation) and 91055 (gastric intubation) are not separately reported when performed as part of an upper endoscopy. Provocative testing (CPT code 91052) can be expedited during GI endoscopy (procurement of gastric specimens). When performed at the same time as GI endoscopy, CPT code 91052 is reported with modifier -52 indicating that a reduced level of service was performed.

Interpretation

An esophageal intubation system includes a main tube that is inserted into the oropharynx. Its distal end extends into the upper esophagus to provide a conduit for esophagoscopes, gastroscopes, and related diagnostic and treatment equipment. Because this is an inherent part of an upper endoscopy, the intubation becomes part of the approach for an upper endoscopy. Approaches cannot be billed in addition to the primary procedure.

Gastric analysis (provocative) is a study of the stomach's contents and requires gastric intubation to obtain the specimen. Because the upper gastrointestinal (GI) endoscopy also includes the gastric intubation, coding the gastric analysis in addition is essentially coding the intubation twice. Therefore, when a gastric analysis is performed with an upper GI endoscopy, a modifier 52 (reduced services) is needed to prevent the gastric intubation from being coded twice.

Ophthalmology and NCCI Guidelines

Excerpt From the Medicine Section of NCCI Guidelines[2(p8)]

General ophthalmological services (e.g., CPT codes 92002-92014) describe components of the ophthalmologic examination. When evaluation and management codes are reported, these general ophthalmological service codes (e.g., CPT codes 92002-92014) are not to be reported; the same services would be represented by both series of codes.

Interpretation

Several categories of CPT codes outside of the E/M section (CPT codes 99201-99499) include E/M services. It would be incorrect to add codes from the E/M section when specific CPT codes include E/M services.

92002 Ophthalmological services: medical examination and evaluation with initiation of diagnostic and treatment program; intermediate, new patient

92004 comprehensive, new patient, 1 or more visits

92012 Ophthalmological services: medical examination and evaluation, with initiation or continuation of diagnostic and treatment program; intermediate, established patient

92014 comprehensive, established patient, 1 or more visits

These codes are for eye examination and include all E/M services related to the examination. Other E/M CPT codes should not be billed in addition to these CPT codes. However, the provider has the choice of using a medical evaluation code from the E/M section of the CPT codebook of the ophthalmologic section of the CPT codebook as long as the documentation supports the code.

Excerpt From the Medicine Section of NCCI Guidelines[2(p8)]

Special ophthalmologic services represent specific services not described as part of a general or routine ophthalmological examination. Special ophthalmological services are recognized as significant, separately identifiable services.

Interpretation

Within the ophthalmology section of medicine section of the CPT codebook is a subsection entitled *Special Ophthalmological Services* (CPT codes 92015-92287). NCCI (and the CPT codebook) instruct that these services are not included in the E/M codes or the general eye examination codes and may be billed separately. If during an eye examination (CPT code 92004), the physician determines that a gonioscopy (eye examination to see if the anterior chamber's drainage angle is open) should also be performed to evaluate the patient for glaucoma, the gonioscopy (CPT code 92020) may be billed in addition to the eye examination.

Excerpt From the Medicine Section of NCCI Guidelines[2(p8-9)]

For procedures requiring intravenous injection of dye or other diagnostic agent, insertion of an intravenous catheter and dye injection are necessary to accomplish the procedure and are included in the procedure.

Interpretation

Procedures that require access or injection into a vessel include in their reimbursement that access. Therefore, the injection or catheterization should not be coded separately. An example would be for fluorescein angiographies, which are performed by injecting a dye into a vein in the arm. Therefore, when coding for fluorescein angiographies, no additional code should be used for the vessel access.

Excerpt From the Medicine Section of NCCI Guidelines[2(p9)]

Fundus photography (CPT code 92250) and scanning ophthalmic computerized diagnostic imaging (CPT code 92135) are generally mutually exclusive of one another in that a provider would use one technique or the other to evaluate fundal disease. However, there are a limited number of clinical conditions where both techniques are medically reasonable and necessary on the ipsilateral eye.

Interpretation

Although these are two clearly distinct services, NCCI guidelines indicate that they bundle because their diagnostic use (fundal disease) often overlaps. If, however, the

documentation within the record supports distinct reasons for each of the services, both may potentially be billed with modifier 59.

Otorhinolaryngologic Services and NCCI Guidelines

Excerpt From the Medicine Section of NCCI Guidelines[2(p9)]

CPT coding for otorhinolaryngologic services includes codes for tests that may be performed qualitatively during physical examination or quantitatively with electrical recording equipment. The procedures described by CPT codes 92552-92557, 92561-92588, and 92597 may be reported only if calibrated electronic equipment is utilized. Qualitative estimation of these tests by the physician is part of the evaluation and management service.

Interpretation

The CPT codebook instructs that in order to code the services of audiometric testing, calibrated electronic equipment must be used, and there must be a written interpretation. Otherwise, these services become incidental to the E/M services performed on the same day. Even if no E/M service was performed on the same day, the CPT codes for audiometric testing could not be used if the calibrated equipment and interpretation were not a part of the service. For example, a patient presents with a headache, and, during the course of the examination, the physician performs a tuning fork hearing assessment along with the rest of the examination. Based on the Centers for Medicare and Medicaid Services (CMS) E/M examination guidelines (see Table 18-1), a tuning fork assessment of hearing is included in the E/M service and not separately coded as an audiometric test because no calibrated equipment or formal interpretation is part of the test.

TABLE 18-1 *Excerpt From the* 1997 Documentation Guidelines for Evaluation and Management Services[3]

Ears, Nose, Mouth, and Throat	• External inspection of ears and nose (eg, overall appearance, scars, lesions, masses)
	• Otoscopic examination of external auditory canals and tympanic membranes
	• Assessment of bearing (eg, whispered voice, finger rub, tuning fork)
	• Inspection of nasal mucosa, septum, and turbinates
	• Inspection of lips, teeth, and gums
	• Examination of oropharynx: oral mucosa, salivary glands, hard and soft palates, tongue, tonsils, and posterior pharynx

Excerpt From the Medicine Section of NCCI Guidelines[2(p9)]

Speech language pathologists may perform services coded as CPT codes 92507, 92508, or 92526. They do not perform services coded as CPT codes 97110, 97112, 97150, 97530, or 97532 which are generally performed by physical or occupational therapists. Speech language pathologists should not report CPT codes 97110, 97112, 97150, 97530, or 97532 as unbundled services included in the services coded as 92507, 92508, or 92526.

Interpretation

92506 Evaluation of speech, language, voice, communication, and/or auditory processing

92507 Treatment of speech, language, voice, communication, and/or auditory processing disorder; individual

92508 group, 2 or more individuals

These codes are for evaluating and treating speech and language conditions and would include all the work necessary to treat or evaluate the condition. Providers should not mislabel speech and language services as either physical or occupational therapy. Remember, the CPT code that is most specific to the encounter or service must be selected over any other code that approximates the service.

In addition, the NCCI edits indicate that speech and language pathologists are supposed to use the CPT codes for speech and language rather than the codes from the physical and occupational therapy section.

If a patient recovering from a stroke is having difficulty in regaining the ability to speak, a speech and language pathologists could be part of the team assisting in this area, whereas occupational therapists might help that same patient with the activities of daily living. Each provider would code from distinct sections of the CPT codebook.

Excerpt From the Medicine Section of NCCI Guidelines[2(p9-10)]

Treatment of swallowing dysfunction and/or oral function for feeding (CPT code 92526) may utilize electrical stimulation. HCPCS code G0283 (electrical stimulation (unattended), to one or more areas for indication(s) other than wound care…) should not be reported with CPT code 92526 for electrical stimulation during the procedure.

Interpretation

When electrical stimulation is used as a part of the treatment for swallowing dysfunction, the stimulation is inherent in CPT 92526 and should not be coded separately. Many speech and language pathologists use electrical stimulation to treat dysphagia or other dysfunctions, and any treatment of swallowing dysfunction is coded to CPT code 92526. Regardless of the type of treatment, CPT code 92526 would be coded for swallowing or oral function treatment.

Excerpt From the Medicine Section of NCCI Guidelines[2(p10)]

CPT code 92502 (otolaryngologic examination under general anesthesia) is not separately reportable with any other otolaryngologic procedure performed under general anesthesia.

Interpretation

As with other E/M services, if an otolaryngologic examination was performed under anesthesia, and any other otolaryngologic procedure was performed during the same encounter under anesthesia, the examination becomes an incidental part of the procedure and is not separately coded. The examination essentially does not provide significant and separately identifiable evaluation from the procedure.

Cardiovascular Services and NCCI Guidelines

Excerpt From the Medicine Section of NCCI Guidelines[2(p10)]

Critical care E&M services (CPT codes 99291 and 99292) and prolonged physician E&M services (CPT codes 99354-99357) are reported based on time. Providers should not include the time devoted to performing separately reportable services when determining the amount of critical care or prolonged physician E&M service time. For example, the time devoted to performing cardiopulmonary resuscitation (CPT code 92950) should not be included in critical care E&M service time.

Interpretation

Time spent in activities that occur outside of the hospital unit or off the hospital floor (eg, telephone calls, whether taken at home, in the office, or elsewhere in the hospital) may not be reported as critical care because the physician is not immediately available to the patient.

Time spent in activities that do not directly contribute to the treatment of the patient may not be reported as critical care, even if they are performed in the critical care unit (eg, participation in administrative meetings or telephone calls to discuss other patients). Time spent performing separately reportable procedures or services should not be included in the time reported as critical care time. The critical care codes 99291 and 99292 are used to report the total duration of time spent by a physician providing critical care services to a critically ill or critically injured patient, even if the time spent by the physician on that date is not continuous. For any given period of time spent providing critical care services, the physician must devote his or her full attention to the patient and, therefore, cannot provide services to any other patient during the same period of time.

Time spent with the individual patient should be recorded in the patient's record. The time that can be reported as critical care time is the time spent engaged in work directly related to the individual patient's care, whether that time was spent at the immediate bedside or elsewhere on the floor or unit.

For example, time spent on the unit or at the nursing station on the hospital floor reviewing test results or imaging studies, discussing the critically ill patient's care with other medical staff, or documenting critical care services in the medical record would be reported as critical care, even though it does not occur at the bedside.

Also, when the patient is unable or clinically incompetent to participate in discussions, time spent on the floor or unit with family members or surrogate decision makers obtaining a medical history, reviewing the patient's condition or prognosis, or discussing treatment or limitation(s) of treatment may be reported as critical care, provided that the conversation bears directly on the management of the patient.

The physician's progress note should include documentation of time involved in performance of separately billable procedures not counted toward critical care time. See Table 18-2 for included and excluded critical care activities.

Only one physician may bill for a given hour of critical care, even if more than one physician is providing care to a critically ill or injured patient.

For example, a 52-year-old woman in route to an emergency department (ED) stops breathing. Paramedics are performing CPR as the patient is brought into the ED. The ED provider takes over CPR, and 20 minutes after arrival, the patient is stabilized and begins to breathe on her own.

TABLE 18-2 *Included and Excluded Critical Care Activities*

Included Activities	Excluded Activities
Time spent on the hospital floor/unit in the care of a critically ill or injured patient	Time spent in activities that do not directly contribute to the care of a critically ill or injured patient
Time spent at the patient's bedside	Time spent on indirect care, such as telephone calls taken at home, the office, or elsewhere in the hospital
Time spent on the hospital floor/unit engaging in work directly related to the patient	Time spent providing care to other patients, either in a critical care unit or elsewhere
Time spent on the hospital floor/unit discussing patient's care with other staff	Time spent with residents on rounds or other venues discussing the patient
Time spent on the hospital floor/unit documenting the performance of specific services, clinical findings, and orders	Time spent performing procedures not bundled in critical care services
Time spent on the hospital floor/unit with family or surrogate decision makers when the discussion bears directly on the medical decision making because the patient is unable to participate	Time spent with family members or other surrogate decision makers when the patient is competent to make medical decisions

One hour later, the patient arrests, and the ED physician performs critical care for another 45 minutes.

The CPR may be billed in addition to the critical care, but the time involved in providing the CPR must be subtracted from the critical care time when coding. Therefore, only 45 minutes would be eligible for critical care time.

Excerpt From the Medicine Section of NCCI Guidelines[2(p10-11)]

A number of therapeutic and diagnostic cardiovascular procedures (e.g., CPT codes 92950-92998, 93501-93545, 93600-93624, 93640-93652) routinely utilize intravenous or intra-arterial vascular access, routinely require electrocardiographic monitoring, and frequently require agents administered by injection or infusion techniques; accordingly, separate codes for routine access, monitoring, injection or infusion services are not to be reported. Fluoroscopic guidance procedures are integral to invasive intravascular procedures and are included in those services.

Interpretation

This guideline requires understanding the component parts of procedures provided. However, NCCI guidelines do specify which CPT codes include vascular access, fluoroscopy, etc. The invasive services within the cardiovascular subsection of the CPT medicine section that include vascular access are the therapeutic procedures (eg, percutaneous transluminal coronary angioplasty [PTCA]), cardiac catheterizations (eg, left heart catheterization), and electrophysiology procedures (eg, bundle of His recording). The vascular access and catheterization should not be coded in addition to these services unless a separate and distinct vascular access was performed. For illustration, take a patient who presents for a left heart catheterization with coronary angiography. The physician inserts a catheter into the femoral artery and manipulates it into the left ventricle. In this case, the catheter insertion is incidental and is an inherent component of the left heart catheterization and would not be coded separately.

Excerpt From the Medicine Section of NCCI Guidelines[2(p11)]

Cardiac output measurement (e.g., CPT codes 93561-93562) is routinely performed during cardiac catheterization procedures per CPT definition and, therefore, CPT codes 93561-93562 are not to be reported with cardiac catheterization codes.

Interpretation

Cardiac catheterization can be used to perform various tests, including angiography, intravascular ultrasonography, measurement of cardiac output, endomyocardial biopsy, and measurements of myocardial metabolism. Cardiac output is measured to determine circulatory adequacy. Because cardiac catheterizations often include this study, the output measurement is incidental to the catheterization and is not to be separately coded.

Excerpt From the Medicine Section of NCCI Guidelines[2(p11)]

CPT codes 93797 and 93798 describe comprehensive services provided by a physician for cardiac rehabilitation. As this includes all services referable to cardiac rehabilitation, it would be inappropriate to bill a separate evaluation and management service code unless an unrelated, separately identifiable, service is performed and documented in the medical record.

Interpretation

Cardiac rehabilitation covers a physician's oversight and supervision of the comprehensive rehabilitation program. Therefore, the cardiac rehabilitation coding would include all related E/M services as well. A separate E/M service could be billed only if there were sufficient documentation that an E/M encounter was unrelated to the cardiac rehabilitation program.

Cardiac Rehabilitation

The American Heart Association[4] defines the services of cardiac rehabilitation as follows:
Cardiac rehabilitation programs include:
- Counseling so the patient can understand and manage the disease process
- Beginning an exercise program
- Counseling on nutrition
- Helping the patient modify risk factors such as high blood pressure, smoking, high blood cholesterol, physical inactivity, obesity and diabetes
- Providing vocational guidance to enable the patient to return to work
- Supplying information on physical limitations
- Lending emotional support
- Counseling on appropriate use of prescribed medications

Excerpt From the Medicine Section of NCCI Guidelines[2(p11)]

If a physician in attendance for a cardiac stress test obtains a history and performs a limited physical examination related to the cardiac stress test, a separate evaluation and management (E&M) code should not be reported separately unless a significant, separately identifiable E&M service is performed unrelated to the performance of the cardiac stress test.

Interpretation

When physician interaction with a patient is necessary to accomplish the cardiac stress test, the interaction generally involves limited inquiry regarding the patient's pertinent history and reasons for the examination, discussion of any patient allergies, acquisition of informed consent, discussion of follow-up, and review of the medical record. In this case, a separate E/M service is not reported. As a rule, if the medical decision making that evolves from procurement of the patient information is limited to whether or not the procedure should be performed or whether comorbidity may impact the procedure or involves discussion and patient education, an E/M code is not reported separately. If a significant, separately identifiable service is rendered, involving taking a history, performing an examination, and making medical decisions distinct from the procedure, the appropriate E/M service may be reported with modifier 25.

Physicians who perform and interpret stress tests often work from an order by the patient's treating provider and, therefore, do not make any clinical determinations as to the efficacy of the ordered service. In this case, because there is no separate E/M service, only the stress test would be billed.

However, if the physician is the one who is medically evaluating the patient and determining a need for the stress test, and the test is performed within that provider's office, both the stress test and E/M service should be billed, as the E/M service determined the need for the test. The E/M service must be documented as separate from the stress test, significant, and medically necessary. For example, a patient's primary care physician orders a cardiac stress test. The cardiologist performs the test and provides the requesting physician with a formal interpretation. In this case, the cardiologist never performs a separate E/M service and cannot bill for a medical visit. However, if another patient's primary care physician refers the patient to a cardiologist for evaluation and consultation for shortness of breath and chest pains, the cardiologist would perform a complete work-up on the patient before deciding to perform a cardiac stress test. If a stress test is completed after the complete work-up, the cardiologist may bill for both the E/M service with modifier 25 and the stress test, as the E/M service was necessary to determine the need for the test.

Excerpt From the Medicine Section of NCCI Guidelines[2(p11)]

CPT codes 93040-93042 describe diagnostic rhythm EKG testing. They should not be reported for cardiac rhythm monitoring in any site of service.

Interpretation

Monitoring is different than diagnosing. If a patient is at risk for cardiac dysrhythmias or other cardiac problems, the provider is likely to do continuous cardiac monitoring on that patient. That is not coded separately from the other services provided the patient. Monitoring is part of the overall care for the patient and not separated from other services being coded. Take a patient being treated in an intensive care unit (ICU) after suffering a myocardial infarction. The hospital has a cardiac monitor on the patient. The cardiac monitor is included in the room rate for the ICU and is not separately coded.

Excerpt From the Medicine Section of NCCI Guidelines[2(p11-12)]

Routine monitoring of EKG rhythm and review of daily hemodynamics including cardiac output are part of critical care evaluation and management services. Separate reporting of EKG rhythm strips and cardiac output measurements…is inappropriate. An exception to this may include a sudden change in patient status associated with a change in cardiac rhythm requiring a return to the ICU or telephonic transmission to review a rhythm strip. If reported separately, time included for this service is not included in the critical care time calculated for the critical care service.

Interpretation

The instructions for critical care in the CPT codebook indicates that the interpretation of cardiac output measurements, electrocardiograms (EKG), and other data that are stored in computers is not separately coded from the critical care coded on that date. However, should the patient experience a change in status and require an individual study, rather than routine monitoring for maintenance, that service may be billed separately from the critical care, as long as the documentation clearly supports what time was spent providing critical care and what time was spent interpreting individual studies. Additionally, the separately billed services would have to be supported as medically necessary.

Excerpt From the Medicine Section of NCCI Guidelines[2(p12)]

…Medicare recognizes three coronary arteries: right coronary artery (modifier -RC), left circumflex coronary artery (modifier -LC) and left anterior descending coronary artery (modifier -LD). For a given coronary artery and its branches, the provider should report only one intervention, the most complex…From a coding perspective, stent placement is considered more complex than an atherectomy which is considered more complex than a balloon angioplasty. These interventions should be reported with the appropriate modifier (-RC, -LC, -LD) indicating in which coronary artery…the procedure(s) was (were) performed. Since Medicare recognizes three coronary arteries (including their branches) for reimbursement purposes, it is possible that a provider will report up to three percutaneous interventions…The first reported procedure must utilize a primary code (CPT codes 92980, 92982, 92995) corresponding to the most complex procedure performed. The procedure(s) performed in the other one or two coronary arteries (including their branches) are reported with the CPT add-on codes (CPT codes 92981, 92984, 92996). Modifier -59 should not be utilized to report percutaneous coronary artery stent placement, atherectomy, or balloon angioplasty.

Interpretation

The upshot here is that only *one intervention, per vessel* should be billed. If multiple interventions are performed in a single vessel, code only the most complex and not the others. To assist in identifying different vessels in coding, Medicare assigned modifiers to each of three coronary arteries and assigned modifiers to each (LC - left circumflex coronary, LD - left descending, RC - right coronary). By using the modifiers, if interventions are performed in different vessels, each may be coded, and the modifier would indicate different vessels.

A surgeon performs an unsuccessful angioplasty of the right coronary artery, which requires the physician to place a stent in the right coronary artery as well as placing a stent in the left circumflex coronary artery. In this example, there are two vessels (the right and left circumflex coronaries); therefore, no more than two interventions may be coded. CPT code 92980-RC for the stent placement in the right coronary artery may be coded, as it is the most extensive service performed on the right coronary artery. However, the angioplasty is unsuccessful and may not be coded in addition. CPT code 92981-LC for the stent placement in the left circumflex coronary artery may be coded, as it is the only service performed on that vessel.

Excerpt From the Medicine Section of NCCI Guidelines[2(p12-13)]

Percutaneous coronary artery interventions (e.g., stent, atherectomy, angioplasty) include coronary artery catheterization, radiopaque dye injections, and fluoroscopic guidance. CPT codes for these procedures… should not be reported separately. If medically reasonable and necessary diagnostic coronary angiography precedes the percutaneous coronary artery intervention, a coronary artery or cardiac catheterization and associated radiopaque dye injections may be reported separately. However, fluoroscopy is not separately reportable with diagnostic coronary angiography or cardiac catheterization.

Interpretation

Diagnostic angiographies performed on the same date of service by the same provider as a percutaneous intravascular interventional procedure should be reported with modifier 59. If a diagnostic angiogram was performed prior to the date of the percutaneous intravascular interventional procedure, a second diagnostic angiogram cannot be reported on the date of the percutaneous intravascular interventional procedure unless it is medically reasonable and necessary to repeat the study to further define the anatomy and pathology. A *diagnostic* study is when a catheter is placed and angiography performed. A diagnostic angiography is an X-ray of arteries and veins achieved by the injection of radiopaque contrast medium to evaluate vessel structure and function.

Diagnostic codes should *not* be used with interventional procedures for the following, because this work is captured in the interventional procedure codes:

- Roadmapping and/or fluoroscopic guidance
- Vessel measurements
- Postangioplasty/stent angiography

Diagnostic codes *are* reported with interventional procedures if either of the following apply:

- No prior catheter-based angiographic study is available, and a full diagnostic study is performed, and the decision to intervene is based on the diagnostic study.
- A prior study is available, however:
  - the patient's condition has changed, or
  - there is inadequate visualization of the anatomy or pathology, or
  - there is a clinical change during the procedure that requires new evaluation.

If there is a medically necessary diagnostic angiography on the same date as a therapeutic angiography, both may be coded, with a modifier 59 on the diagnostic study.

Take, for example, a patient who presents with a *diagnosed* right internal coronary lesion, and the interventional cardiologist plans to perform a PTCA with stent placement and performs an angiography for roadmapping the site. In this case, the angiography does not appear to be diagnostic and, therefore, would not be coded in addition to the stent placement.

On the other hand, a patient who presents with a *suspected* right internal coronary lesion, and the interventional cardiologist performs a coronary angiography, establishing the need for a PTCA with adjunctive stent angioplasty. In this case, the angiography appears to be diagnostic and, therefore, would be coded in addition to the stent placement.

Notice that, in the first example, the procedure and diagnosis are known, whereas in the second example, they are not known, and the angiographies are used to establish what type of treatment was needed.

Excerpt From the Medicine Section of NCCI Guidelines[2(p13)]

Many Pacemaker/Pacing Cardioverter-Defibrillator procedures (HCPCS/CPT codes 33202-33249, G0297-G0300) and Intracardiac Electrophysiology procedures (CPT codes 93600-93662) require intravascular placement of catheters into coronary vessels or cardiac chambers under fluoroscopic guidance. Physicians should not separately report cardiac catheterization or selective vascular catheterization CPT codes for placement of these catheters. A cardiac catheterization CPT code is separately reportable if it is a medically reasonable, necessary, and distinct service performed at the same or different patient encounter. Fluoroscopy codes are not separately reportable with the procedures described by HCPCS/CPT codes 33202-33249, G0297-G0300, and 93600-93662. Similarly, ultrasound guidance is not separately reportable with these HCPCS/CPT codes.

Interpretation

As indicated throughout the NCCI guidelines, there are certain procedures that require and include vascular access, fluoroscopy, ultrasound guidance, and so forth. The invasive procedures that are cardiovascular in nature, which would include cardiac catheterization and fluoroscopy, are pacemakers, cardiodefibrillators, and electrophysiology procedures. The cardiac catheterization and fluoroscopy are incidental to the pacemakers, cardiodefibrillators, and electrophysiology procedures.

Cardiac catheterization and coronary angioplasty, atherectomy, or stenting procedures include insertion of a needle and/or catheter, infusion, fluoroscopy and EKG strips … All are components of performing a cardiac catheterization or coronary artery angioplasty, atherectomy, or stenting.

Interpretation

As indicated throughout the NCCI edits, services that are inherent components of more comprehensive services may not be coded separately. For cardiac catheterizations or other percutaneous coronary interventions, the access (via needle or catheter insertion), infusion (of contrast or other media), fluoroscopy (for guidance), and EKG strips (for monitoring during the procedure) are all included components that may not be coded separately. The reimbursement for the comprehensive service (cardiac catheterization, other percutaneous interventions) includes the reimbursement for these inherent services. For example, a patient presents for a cardiac catheterization during which the physician inserts a catheter through the brachial artery into the heart and then injects dye to determine the number and locations of blockages. In this case, the catheter insertion and dye are inherent parts of the catheterization and would not be coded separately from the cardiac catheterization.

Cardiac catheterization procedures may require procurement of EKG tracings during the procedure to assess chest pain during catheterization and angioplasty; when performed in this fashion, these EKG tracings are not separately reported. EKGs procured prior to, or after, the procedure may be separately reported with modifier -59.

Interpretation

EKG tracings during a cardiac catheterization serve to monitor the patient's condition during the procedure, and the tracings are incidental to the cardiac catheterization. However, if an EKG was performed as a diagnostic tool prior to the procedure or after the procedure, that would not be for monitoring during the procedure and could be billed separately from the cardiac catheterization with a modifier 59. Take the patient who presents to an ED with chest pain, and the physician orders an EKG as well as other diagnostic studies (eg, troponin, chest X-ray). The physician then performs a cardiac catheterization. During the catheterization, the physician continuously monitors the patient's EKG rhythm. In this case, the initial EKG is separate and distinct from the cardiac catheterization and would be billed with a modifier 59. However, the monitoring during the catheterization would not be coded separately from the procedure.

Placement of an occlusive device such as an angio seal or vascular plug into an arterial or venous access site after cardiac catheterization or other diagnostic or interventional procedure should be reported as HCPCS code G0269. Providers should not report an associated imaging code such as CPT code 75710 or HCPCS code G0278.

Interpretation

Often at the end of a percutaneous procedure, the artery puncture site is closed with an Angio-Seal or other vascular plug to quickly seal the site. There should be no additional code used for an angiography related to the Angio-Seal. However, because the Angio-Seal is used after percutaneous vascular procedures, it is very likely that other angiographies will be coded for the procedure. Do not code any angiography specifically related to the Angio-Seal procedure.

G0269 Placement of occlusive device into either a venous or arterial access site, post surgical or interventional procedure (e.g. angioseal plug, vascular plug)

75710 Angiography, extremity, unilateral, radiological supervision and interpretation

G0278 Iliac and/or femoral artery angiography, non-selective, bilateral or ipsilateral to catheter insertion, performed at the same time as cardiac catheterization and/or coronary angiography, includes positioning or placement of the catheter in the distal aorta or ipsilateral femoral or iliac artery, injection of dye, production of permanent images, and radiologic supervision and interpretation (List separately in addition to primary procedure)

To illustrate the point, consider the patient who presents for a cerebral angiography and vertebral stenting. At the conclusion of the procedure, the catheter is removed, and an angiogram is performed through the previously placed sheath to determine whether the common femoral artery is patent and suitable in size and morphology for use of a vascular closure device. There is sufficient patency, and a vascular plug is used to close the vessel.

The diagnostic and therapeutic angiographies and procedures would be coded; however, the final angiography to determine whether the vessel is suitable for the vascular plug should not be coded in addition to the vascular plug procedure itself.

Excerpt From the Medicine Section of NCCI Guidelines[2(p14)]

Renal artery angiography at the time of cardiac catheterization should be reported as HCPCS code G0275 if selective catheterization of the renal artery is not performed. HCPCS code G0275 should not be reported with CPT code 36245 for selective renal artery catheterization or CPT codes 75722 or 75724 for renal angiography. If it is medically necessary to perform selective renal artery catheterization and renal angiography, HCPCS code G0275 should not be additionally reported.

Interpretation

Selective catheterization of the renal artery is when the catheter is manipulated to the renal artery. When the renal artery is selectively catheterized, the catheterization should be coded with CPT code 36245, and the complementary renal angiography would be coded with CPT code 75722 or 75724. When a nonselective renal artery angiography is performed concomitantly with a cardiac catheterization, HCPCS code G0275 would be used instead of the selective catheter and angiography codes. The documentation should specify whether or not the renal artery was selectively catheterized (the catheter must be in the renal artery).

Excerpt From the Medicine Section of NCCI Guidelines[2(p14)]

Cardiovascular stress tests include insertion of needle and/or catheter, infusion (pharmacologic stress tests) and EKG strips.

Interpretation

Cardiovascular stress tests require stressing the body through exercise, pharmacologic agents, or a combination of both. For those stress tests using pharmacologic agents, the administration (injection or infusion) of those agents is an inherent part of the test and should not be coded separately.

Key to performing a cardiovascular stress test is continuous EKG monitoring. Actually, that is the whole point of the test. Therefore, EKGs, EKG rhythm strips, and other cardiac monitoring are all included in the code for the stress test. Do not code these services separately.

Take the 85-year-old man presenting for a cardiovascular stress test to determine whether he has coronary artery disease. Because of the patient's advanced age and medical condition, an exercise stress test is contraindicated. A vasodilator pharmaceutical is infused to induce the stress. During the procedure, a baseline EKG is done, and any changes related to positioning (lying, standing, sitting) and during recovery are noted. Increases and decreases in blood pressure are also noted. In this case, the cardiovascular stress test may be coded, but the vasodilator administration and EKG monitoring are component parts to the stress test and should not be coded separately.

Excerpt From the Medicine Section of NCCI Guidelines[2(p15)]

CPT code 93503 (insertion and placement of flow directed catheter (e.g., Swan Ganz)) should not be reported with CPT codes 36555-36556 (insertion of non-tunneled centrally inserted central venous catheter) or CPT codes 36568-36569 (insertion of peripherally inserted central venous catheter) for the insertion of a single catheter. If a physician does not complete the insertion of one type of catheter and subsequently inserts another at the same patient encounter, only the completed procedure may be reported.

Interpretation

Failed procedures are incidental to successful procedures when they are performed during the same surgical session. CMS provides several examples for the more complex guideline, including the following:

Incomplete procedures are included in *complete* procedures when they are performed at the same encounter of the same anatomic site. If these services were performed at different anatomic sites and for different medically necessary reasons, both may be coded. A 61-year-old man with ischemic cardiomyopathy has congestive heart failure despite chronic milrinone infusion and the physician attempts placement of a Swan-Ganz catheter via the right internal jugular vein. Attempts to place the catheter are unsuccessful because of anatomic distortion. The attempt is then converted to a subclavian-directed central line placement, with success. Only the subclavian central line procedure would be coded, because the Swan-Ganz catheter attempt was unsuccessful.

Pulmonary Services and NCCI Guidelines

Excerpt From the Medicine Section of NCCI Guidelines[2(p15)]

Alternate methods of reporting data obtained during a spirometry or other pulmonary function session cannot be separately reported. Specifically, the flow volume loop is an alternative method of calculating a standard spirometric parameter. The CPT code 94375 is included in standard spirometry (rest and exercise) studies.

Interpretation

Spirometry is the most basic and frequently performed test of pulmonary (lung) function. A device called a spirometer is used to measure how much air the lungs can hold and how well the respiratory system is able to move air into and out of the lungs. A flow-volume loop measures the rate of airflow as a function of lung volume during a respiratory cycle. If essentially the same data is obtained via different methods, only one method of data collection may be coded; therefore, NCCI bundles the flow-volume loop into the spirometry service and does not allow a modifier to bypass the edit.

Excerpt From the Medicine Section of NCCI Guidelines[2(p15)]

When a physician who is in attendance for a pulmonary function study, obtains a limited history, and performs a limited examination referable specifically to the pulmonary function testing, separately coding for an evaluation and management service is not appropriate. If a significant, separately identifiable service is performed unrelated to the technical performance of the pulmonary function test, an evaluation and management service may be reported.

Interpretation

When physician interaction with a patient is necessary to accomplish the pulmonary function study, the interaction generally involves a limited inquiry and limited examination. In this case, a separate E/M service is not reported. As a rule, if the medical decision making that evolves from the procurement of the information from the patient is limited to whether or not the procedure should be performed or whether comorbidity may impact the procedure or involves discussion and patient education, an E/M code is not reported separately. If a significant, separately identifiable service is rendered, involving taking a history, performing an examination, and making medical decisions distinct from the procedure, the appropriate E/M service may be reported.

Physicians performing pulmonary function studies often work from an order by the patient's treating provider and, therefore, are not making clinical determinations as to the efficacy of the ordered service. In this case, because there is no distinguished E/M service, only the pulmonary function study would be billed.

However, if the physician is the one who medically evaluated the patient and determined a need for the pulmonary function study, and the study was performed within that provider's office, both the study and E/M service should be billed, as the E/M determined the need for the test. The E/M service must be documented as separate from the pulmonary function test, significant, and medically necessary.

Therefore, if a patient's primary care physician orders a pulmonary function study and the pulmonologist performs the test providing the requesting physician with an interpretation, the pulmonologist never performs a separate E/M service and cannot bill a medical visit.

However, if a patient's primary care physician refers the patient to a pulmonologist for evaluation and consultation regarding shortness of breath and the pulmonologist performs a complete work-up on the patient and decides to perform a pulmonary function study, the pulmonologist may bill both the E/M service with a modifier 25 and the pulmonary function study, as the E/M service was necessary to determine the need for the test.

Excerpt From the Medicine Section of NCCI Guidelines[2(p15)]

When multiple spirometric determinations are necessary (e.g., CPT code 94070) to complete the service described in the CPT code, only one unit of service is reported.

Interpretation

CPT code 94070 includes multiple determinations. Because the code specifies multiple determinations, only one unit of service is necessary, as the code inherently includes the multiple services. This would be true of any CPT codes that indicate *multiple* within the code nomenclature. CPT codes with *multiple* in the description usually have a medically unlikely edit of one.

94760   Noninvasive ear or pulse oximetry for oxygen saturation; single determination

94761   multiple determinations (eg, during exercise)

If multiple determinations were made for pulse oximetry, CPT code 94761 would be the appropriate code, with a single unit of service. If CPT code 94760 was billed with multiple units of service, it would be a coding and bundling error.

Excerpt From the Medicine Section of NCCI Guidelines[2(p15-16)]

Complex pulmonary stress testing (e.g., CPT code 94621) is a comprehensive stress test with a number of component tests separately defined in the *CPT Manual*. It is inappropriate to separately code venous access, EKG monitoring, spirometric parameters performed before, during and after exercise, oximetry, O2 consumption, CO2 production, rebreathing cardiac output calculations, etc., when performed as part of a complex pulmonary stress test. It is also inappropriate to bill for a cardiac stress test and the component codes used to perform a simple pulmonary stress test (CPT code 94620), when a complex pulmonary stress test is performed. If using a standard exercise protocol, serial electrocardiograms are obtained, and a separate report describing a cardiac stress test (professional component) is included in the medical record, the professional components for both a cardiac and pulmonary stress test may be reported.

Interpretation

There are three guidelines here:

1. Do not bill component services in addition to the comprehensive service. Since CPT code 94621 includes electrocardiographic monitoring, venous access, etc, it would be incorrect to code those services in addition to CPT 94621.
2. Do not downcode one service in order to add component codes separately. If the complex pulmonary stress test is the service performed, it would be incorrect to

code a simple pulmonary stress test in order to add the EKG monitoring or other component service.
3. If a separate and true cardiac stress test is performed with a separate interpretation, both the cardiac stress test and pulmonary stress test may be coded for professional fee services. There would be no additional code for the technical component.

Excerpt From the Medicine Section of NCCI Guidelines[2(p16)]

Pursuant to the *Federal Register* (Volume 58, Number 230, 12/2/1993, pages 63640-63641), ventilation management CPT codes (94002-94004 and 94660-94662) are not separately reportable with evaluation and management (E&M) CPT codes. If an E&M code and a ventilation management code are reported, only the E&M code is payable.

Interpretation

This is not complicated; do not code ventilation management in addition to an E/M service performed on the same day. Choose the code that most closely matches the documentation. Often there is substantial documentation of an E/M service, which would be coded. Mechanical ventilation is used when patients are unable to breathe adequately on their own. The ventilation management breathes for them until they are sufficiently recovered to initiate respiration.

Take, for example, an inpatient trauma patient who requires ventilation management. Her ICU provider visits the patient daily since her transfer out of ICU and, during the visits, provides ventilation management care. Because there is most likely sufficient documentation for a subsequent care hospital visit, the visit would be coded, rather than the ventilation management. The ventilation management becomes incidental to the visit.

Excerpt From the Medicine Section of NCCI Guidelines[2(p16)]

The procedure described by CPT code 94644 (continuous inhalation treatment with aerosol medication for acute airway obstruction, first hour) does not include any physician work RVUs. When performed in a facility, the procedure utilizes facility staff and supplies, and the physician does not have any practice expenses related to the procedure. Thus, a physician should not report this code when the physician orders it in a facility.

Interpretation

Medicare's reimbursement for CPT code 94644 is for the facility and malpractice costs and does not recognize any professional fee. Therefore, this code is used (and only requires) when a nonphysician (eg, nurse) provides the service. Because use of this code does not require that the service be performed by a physician, the physician may not bill for this service when it is performed in a setting other than the physician's office or clinic. The physician must have responsibility for the overhead costs (eg, staff performing, materials) before this code can be used. Because the physician would not incur any costs or expend any effort for this service in a facility setting, physicians should not bill for this CPT code in that setting.

Excerpt From the Medicine Section of NCCI Guidelines[2(p16)]

CPT code 94640 (pressurized or nonpressurized inhalation treatment for acute airway obstruction…) and CPT code 94664 (demonstration and/or evaluation of patient utilization of an aerosol generator…) should not be reported for the same patient encounter. If performed at separate patient encounters on the same date of service, the two services may be reported separately.

Interpretation

In contrast with instructions provided in the April 2000 issue of *CPT Assistant*,[5] the NCCI edits do not allow CPT codes 94640 and 94664 to be billed together when the procedures are performed during a single encounter. However, should there be separate encounters on a single date of service, both codes may be reported together by appending modifier 59 to one of the encounters.

CPT code 94664 is used to report demonstrating the use of an aerosol generator to a patient and/or to observe the use of an aerosol generator by the patient. It is an instructional encounter, whereas CPT code 94640 is for treatment or inducing sputum for diagnosis. If a patient presents for treatment of bronchospasm and the respiratory therapist demonstrates the use of a nebulizer and observes as the patient attempts to use the nebulizer, then the encounter should be CPT code 94640. No additional code would be used for the demonstration.

Allergy Testing and Immunotherapy and NCCI Guidelines

Excerpt From the Medicine Section of NCCI Guidelines[2(p16-17)]

If percutaneous or intracutaneous (intradermal) single test (CPT codes 95004 or 95024) and "sequential and incremental" tests (CPT codes 95010, 95015, or 95027) are performed on the same date of service, both the "sequential and incremental" test and single test codes may be reported if the tests are for different allergens or different dilutions of the same allergen. The unit of service to report is the number of separate tests. Do not report both a single test and a "sequential and incremental" test for the same dilution of an allergen. For example, if the single test for an antigen is positive and the provider proceeds to "sequential and incremental" tests with three additional *different* dilutions of the same antigen, the provider may report one unit of service for the single test code and three units of service for the "sequential and incremental" test code.

Interpretation

The single tests are bundled into the sequential/incremental tests. Because the sequential/incremental tests are the more extensive service, they would be coded over the single tests when performed on one antigen or one dilution. Only the most extensive service may be billed per allergen or per dilution. The bundling edit may be bypassed if the documentation clearly supports that the single test was performed on different allergens or different dilutions.

Neurology and Neuromuscular Procedures and NCCI Guidelines

Excerpt From the Medicine Section of NCCI Guidelines[2(p18)]

Sleep testing differs from polysomnography in that the latter requires the presence of sleep staging. Sleep staging includes a qualitative and quantitative assessment of sleep as determined by standard sleep scoring techniques. Accordingly, at the same session, a "sleep study" and "polysomnography" are not reported together.

Interpretation

Polysomnography is a sleep study that incorporates multiple parameters by measuring sleep cycles and stages by recording brain waves, electrical activity of muscles, eye movement, breathing rate, blood pressure, blood oxygen saturation, and heart rhythm. Because the polysomnography means multiple sleep studies, it would be duplicative to code a sleep study in addition to a polysomnography. Polysomnographies are the more commonly performed services.

Excerpt From the Medicine Section of NCCI Guidelines[2(p18)]

Polysomnography requires at least one central and usually several other EEG electrodes. EEG procurement for polysomnography (sleep staging) differs greatly from that required for diagnostic EEG testing (i.e., speed of paper, number of channels, etc.). Accordingly, EEG testing is not to be reported with polysomnography unless performed separately…

Continuous electroencephalographic monitoring services (CPT codes 95950-95962) represent different services than those provided during sleep testing; accordingly these codes are only to be reported when a separately identifiable service is performed and documented.

Interpretation

Since EEG recordings are an inherent part of a polysomnography, the EEG should not be billed in addition to the polysomnography unless a distinct and separate EEG was performed for a medically indicated reason. When the EEG is performed independent of the polysomnography for a separate diagnostic purpose, both may be coded. The documentation must support a separate written interpretation for the EEG to be billed, and it must support the need for a separate EEG.

Excerpt From the Medicine Section of NCCI Guidelines[2(p18)]

When nerve testing (EMG, nerve conduction velocity, etc.) is performed to assess the level of paralysis during anesthesia or during mechanical ventilation, the series of CPT codes 95851-95937 are not to be separately reported; these codes reflect significant, separately identifiable diagnostic services requiring a formal report in the medical record. Additionally, electrical stimulation used to identify or locate nerves as part of a procedure involving treatment of a cranial or peripheral nerve (e.g., nerve block, nerve destruction, neuroplasty, transection, excision, repair, etc.) is part of the primary procedure.

Interpretation

It makes sense that nerve testing would be included in the anesthesia if the test is performed to confirm the patient's paralysis; therefore, the nerve testing would not be coded in addition to the anesthesia services performed. However, if the nerve testing is truly diagnostic and a separate interpretation is documented, it may be coded in addition to the anesthesia. The medical necessity must be apparent within the documentation.

Excerpt From the Medicine Section of NCCI Guidelines[2(p19)]

Intraoperative neurophysiology testing (CPT code 95920) should not be reported by the physician performing an operative procedure since it is included in the global package. However, when performed by a different physician during the procedure, it is separately reportable by the second physician. The physician performing an operative procedure should not bill other 90000 neurophysiology testing codes for intraoperative neurophysiology testing…since they are also included in the global package.

Interpretation

Intraoperative neurophysiology monitoring is where a neurophysiologist performs testing and monitoring of the nervous system during surgery to assist the surgeons in avoiding or reducing complications such as paralysis or stroke. This monitoring also provides information to the surgeon for use in intraoperative decision-making.

The NCCI guideline is relatively simple: If the surgeon performed intraoperative neurophysiology testing, the testing is part of global surgery reimbursement and cannot be billed separately. However, if a provider other than the surgeon performs testing, the service may be billed by the performing provider.

Essentially, for this code to be used, a physician other than the surgeon must have performed the intraoperative monitoring. The monitoring physician would bill the specific testing performed in addition to the intraoperative monitoring time (CPT code 95920).

An important note here is that the time to interpret the base study is excluded from the time used to bill the intraoperative monitoring.

In order to bill this monitoring, these requirements must be met:

- The operating surgeon must request this test.
- The monitoring physician must perform intraoperative testing in real time.
- The physician's time must be solely dedicated to performing this service.
- There must be continuous or immediate contact with the surgeon to report changes.

To bill, the monitoring physician should bill for the actual time (1 unit of service per hour) spent monitoring the electrical activity during the surgical procedure. The provider performing the baseline test is the provider who provides the monitoring. The actual time of monitoring (CPT code 95920) begins immediately after the surgery has started.

For example, a surgeon is performing a single-level C6-C7 anterior cervical diskectomy with anterior cervical fusion, anterior cervical instrumentation, and structural allograft bone graft. During the operation, the surgeon requests that a neurophysiologist perform neural integrity monitoring. Because the surgeon requests the monitoring, and a physician other than the surgeon provides the service, the neurophysiologist could bill for the monitoring and base modality.

However, if a surgeon is performing a tympanomastoidectomy, and, during the procedure, the surgeon also performs facial nerve monitoring, because the surgeon performs the monitoring, the monitoring could not be coded in addition to the surgery.

Excerpt From the Medicine Section of NCCI Guidelines[2(p19)]

The NCCI edit with column one CPT code 95903 (Motor nerve conduction studies with F-wave study, each nerve) and column two CPT code 95900 (Motor nerve conduction studies without F-wave study, each nerve) is often bypassed by utilizing modifier -59. Use of modifier -59 with the column two CPT code 95900 of this NCCI edit is only appropriate if the two procedures are performed on different nerves or in separate patient encounters.

Interpretation

Since CPT code 95903 is for the more complete study (with F-wave), CPT code 95900 becomes a component to 95903 and should not be reported in addition to 95900. However, if multiple nerves are involved and one has an F-wave and one does not, both codes may be billed with a modifier 59. Of course, if the tests were performed at different patient encounters (medically necessary and well documented), then both tests may be coded.

So, if the procedures were performed at separate patient encounters or multiple/different nerves were tested, some with and some without F-waves, a modifier 59 may be used to bypass the bundling edit. If one nerve is studied during a single encounter, only one code (the more extensive) should be billed. For example, a patient with suspected carpal tunnel syndrome presents for nerve conduction studies of the ulnar nerve. Specifically, the following nerve conduction studies are performed:

- Ulnar motor nerve to the abductor digiti minimi with F-wave
- Ulnar motor nerve to the palmar interosseous without F-wave
- Ulnar motor nerve to the first dorsal interosseous without and with F-wave

Three motor nerve conduction studies may be coded:

95900 Nerve conduction, amplitude and latency/velocity study, each nerve; motor, without F-wave study

95903 motor, with F-wave study

CPT code 95903x2 for the (1) abductor digit minimi and (2) first dorsal interosseous
CPT code 95900-59x1 for the palmar interosseous
Modifier 59 is to bypass the bundling edit.

Central Nervous System Assessments/Tests and NCCI Guidelines

Excerpt From the Medicine Section of NCCI Guidelines[2(p19)]

Neurobehavioral status exam (CPT code 96116) should not be reported when a mini-mental status examination is performed. CPT code 96116 may never be reported with psychiatric diagnostic examinations (CPT codes 90801 or 90802). CPT code 96116 may be reported with other psychiatric services or evaluation and management services only if a complete neurobehavioral status exam is performed. If a mini-mental status examination is performed by a physician, it is included in the evaluation and management service.

Interpretation

A mini-mental status exam is a brief assessment of the patient's:

- orientation to time, place, person
- recent and remote memory
- mood and affect

The mini-mental status is not as extensive as the neurobehavioral status exam, which is an assessment of thinking, reasoning, etc., requiring much more in-depth an assessment by the physician.

In addition, everything assessed in the neurobehavioral status exam is included in the psychiatric diagnostic examination (CPT code 90801 and 90802) and is not to be coded separately. Because physicians who provide psychotherapy assess the specific areas identified in the neurobehavioral status examination, it would be duplicative to code both services.

96116 Neurobehavioral status exam (clinical assessment of thinking, reasoning and judgment, eg, acquired knowledge, attention, language, memory, planning and problem solving, and visual spatial abilities), per hour of the psychologist's or physician's time, both face-to-face time with the patient and time interpreting test results and preparing the report

Special Dermatological Procedures and NCCI Guidelines

Excerpt From the Medicine Section of NCCI Guidelines[2(p22)]

Medicare does not allow separate payment of E&M CPT code 99211 with photochemotherapy procedures (CPT codes 96910-96913) for services performed by a nurse or technician such as examining a patient prior to a subsequent procedure for burns or reactions to the prior treatment. If a physician performs a significant separately identifiable medically reasonable and necessary E&M service on the same date of service, it may be reported with modifier -25.

Interpretation

Usually, when a procedure is performed, the low level E/M code (CPT code 99211) is not separately billable; however, higher levels of E/M (Level 2-5) documented and supported as medically necessary may be coded by appending a modifier 25 to the E/M service. For example, a patient presents for a photochemotherapy procedure, and the nurse checks the patient's vital signs, asks if there have been any problems with the prior treatment, and obtains a consent form. In this scenario, only the photochemotherapy should be coded, as the nurse's work is simply part of prepping the patient for the procedure. On the other hand, take the same patient presenting one month later for treatment, but this time the patient is complaining of a reaction after the last treatment as well as a severe flare-up of her atopic dermatitis. The physician evaluates the patient; performs a detailed history; does an expanded, problem-focused examination; and performs medical decision making of moderate complexity. The physician determines that the patient could safely undergo the photochemotherapy treatment. In this scenario, both the photochemotherapy and E/M service with modifier 25 may be coded.

Physical Medicine and Rehabilitation and NCCI Guidelines

Interpretation

Supervised modalities (CPT code range 97010-97028) do not require the billing provider to work one-on-one with the patient. Physicians may be supervising several patients' treatments during a single 15-minute period. However, there are other CPT codes that specify that one-on-one contact between the provider and patient is necessary (eg, constant attendance CPT codes) and are billed in 15-minute increments. For constant attendance modalities, only one service and one patient may be attended to during the 15-minute time period. Two patients may not be constantly attended at the same time. To illustrate this guideline, the CMS web site[6] has much information on appropriate billing for physical therapy. Here is an excerpt:

1. Billing - CPT Codes: Not Permitted
   In the same 15-minute (or other) time period, a therapist cannot bill any of the following pairs of CPT codes for outpatient therapy services provided to the same, or to different patients. Examples include:
   a. Any two CPT codes for "therapeutic procedures" requiring direct one-on-one patient contact (CPT codes 97110-97542);
   b. Any two CPT codes for modalities requiring "constant attendance" and direct one-on-one patient contact (CPT codes 97032 - 97039);
   c. Any two CPT codes requiring either constant attendance or direct one-on-one patient contact - as described in (a) and (b) above — (CPT codes 97032- 97542). For example: any CPT code for a therapeutic procedure (eg. 97116-gait training) with any attended modality CPT code (eg. 97035-ultrasound);

d. Any CPT code for therapeutic procedures requiring direct one-on-one patient contact (CPT codes 97110 - 97542) with the group therapy CPT code (97150) requiring constant attendance. For example: group therapy (97150) with neuromuscular reeducation (97112);

e. Any CPT code for modalities requiring constant attendance (CPT codes 97032 - 97039) with the group therapy CPT code (97150). For example: group therapy (97150) with ultrasound (97035);

f. Any untimed evaluation or reevaluation code (CPT codes 97001-97004) with any other timed or untimed CPT codes, including constant attendance modalities (CPT codes 97032 - 97039), therapeutic procedures (CPT codes 97110-97542) and group therapy (CPT code 97150)

2. Billing - CPT Codes: Permitted
   In the same 15-minute time period, one therapist may bill for more than one therapy service occurring in the same 15-minute time period where "supervised modalities" are defined by CPT as untimed and unattended—not requiring the presence of the therapist (CPT codes 97010 - 97028). One or more supervised modalities may be billed in the same 15-minute time period with any other CPT code, timed or untimed, requiring constant attendance or direct one-on-one patient contact. However, any actual time the therapist uses to attend one-on-one to a patient receiving a supervised modality cannot be counted for any other service provided by the therapist.
   a. One-on-One Example: In a 45-minute period, a therapist works with 3 patients - A, B, and C - providing therapeutic exercises to each patient with direct one-on-one contact in the following sequence: Patient A receives 8 minutes, patient B receives 8 minutes and patient C receives 8 minutes. After this initial 24-minute period, the therapist returns to work with patient A for 10 more minutes (18 minutes total), then patient B for 5 more minutes (13 minutes total), and finally patient C for 6 additional minutes (14 minutes total). During the times the patients are not receiving direct one-on-one contact with the therapist, they are each exercising independently. The therapist appropriately bills each patient one 15 minute unit of therapeutic exercise (97110) corresponding to the time of the skilled intervention with each patient.
   b. Group Example: In a 25-minute period, a therapist works with two patients, A and B, and divides his/her time between two patients. The therapist moves back and forth between the two patients, spending a minute or two at a time, and provides occasional assistance and modifications

to patient A's exercise program and offers verbal cues for patient B's gait training and balance activities in the parallel bars. The therapist does not track continuous or notable, identifiable episodes of direct one-on-one contact with either patient and would bill each patient one unit of group therapy (97150) corresponding to the time of the skilled intervention with each patient.

Excerpt From the Medicine Section of NCCI Guidelines[2(p22-23)]

NCCI contains edits with column one codes of the physical medicine and rehabilitation therapy services and column two codes of the physical therapy and occupational therapy re-evaluation CPT codes of 97002 and 97004 respectively. The re-evaluation services should not be routinely reported during a planned course of physical or occupational therapy. However, if the patient's status should change and a re-evaluation is warranted, it may be reported with modifier -59 appended to CPT code 97002 or 97004 as appropriate.

Interpretation

The intent of a re-evaluation is to assess progress and modify or redirect future interventions. If a new problem or abnormality is encountered, then initial assessment would be coded rather than a re-evaluation. The re-evaluations should be fairly limited during a course of treatment, but when medically necessary, may be billed. If the re-evaluation falls on the same date as physical therapy, a modifier 59 should be appended to indicate that the re-evaluation was separate and distinct from the therapy.

SUMMARY

- The entire medicine section from the NCCI manual should be read.

- Because the Medicine section of the CPT codebook is so diverse, the clinical examples CPT codebook offers are very helpful.

- The hydration, infusion, injection, and chemotherapy administration services can be quite confusing. When coding these services, refer to the CPT codebook instructions, the NCCI edit guidelines, and payer-specific information.

Definitions and Acronyms Important to Chapter 18

cardiac catheterization: This is an invasive medical procedure that is used for diagnostic and therapeutic reasons. A catheter is introduced into a blood vessel and manipulated to the heart.

cardiac rehabilitation: The American Heart Association defines the services of cardiac rehabilitation as a medically supervised program to help heart patients recover quickly and improve their overall physical, mental, and social functioning.

central venous access: Central venous access is the introduction of a catheter into a vein that leads to the heart. It is often used as a means for administering drugs or assessing pressures.

spirometry: Spirometry is the most basic and frequently performed test of pulmonary (lung) function. A device (spirometer) is used to measure how much air the lungs can hold and how well the respiratory system is able to move air into and out of the lungs.

CHAPTER EXERCISES

EXERCISE 1
A hospital intensive care provider was called to the ICU because a patient underwent cardiac arrest. In attempting to stabilize the patient, the intensive care provider performed the following procedures during 48 minutes of critical care:
a. CPR
b. Nasogastric tube placement
c. Chest x-ray to check placement of the tube

What services can be coded?

EXERCISE 2
In a hospital outpatient setting, a patient was being infused with Taxol for chemotherapy. Before the chemotherapy was started, an infusion of normal saline and Decadron was given (first the saline, then the Decadron) to assist with line patency and post-chemotherapy nausea.

What services could the physician bill?

ANSWERS TO CHAPTER EXERCISES

EXERCISE 1: Because the critical care time is not delineated from the separately coded services, the case cannot be coded. Additional documentation is needed. If the critical care was for 48 minutes aside from these services, the CPR could be coded separately.

EXERCISE 2: None. In the hospital setting, if the physician is supervising the staff, rather than personally performing the service, no administration services may be coded on the professional fee side.

REFERENCES

1. American Medical Association. *Current Procedural Terminology (CPT®) Professional Edition 2009*. Chicago, IL: American Medical Association; 2008.

2. Centers for Medicare and Medicaid Services. "Chapter XI Medicine, Evaluation and Management Services." In: NCCI Policy Manual for Medicare Services. www.cms.hhs.gov/ NationalCorrectCodInitEd/01_overview.asp#TopOfPage. Accessed June 14, 2009.

3. Centers for Medicare and Medicaid Services. *1997 Documentation Guidelines for Evaluation and Management Services*. General multi-system examination. Page 14.

4. American Heart Association. *Cardiac Rehabilitation Guidelines*. www.americanheart.org/presenter.jhtml?identifier=4490. Accessed February 25, 2009.

5. American Medical Association. "Coding consultation, pulmonary, medicine 94640, 94664, 97535 (Q&A)." *CPT Assistant*, 2000;10(4):11.

6. Centers for Medicare and Medicaid Services. *Part B Billing Scenarios for PTs and OTs*. www.cms.hhs.gov/TherapyServices/02_ billing_scenarios.asp. Accessed June 14, 2009.

HCPCS Level II NCCI Edits

Chapter 19 provides background about services in the Healthcare Common Procedure Coding System (HCPCS) Level II codes, reviews the National Correct Coding Initiative (NCCI) guidelines for HCPCS Level II codes, and provides examples to reflect the logic behind the edits. As do the other chapters, this chapter provides an NCCI guideline followed by our interpretation, an example, or both. The HCPCS Level II codes include services, supplies, equipment, and pharmaceuticals. This chapter addresses the codes with NCCI guidelines.

Introduction Section of HCPCS NCCI Guidelines

> **Excerpt From the HCPCS Level II Section of NCCI Guidelines[2(p2)]**
>
> Introduction
> The principles of correct coding discussed in Chapter I apply to the CPT codes in the range A0000-V9999. Several general guidelines are repeated in this Chapter. However, those general guidelines from Chapter I not discussed in this chapter are nonetheless applicable.

Interpretation

This instruction indicates that the overall NCCI guidelines apply to each section of *Current Procedural Terminology (CPT®)*[1] codebook and, even if they are not repeated within a chapter, they are nonetheless a guideline to be followed. The introductory guidelines were covered comprehensively in Chapter 2 of this book; those introductory guidelines that have clear application within the HCPCS Level II codes are reiterated in this chapter.

> **Excerpt From the HCPCS Level II Section of NCCI Guidelines[2(p3-4)]**
>
> All procedures on the Medicare Physician Fee Schedule are assigned a Global period of 000, 010, 090, XXX, YYY, or ZZZ. The global concept does not apply to XXX procedures. The global period for YYY procedures is defined by the Carrier. All procedures with a global period of ZZZ are related to another procedure, and the applicable global period for the ZZZ code is determined by the related procedure.

Interpretation

Many Level II HCPCS codes are designated as XXX procedures with no global surgery relationship. However, there still could be bundling issues for a Level II code and E/M services when services are performed on a single date for a single patient. Each code edit must be reviewed to determine whether there is a bundling issue.

The XXX procedures may include some preprocedure/intraprocedure/postprocedure work performed each time the procedure is provided. If so, do not code that usual work in addition to the XXX procedure.

If the provider does indeed provide a medically necessary and well-documented E/M service on the same date as the XXX procedure, it may be coded separately. A modifier 25 may be appended to the E/M service, but, remember, many HCPCS Level II codes do not bundle with the E/M, so the modifier might not be necessary.

For example, HCPCS code A4206 Syringe with needle, sterile, 1 cc or less, each

This code is for a supply (syringe) and is designated as an XXX procedure. There are no E/M bundling issues for this code.

On the other hand, HCPCS code G0027 Semen analysis; presence and/or motility of sperm excluding huhner. This code is for a procedure (semen analysis) and is designated as an XXX procedure. It does not bundle into E/M CPT codes and may be coded in addition to E/M services when both are performed and documented on the same date.

HCPCS code G0101 Cervical or vaginal cancer screening; pelvic and clinical breast examination

This code is for a procedure (cancer screening) and is designated as an XXX procedure. E/M codes bundle into this procedure. The documentation would have to support that the E/M service was unrelated to the cancer screening service. A modifier 25 would be needed on the E/M code if both services were clearly supported.

Excerpt From the HCPCS Level II Section of NCCI Guidelines[2(p3)]

Since NCCI edits are applied to same day services by the same provider to the same beneficiary, certain Global Surgery Rules are applicable to NCCI. An E&M service is separately reportable on the same date of service as a procedure with a global period of 000, 010, or 090 under limited circumstances.

If a procedure has a global period of 090 days, it is defined as a major surgical procedure. If an E&M is performed on the same date of service as a major surgical procedure for the purpose of deciding whether to perform this surgical procedure, the E&M service is separately reportable with modifier -57. Other E&M services on the same date of service as a major surgical procedure are included in the global payment for the procedure and are not separately reportable. NCCI does not contain edits based on this rule because Medicare Carriers have separate edits.

Interpretation

There are HCPCS Level II codes that have global periods of 90 days, but the NCCI edits are not based on the global surgery policy; therefore, there would be no NCCI edit. However, remember that the global surgery guidelines must be followed (see Chapter 3 for more information on the global surgery policy). For instance, consider HCPCS code G0343:

G0343 Laparotomy for islet cell transplant, includes portal vein catheterization and infusion

This HCPCS code has a 90-day global period attached. E/M services by the surgeon the day of or the day before are billable if modifier 57 is appended, based on the global surgery guidelines found within the *Medicare Claims Processing Manual*,[3] Chapter 12 - Physicians/Nonphysician Practitioners, Section 30.6.6, and as outlined in Chapter 3 of this book. This is not an NCCI edit.

Excerpt From the HCPCS Level II Section of NCCI Guidelines[2(p3-4)]

If a procedure has a global period of 000 or 010 days, it is defined as a minor surgical procedure. The decision to perform a minor surgical procedure is included in the payment for the minor surgical procedure and should not be reported separately as an E&M service. However, a significant and separately identifiable E&M service unrelated to the decision to perform the minor surgical procedure is separately reportable with modifier -25. NCCI does contain some edits based on these principles, but the Medicare Carriers have separate edits. Neither the NCCI nor Carriers have all possible edits based on these principles.

Interpretation

There are HCPCS Level II codes that have global periods of zero to 10 days. Even though the NCCI edits do not bundle E/M services based on the global surgery policy, there are some codes that bundle E/M services and the HCPCS Level II code.

HCPCS code G0341 Percutaneous islet cell transplant, includes portal vein catheterization and infusion

This HCPCS code has a zero-day global period attached, and there are no NCCI edits bundling an E/M service with this procedure. However, based on the global surgery policy, E/M services by the surgeon the day of the procedure should be billed with modifier 25 if the documentation supports a separate and significant medical visit. Otherwise, the E/M service would be included in the reimbursement for the transplant.

Medically Unlikely Edits and HCPCS Level II NCCI Guidelines

Chapter 2 of this book reviews in detail Centers for Medicare and Medicaid Services (CMS) guidelines related to medically unlikely edits (MUEs). Table 19-1 shows examples of MUEs for HCPCS Level II codes. The entire list of MUEs should be referred to during coding.

TABLE 19-1 *Medically Unlikely Edits (MUE) Examples for HCPCS Level II Codes*

HCPCS\CPT Code	Practitioner DME Supplier MUE
A4221	1
A4561	2
A6503	2
A9502	3
A9503	1
A9504	1
B4222	1
E0110	1
E0111	2
G0291	2
G0293	1
G0294	1
K0455	1
K0462	1
K0606	1
K0607	1
K0608	1

Abbreviation: DME indicates durable medical equipment.

General Policy Statements for HCPCS Level II NCCI Guidelines

Excerpt From the HCPCS Level II Section of NCCI Guidelines[2(p5)]

HCPCS code M0064 is not to be reported separately from CPT codes 90801-90857 (psychiatric services). This code describes a brief office visit for the sole purpose of monitoring or changing drug prescriptions used in the treatment of mental psychoneurotic and personality disorders.

Interpretation

There are two codes for psychotropic medication management: HCPCS M0064 and 90862. M0064 is for a brief office visit for the sole purpose of monitoring or changing drug prescriptions used in treatment of mental, psychoneurotic,

and personality disorders, whereas CPT code 90862 involves managing, observing responses, and regulating psychotropic prescription medicines. This code is for an in-depth management of psychotropic agents and requires a very skilled aspect of patient care. The effects and side effects of the drugs may be evaluated, the medications may be modified or renewed, and some psychotherapy, usually supportive, may be rendered but is not required.

If the physician supplied other medical E/M services in addition to pharmacologic management at the visit, an E/M code may be used, and the E/M service will include CPT 90862. Do not code 90862 in addition to the E/M service. On the other hand, if the patient received psychotherapy and pharmacologic management at the same visit, the psychotherapy codes (with or without medical E/M services) should be used. The pharmacologic management is included as part of the psychotherapy service, and CPT code 90862 should not be billed in addition to the psychotherapy codes.

Code 90862 is not intended to refer to a brief evaluation of the patient's state or simple dosage adjustment of long-term medication. The code refers to the in-depth management of psychopharmacologic agents, which are potent medications with frequent serious side effects, and represents a very skilled aspect of patient care.

HCPCS code M0064 should be used for the lesser level of drug monitoring such as simple dosage adjustment.

M0064 should not be billed in addition to other E/M services or psychotherapy, as M0064 would be incidental to those other services.

Excerpt From the HCPCS Level II Section of NCCI Guidelines[2(p5-6)]

HCPCS code Q0091, for screening pap smears includes the services necessary to procure and transport the specimen to the laboratory. If an evaluation and management service is performed at the same visit solely for the purpose of performing a screening pap smear, then the evaluation and management service is not reported separately. If a significant, separately identifiable evaluation and management service is performed to evaluate other medical problems, then both the screening pap smear and the evaluation and management service are reported.

Interpretation

HCPCS code Q0091 represents the obtaining, preparing, and conveying of a Pap smear. If the patient presented for screening, and the provider's service was solely for obtaining a Pap smear, Q0091 would be the only code used.

However, when an E/M service was significant and separate from the screening Pap smear procurement, both the visit and Q0091 may be coded, with a modifier 25 appended to the E/M service.

For example, a patient presents to her gynecologist with a suspected lump in her breast, for which the physician performs an E/M service. Additionally, the physician obtained a Pap smear for screening purposes. For this scenario, the E/M with a modifier 25 may be billed in addition to the Q0091 (Pap smear) as long as the documentation was clear.

Interpretation

HCPCS code G0101 represents a cervical or vaginal cancer screening; pelvic and clinical breast examination. This NCCI guideline states that HCPCS G0101 may be coded in addition to an E/M service if the E/M is unrelated to the G0101. For example, if a screening examination was performed, and the patient also had allergic rhinitis that was addressed through an E/M service, both may be coded, with modifier 25 appended to the E/M code. The documentation would have to clearly support both services being performed.

Take a patient who presents to her gynecologist for an annual examination. During the preventive visit, the patient discusses episodic syncope over the previous six months. The gynecologist obtains additional history relating to the new symptoms and extends the exam to include a neurological element. Additionally, the gynecologist orders additional diagnostic studies related to the syncope. The routine gynecologic examination would be coded as G0101, along with the E/M service for the syncope work-up.

Interpretation

CMS states that a digital rectal examination (DRE) should never be separately reported from an E/M service when both services are performed on a single date of service. Coders may make a note in the CPT codebook to make certain these services are not erroneously unbundled.

HCPCS code G0102 (DRE) bundles into the E/M CPT codes, and the edit cannot be bypassed with a modifier. See Table 19-2 for examples of edits for DRE services with E/M codes. CMS does have a correct coding modifier of zero for this procedure, which means the DRE services should never be coded in addition to the E/M CPT code.

TABLE 19-2 *Digital Rectal Examination Edit Examples With Evaluation and Management Services*

Column 1/Column 2 Edits		
Column 1	Column 2	Modifier 0 = not allowed 1 = allowed 9 = not applicable
99195	99344	9
99201	G0101	9
99201	G0102	0
99201	G0104	9
99202	G0101	9
99202	G0102	0
99202	G0104	9
99203	G0101	9
99203	G0102	0
99203	G0104	9
99203	G0105	9
99204	G0101	9
99204	G0102	0
99204	G0104	9
99205	G0101	9
99205	G0102	0
99205	G0104	9
99205	G0105	9
99205	G0106	9

SUMMARY

- The entire HCPCS Level II section from the NCCI manual should be read.

- A review of Medicare *HCPCS General Information*[4] for HCPCS Level II codes is helpful in understanding the HCPCS coding system more completely.

- Overall, the guidelines for HCPCS mimic those for HCPCS Level I (CPT) codes; however, many of the services, items, and so forth are not found within the Level I system, so each code edit must be reviewed on a claim-by-claim basis.

Definitions and Acronyms

Healthcare Common Procedure Coding System (HCPCS): This is the tiered system of procedural, surgery, supplies, and equipment coding implemented by CMS. The system includes CPT (HCPCS Level I) and HCPCS Level II codes.

HCPCS Level II codes: Codes created and maintained by CMS to supplement Level I HCPCS (CPT) codes. Level II codes include many services and supplies not included in the CPT coding system and temporary codes for which CMS has special guidelines for use.

HCPCS temporary codes for the Outpatient Prospective Payment System (OPPS): These are Level II C codes that are temporary codes established specifically for the OPPS. These C codes represent items or services that might support additional payment and services for which there is no other code.

HCPCS temporary codes for services: These are codes for services for which CMS has specific criteria for coverage and payment. An example would be a HCPCS Level II temporary code for a screening colonoscopy. There is a CPT code for colonoscopy, but the screening colonoscopy has specific frequency and coverage criteria that require a different code from that of the diagnostic service.

CHAPTER EXERCISES

EXERCISES

Would there be an NCCI edit for the following scenarios (look up the edit, if necessary, to answer)?

a. HCPCS G0105 on the same day as an E/M service. Would these edit against each other? Why? Is it possible to bypass the edit?

b. HCPCS G0237 on the same day as an E/M service. Would these edit against each other? Why? Is it possible to bypass the edit?

ANSWERS TO CHAPTER EXERCISES

a. HCPCS G0105 (screening colonoscopy) has a global period of zero days, and even though NCCI edits do not bundle based on global days, any E/M performed on the same day does bundle into the screening colonoscopy code. Documentation would have to clearly support that the E/M service was necessary and significantly separate (more than normal periprocedure care for the colonoscopy) in order for the service to be separately reported with modifier 25.

b. HCPCS G0237 (exercises) has a global period of XXX, and there are no NCCI edits bundling this service with an E/M service. However, the E/M service would still need to be documented and medically necessary in order to be billed.

REFERENCES

1. American Medical Association. *Current Procedural Terminology (CPT®) Professional Edition 2009*. Chicago, IL: American Medical Association; 2008.

2. Centers for Medicare and Medicaid Services. "Chapter XII Supplemental Serices HCPCS Level II Codes." In: NCCI Policy Manual for Medicare Services. www.cms.hhs.gov/NationalCorrectCodInitEd/01_overview.asp#TopOfPage. Accessed June 15, 2009.

3. Centers for Medicare and Medicaid Services. *Medicare Claims Processing Manual*. Chapter 12 - Physicians/Nonphysician Practitioners. Section 30.6.6. www.cms.hhs.gov/manuals/downloads/clm104c12.pdf. Accessed June 15, 2009.

4. Centers for Medicare and Medicaid Services. Medicare *HCPCS General Information*. www.cms.hhs.gov/MedHCPCSGenInfo/. Accessed June 15, 2009.

Category III NCCI Edits

Chapter 20 provides background about services in the Category III section of the CPT® codebook[1], reviews the National Correct Coding Initiative (NCCI) coding guidelines for Category III services, and provides examples to reflect the logic behind the edits. As do the other chapters, this chapter provides an NCCI guideline followed by our interpretation, an example, or both.

Category III codes are temporary codes for emerging technology, services, and procedures to allow data collection for these specific services or procedures. When a code exists in Category III, it should be used instead of a Category I CPT code. Because unlisted codes are nonspecific, they do not allow for the needed data collection.

Introduction Section of Category III NCCI Guidelines

> **Excerpt From the Category III Section of NCCI Guidelines[2(p2)]**
>
> Introduction
> The principles of correct coding discussed in Chapter I apply to the CPT codes in the range 0001T-0199T. Several general guidelines are repeated in this Chapter. However, those general guidelines from Chapter I not discussed in this chapter are nonetheless applicable.

Interpretation

This instruction indicates that the overall NCCI guidelines apply to each section of the CPT codebook, and, even if they are not repeated within a chapter, they are nonetheless a guideline to be followed. The introductory guidelines were covered comprehensively in Chapter 2 of this book; those introductory guidelines that have clear application within the Category III codes are reiterated in this chapter.

Evaluation and Management Services for Category III NCCI Guidelines

CPT Category III is a section of temporary CPT codes to capture health care related to emerging technology, services, and procedures. Because the Category III codes include services related to each section of CPT Category I codes, the evaluation and management (E/M) guidelines are hard to generalize to the entire section. The Centers for Medicare and Medicaid Services (CMS) states that the Medicare global surgery care guidelines are not applicable to NCCI edits; however, there are services that could potentially be bundled into the E/M service when the services are performed on a single date for a single patient. Each code edit must be reviewed to determine whether there is a bundling issue.

> **Excerpt From the Category III Section of NCCI Guidelines[2(p3-4)]**
>
> All procedures on the Medicare Physician Fee Schedule are assigned a Global period of 000, 010, 090, XXX, YYY, or ZZZ. ...
>
> Procedures with a global surgery indicator of "XXX" are not covered by these rules. Many of these "XXX" procedures are performed by physicians and have inherent pre-procedure, intra-procedure, and post-procedure work usually performed each time the procedure is completed. This work should never be reported as a separate E&M code. Other "XXX" procedures are not usually performed by a physician and have no physician work relative value units associated with them. A physician should never report a separate E&M code with these procedures for the supervision of others performing the procedure or for the interpretation of the procedure.

Interpretation

Currently, the Category III codes are designated as XXX procedures. If the provider does indeed provide a medically necessary and well-documented E/M service, making it separate and distinct from the Category III procedure, the E/M service may be coded separately.

Medically Unlikely Edits and Category III NCCI Guidelines

Chapter 2 of this book reviews in detail the CMS guidelines related to medically unlikely edits (MUEs). Table 20-1 shows examples of MUEs for Category III codes. The entire list of MUEs should be referred to when coding.

TABLE 20-1 *Medically Unlikely Edits (MUE) Examples for Category III Codes*

HCPCS\CPT Code	Practitioner DME Supplier MUE
0016T	2
0017T	2
0026T	1
0027T	1
0028T	1
0031T	1
0032T	1
0041T	1
0042T	1
0043T	1
0046T	2
0047T	2
0048T	1
0049T	1
0050T	1
0051T	1

General Policy Statements for Category III NCCI Guidelines

Excerpt From the Category III Section of NCCI Guidelines[2(5)]

With few exceptions the payment for a surgical procedure includes payment for dressings, supplies, and local anesthesia. These items are not separately reportable under their own HCPCS/CPT codes. Wound closures utilizing adhesive strips, topical skin adhesive, or tape alone are not separately reportable. In the absence of an operative procedure, these types of wound closures are included in an E&M service.

Interpretation

Recall that within the NCCI introductory guidelines, specifically the Standards of Medical/Surgical Practice section, that necessary surgical closure and dressing are included in the code for the primary procedure and should not be coded separately from the root operation. As a necessary component of a primary procedure, the surgical closure is what the physician had to perform in order to successfully accomplish the comprehensive service. It should not be separated from the comprehensive service when being coded. Additionally, as addressed in Chapters 2 and 4 of this book, anesthesia performed by the surgeon is included in the surgical CPT code and is not to be coded separately from the procedure.

For example, an implantation of an artificial heart (Category III code 0051T) always includes closure of the surgery site. Because this is a usual part of the procedure, no additional coding for closure should be provided.

Excerpt From the Category III Section of NCCI Guidelines[2(p5)]

With limited exceptions Medicare Anesthesia Rules prevent separate payment for anesthesia for a medical or surgical service when provided by the physician performing the service.... Additionally, the physician should not unbundle the anesthesia procedure and report component codes individually. For example, introduction of a needle or intracatheter into a vein (CPT code 36000), venipuncture (CPT code 36410), or drug administration...should not be reported when these services are related to the delivery of an anesthetic agent.

Interpretation

If the physician who performed a surgery also provided the anesthesia services for the surgery, separate CPT codes for the anesthesia may not be used. The anesthesia is included in the surgery when both services are performed by the same physician. Also, when a provider codes for the anesthesia, all aspects of the anesthesia are included in the anesthesia CPT code. Services inherent in performing anesthesia are not separately billable unless clearly unrelated to the anesthesia service.

Excerpt From the Category III Section of NCCI Guidelines[2(p5-6)]

Medicare may allow separate payment for moderate conscious sedation services (CPT codes 99143-99145) when provided by the same physician performing the medical or surgical procedure except for those procedures listed in Appendix G of the *CPT Manual*.[1]

Interpretation

Moderate sedation is a drug-induced depression of consciousness during which patients respond purposefully to verbal commands and perhaps some tactile stimulation. There are no interventions required to maintain the patient's airway because spontaneous ventilation is adequate.

If the physician who performed the procedure also provided the moderate sedation for the procedure, payment may be made for the conscious sedation services using CPT codes 99143 through 99145. However, please be sure to check Appendix G of the CPT codebook for a listing of services for which conscious sedation may not be separately billed.

 CPT Coding Tip: *Appendix G includes CPT codes that include moderate sedation. Additionally, the CPT codebook identifies those procedures that include moderate sedation with this symbol ⊙ preceding the code. There are no current Category III CPT codes that fall within Appendix G.*

CPT Codebook[1(p447)] Moderate (Conscious) Sedation Guidelines

When moderate sedation is provided, the following services are included and *not* reported separately:

Assessment of the patient (not included in intraservice time)

Establishment of intravenous access and fluids to maintain patency, when performed

Administration of agent(s)

Maintenance of sedation

Monitoring of oxygen saturation, heart rate, and blood pressure

Recovery (not included in intraservice time)

99143 Moderate sedation services (other than those services described by codes 00100-01999) provided by the same physician performing the diagnostic or therapeutic service that the sedation supports, requiring the presence of an independent trained observer to assist in the monitoring of the patient's level of consciousness and physiological status; younger than 5 years of age, first 30 minutes intra-service time

99144 age 5 years or older, first 30 minutes intra-service time

+99145 each additional 15 minutes intra-service time (List separately in addition to code for primary service)

These codes (99143, 99144, and 99145) describe the scenario in which the same physician who performed the diagnostic or therapeutic procedure provided the moderate sedation, and an independent trained observer's presence was required to assist in monitoring the patient's level of consciousness and physiological status.

For example, if a patient presents for placement of a retinal prosthesis receiver and generator placed subconjunctivally (Category III code 0100T), and the physician who performs the procedure also provides monitored anesthesia, both the Category III code and monitoring anesthesia care may be billed.

Excerpt From the Category III Section of NCCI Guidelines[2(p6)]

Under Medicare Global Surgery Rules, drug administration services…are not separately reportable by the physician performing a procedure for drug administration services related to the procedure.

Interpretation

If administering a drug is an inherent part of a procedure, the drug administration is inherent in the procedure code and should not be coded separately. The pharmaceutical used may be coded additionally, but not the administration. A case in point would be a patient who presents for a computed tomography (CT) scan of the heart with contrast material. The contrast material administration, if given intravascularly, is included in the CT code (0145T).

Excerpt From the Category III Section of NCCI Guidelines[2(p6)]

Medicare Global Surgery Rules prevent separate payment for postoperative pain management when provided by the physician performing an operative procedure. … The services described by these codes may be reported by the physician performing the operative procedure only if provided for purposes unrelated to the postoperative pain management, the operative procedure, or anesthesia for the procedure.

Interpretation

The Medicare approved amount for surgeries includes payment for the following services related to the surgery when they are furnished by the surgeon. Note that postoperative pain management is included in the surgery reimbursement and should not be billed separately.

- **Preoperative visits** after the decision is made to operate beginning with the day before the day of surgery for major procedures and the day of surgery for minor procedures
- **Intraoperative services** that are a usual and necessary part of a surgical procedure
- **Complications following surgery** that do not require additional trips to the operating room
- **Postoperative visits** that are related to recovery from the surgery
- **Postsurgical pain management** by the surgeon
- **Supplies**
- **Miscellaneous services**: Items such as dressing changes; local incisional care; removal of an operative pack; removal of cutaneous sutures and staples, lines, wires, tubes, drains, casts, and splints; insertion, irrigation, and removal of urinary catheters, routine peripheral intravenous lines, nasogastric and rectal tubes; and changes and removal of tracheostomy tubes

Take the example of a patient presenting for implantation of a cerebral thermal perfusion probe via a burr hole. Several hours postoperatively, the patient complains of severe pain. If the surgeon manages the pain, no additional service should be coded.

SUMMARY

- The entire Category III section from the NCCI manual should be read.
- When there is no CPT Category I code for the service being billed, check the Category III codes before assigning an unlisted code.
- Overall, the guidelines for Category III codes mimic those for Category I codes; however, each code edit must be reviewed on a claim-by-claim basis.

Definitions Important to Chapter 20

CPT Category III codes: Temporary *Current Procedural Terminology (CPT®)*[1] codes developed by the American Medical Association for data collection. These codes are for services that use emerging technology.

moderate (conscious) sedation: Drug-induced depression of consciousness during which patients respond purposefully to verbal commands, either alone or accompanied by light tactile stimulation. It does not include minimal sedation, deep sedation, or monitored anesthesia care.

CHAPTER EXERCISES

EXERCISE 1
A physician performs a Category III procedure under a local anesthetic. Can the local anesthetic be separately coded?

EXERCISE 2
A physician performs a laparotomy with removal of gastric stimulation electrodes (CPT Category III code 0158T) and closes the incision in layers. Can the closure be separately coded?

ANSWERS TO CHAPTER EXERCISES

EXERCISE 1: No, not if the physician who performed the procedure also administered the local anesthetic. Anesthesia administered by the surgeon (or physician performing the procedure) is incidental to the procedure code and should not be separately reported.

EXERCISE 2: No. Closure of the surgical approach (incision) is incidental to and included in the surgery code. The layered closure should not be coded separately.

REFERENCES

1. American Medical Association. *Current Procedural Terminology (CPT®) 2009.* Chicago, IL: American Medical Association; 2008.
2. Centers for Medicare and Medicaid Services. "Chapter XII Category III Codes." In: NCCI Policy Manual for Medicare Services. www.cms.hhs.gov/NationalCorrectCodInitEd/01_overview.asp#TopOfPage. Accessed June 15, 2009.

The Outpatient Hospital Setting

Chapter 21 serves as an overview of the subtle differences between outpatient facility bundling guidelines and the physician professional service bundling guidelines. There are few differences between the two provider categories, but important distinctions should be made. Many facilities bill for both the professional component and the facility component, and understanding these few differences becomes critical in accurate coding.

For coding of outpatient hospital services, this chapter becomes critical in the overall consideration of the edits and how they impact facility coding. The guidelines that are consistent between the professional fee and facility fee are not restated here, only the guidelines that differ. Therefore, all the chapters are important to review.

Introduction to Hospital Outpatient Prospective Payment

In the 1997 Balanced Budget Act and the 1999 Balanced Budget Refinement Act, Congress instructed the Centers for Medicare and Medicaid Services (CMS) to create a prospective payment system for outpatient services, similar to the diagnosis-related group (DRG) system implemented for inpatient services.

All services paid under the Outpatient Prospective Payment (OPPS) system are classified into groups called Ambulatory Payment Classifications (APCs). Each APC groups services that are similar clinically and in resource consumption and are driven by *Current Procedural Terminology* (CPT®)[1]/Healthcare Common Procedure Coding System (HCPCS) coding. A payment rate is established for each APC. The CMS final rule for the new system was published in the *Federal Register*[3], on April 7, 2000 (65 FR 18434). The new system went into effect on August 1, 2000, and is formally updated annually.

Multiple APCs could be paid on a single claim in the outpatient setting driven by multiple CPT/HCPCS codes. Because multiple codes are billed for a single outpatient encounter, the NCCI edits become a necessary part of the CMS editing of these claims.

Outpatient Prospective Payment System NCCI Edit Resources

As indicated in Chapter 1, it is helpful to have access to as many NCCI resources as possible. Refer back to those resources, and review the additional OPPS-specific resources shared here.

CMS Web Site

Although they were reviewed thoroughly in Chapter 1, CMS resources are briefly covered in this chapter, because the layout is slightly different for OPPS-specific services. The following four steps explain how to access the NCCI edits on the CMS web site:

Step 1. Visit the CMS web site at www.cms.hhs.gov[4], and select the Medicare category.

Step 2. Scroll down to the Provider Type category, and select Hospital Center.

Step 3. Scroll down to the Billing or Coding category, and select National Correct Coding Edits Hospitals.

In this section, review all the appropriate information. This will aid in understanding where to look for additional instruction. Look at the Overview section first, which provides the background for the NCCI edits as well as several downloadable transmittals, the policy manual (a must read), the section of the Medicare manual addressing NCCI edits, articles, and frequently asked questions relative to the NCCI. Most of these are discussed within this book, but it is helpful to know where the resource is accessed.

Step 4. Look then at the other categories of information, which include the following:

- Hospital Outpatient PPS and therapy NCCI
- Medically Unlikely Edits
- NCCI Edits—Physicians
- NCCI Edits—Hospital Outpatient PPS
- NCCI Transmittals

Those edits important to each claim should be accessed. Billing for a physician's service would require accessing the NCCI Edits for Physicians, billing for outpatient hospital services would require review of those edits, and so on. Refer back to Figure 1.2 for screen shots of the four-step process.

Variations in NCCI Edits for Outpatient Hospital Services

There are differences, albeit few, between the professional fee and facility NCCI edits and guidelines. The CMS developed the NCCI for implementation January 1, 1996, to promote correct coding by physicians and facilities and to ensure that appropriate payments are made for health care services, and they expanded the edits to include outpatient hospital services in 2000. The NCCI edits are part of the Outpatient Code Editor (OCE) that edits all outpatient claims and assigns APCs for outpatient Prospective Payment System services. In the past, the OCE did not include NCCI edits for anesthesiology, evaluation and management (E/M), and mental health services, but as of January 1, 2009, the NCCI edits no longer exclude any category of service. Bypass modifiers and coding pairs in the OCE may differ from those in the NCCI because of differences between facility and professional services. The OCE generates NCCI edits when OPPS claims are processed for payment.

General Guideline Differences

Excerpt from the Introduction Section of NCCI Edits[5(p2)]

Although the NCCI was initially developed for use by Medicare Carriers to process Part B claims, many of the edits were added to the Outpatient Code Editor (OCE) in August 2000, for use by Fiscal Intermediaries to process claims for Part B outpatient hospital services. Some of the edits applied to outpatient hospital claims through OCE differ from the comparable edits in NCCI. Effective January 2006, all therapy claims paid by Fiscal Intermediaries were also subject to NCCI edits in the OCE.

Interpretation

There are differences in the actual edits between the physician edits and hospital edits. Some overlap, others do not. Also, the OCE edits include more than NCCI edits. Regardless, hospitals are responsible for making sure they abide by the guidelines and edits applicable to them for the specific date of service.

 Tip: If one software program is used for editing claims, make sure that the differences between the two sets of edits (physician and hospital) are easily accessible. Another alternative that would be very time consuming would be to always check the CMS web site for the most current edits. However, the editing software should make allowances for any differences in edits.

In this Manual many policies are described utilizing the term "physician." Unless indicated differently the usage of this term does not restrict the policies to physicians only but applies to all practitioners, hospitals, providers, or suppliers eligible to bill the relevant HCPCS/CPT codes pursuant to applicable portions of the Social Security Act (SSA) of 1965, the Code of Federal Regulations (CFR), and Medicare rules. In some sections of this Manual, the term "physician" would not include some of these entities because specific rules do not apply to them. For example, Anesthesia Rules and Global Surgery Rules do not apply to hospitals.

Interpretation

Because the guidelines apply to both facility and professional fee services, the NCCI edits are clarifying that point within this statement. When the term *physician* is used, it should be interpreted as *provider*. Within several sections of NCCI guidelines, the instruction reads:

Physicians should report the HCPCS/CPT code that describes the procedure performed to the greatest specificity possible. A HCPCS/CPT code should be reported only if all services described by the code are performed. A physician should not report multiple HCPCS/CPT codes if a single HCPCS/CPT code exists that describes the services. This type of unbundling is incorrect coding.

For facility billing, this guideline still applies, even though the instruction reads *physician*.

Under OPPS, the administration of fluids and drugs during or for an operative procedure are included services and are not separately reportable....

Interpretation

For OPPS billing, this guideline is instructing that the *administration* of agents for an operative procedure becomes inherent in the surgery coding and should not be billed separately. Any substances used during the administration can be billed.

Coding Tip: *For OPPS, certain drugs and other agents (not the administration of the agent) have HCPCS Level II codes that may be billed separately from the procedure. Even though the administration is included in the procedure, these substances may be billed separately. Even if the substance does not have a separately paid HCPCS code, the charge for the drugs can be billed separately from the procedure under a revenue code without a HCPCS code.*

Under OPPS, anesthesia for a surgical procedure is an included service and is not separately reportable. For example, a provider should not report CPT codes ... for anesthesia services.

Interpretation

This guideline is somewhat different from the last one. In OPPS, anesthesia can be a separate line item on the UB-04 under an anesthesia revenue code, but there should be *no* HCPCS/CPT code assigned to the anesthesia service, as the reimbursement bundles the anesthesia in with the surgery APC. For example, during a surgery for removal of a pterygium, intravenous anesthesia is started. Administration of fentanyl and pentothal is inherent in the surgery anesthesia code and is not coded separately as an intravenous injection. Also, if, during a cholecystectomy, general anesthesia is used, the anesthesia administration would not be coded with an anesthesia CPT code. However, the hospital may bill an anesthesia revenue code (37x) without an anesthesia CPT code. This ensures that the charges accurately reflect the costs to the facility.

Tip: *There might be a professional fee code for the anesthesia, but that would not be on the hospital's UB claim. Rather, the anesthesiologist would bill professional fee services separately from the hospital bill.*

Musculoskeletal Guideline Differences

Excerpt From Musculoskeletal System NCCI Edits[7(p6)]

For OPPS, if a hospital treated a fracture, dislocation, or injury with a cast, splint, or strap as an initial service without any other definitive procedure or treatment, the hospital should report the appropriate casting/splinting/strapping CPT code. Payment for the cast/splint/strap supplies is included in the payment for the procedure reported.

Interpretation

This instruction from NCCI basically states that when a cast or strapping is applied to immobilize the site for the patient to see a specialist for definitive treatment later, the cast/strapping CPT codes should be used. The provider is essentially not repairing the fracture but rather stabilizing the fracture for further treatment later. Therefore, if a patient presents to an emergency department (ED) with a broken finger. The ED clinician applies a cast and advises the patient to see an orthopaedic surgeon the next day. The ED treatment is for immobilization only and should not be coded as a fracture repair. Another example would be a patient presenting to the ED with a broken finger. The ED clinician manipulates the finger back into alignment and buddy-tapes the finger to an adjoining finger. He prescribes pain medication and advises the patient to return to the ED as needed or go to his primary care physician if necessary.

This example is somewhat tricky, but basically, the physician is performing restorative treatment, and this would be coded as fracture care, with no code added for the taping. Also, it is likely that an E/M service would also be coded, depending on the level of documentation.

Radiology Guideline Differences

Excerpt From Radiology NCCI Edits[8(p5)]

When limited comparative radiographic studies are performed (e.g., post-reduction radiographs, post-intubation, post-catheter placement, etc.), the CPT code for the radiographic series should be reported with modifier -52, indicating that a reduced level of interpretive service was provided. This requirement does not apply to OPPS services reported by hospitals.

Interpretation

This guideline indicates that the interpretation is the reduced service, and because the hospital is billing for the technical component (actually taking the film), there is no reduction in work or cost, and, therefore, modifier 52 would not be needed.

Often, a second image is necessary to see if the treatment provided was successful. For example, for fractures, a post-reduction film often would be made to determine whether proper alignment was obtained through the manipulation.

Pathology/Laboratory Guideline Differences

Medicine Section Guideline Differences

Excerpt From Pathology/Laboratory Service NCCI Edits[9(p13)]

When a physician (limited to M.D./D.O.) reads/quantitates (CPT codes 88367, 88368) and interprets (CPT codes 88365-88368) the tissues/cells stained with the probe(s), the provider may report the global code or professional component (modifier -26) as appropriate. When the professional component of CPT codes 88365-88368 is reported by the physician (limited to M.D./D.O.), the laboratory may report the technical component (modifier -TC), and a hospital reporting an outpatient laboratory test may report the appropriate CPT code. If a non-physician (provider other than M.D./D.O.) reads and quantitates the tissues/cells stained with the probe(s), the laboratory should not report the technical component (-TC) of CPT codes 88367-88368, and a hospital reporting an outpatient laboratory test should not report CPT codes 88367 or 88368. The laboratory or hospital may report these services with CPT codes 88271-88275.

Excerpt From Medicine Section NCCI Edits[10(p5)]

CPT code 96522 (refilling and maintenance of implantable pump or reservoir) and CPT code 96521 (refilling and maintenance of portable pump) should not be reported with CPT code 96416 (initiation of prolonged intra-venous chemotherapy infusion (more than eight hours), requiring use of a portable or implantable pump) or CPT code 96425 (chemotherapy administration, intra-arterial; infusion technique, initiation of prolonged infusion (more than eight hours) requiring the use of a portable or implantable pump). CPT codes 96416 and 96425 include the initial filling and maintenance of a portable or implantable pump. CPT codes 96521 and 96522 are used to report subsequent refilling of the pump. Similarly under the OPPS, CPT codes 96521 (refilling and maintenance of portable pump) and 96522 (refilling and maintenance of portable or implantable pump or reservoir) should not be reported with HCPCS/CPT code C8957 (initiation of prolonged intravenous infusion (more than 8 hours)).

Interpretation

This guideline is merely noting current correct CPT coding for these services; however, an extra comment here is that in order for these codes to be used, the services *must* be performed by a physician. Even for hospital coding (which is coding for the hospital's overhead, not the professional component), this guideline applies. A notation in the CPT codebook next to these services might be warranted as a reminder.

Interpretation

C8957 Intravenous infusion for therapy/diagnosis; initiation of prolonged infusion (more than 8 hours), requiring use of portable or implantable pump

96521 Refilling and maintenance of portable pump

96522 Refilling and maintenance of implantable pump or reservoir for drug delivery, systemic (eg, intravenous, intra-arterial)

CPT codes 96521 and 96522 state that they are for refilling, not initial filling; therefore, this clarifies that the initiation services for prolonged infusion include the initial filling and maintenance of the pump. Coding the refilling and maintenance (CPT code 96522 or 96521) in addition to the initiation would be double billing for the refilling and maintenance portion.

For example, a patient presents for chemotherapy at the conclusion of which an infusion pump is initiated to pump fluorouracil for four days thereafter. The C8957 code would include the initial filling of the pump. Only if the patient presents for *refilling* would CPT code 96521 or 96522 be used.

Excerpt From Medicine Section NCCI Edits[10(p9-10)]

Treatment of swallowing dysfunction and/or oral function for feeding (CPT code 92526) may utilize electrical stimulation. HCPCS Level II code G0283 (electrical stimulation (unattended), to one or more areas for indication(s) other than wound care....) should not be reported with CPT code 92526 for electrical stimulation during the procedure. The NCCI edit (92526/G0283) for Medicare Carriers does not allow use of NCCI-associated modifiers with this edit because the same provider would never perform both of these services on the same date of service. However, the same edit in OCE for Fiscal Intermediaries does allow use of NCCI-associated modifiers because two separate practitioners in the same outpatient hospital facility or institutional therapy provider might perform the two procedures for different purposes at different patient encounters on the same date of service.

Interpretation

This guideline must be read completely for understanding of the logic. First, if the treating physician is billing for the electrical stimulation and the treatment of swallowing dysfunction, the likelihood is that the services are performed together. However, because outpatient hospitals can have many different clinics, providers, and specialists all providing care to a single patient on one date of service, they can *potentially* bypass the edit. In order to do so, the services would need to be at distinct (separate) encounters for different reasons. For example, a patient presents to an outpatient hospital clinic complaining of difficulty in swallowing. The physician treats the dysfunction with electrical stimulation. Because this is done in one session for one condition, only CPT code 92526 should be coded. On the other hand, consider another patient who is treated at one hospital-owned clinic for difficulty in swallowing and, later that day, has a planned electrical stimulation treatment in the physical therapy department of the hospital for an injury unrelated to the difficulty swallowing. Because these visits were completely unrelated (distinct diagnoses and separate departments) and appear to both be medically necessary, both the visit and the electrical stimulation may be coded.

Excerpt From Medicine Section NCCI Edits[10(p20)]

...drug administration services performed in hospital facilities including emergency departments are not separately reportable by physicians. Drug administration services performed in an Ambulatory Surgical Center (ASC) related to a Medicare approved ASC payable procedure are not separately reportable by physicians. Hospital outpatient facilities may bill separately for drug administration services when appropriate. For purposes of this paragraph, the term "physician" refers to M.D.'s, D.O.'s, and other practitioners who bill Medicare carriers for services payable on the "Medicare Physician Fee Schedule."

Interpretation

Usually, the administration of drugs is not personally performed by a physician. Rather, the physician supervises the administration. Because the physician's staff performed the administration in the office, the physician may bill these services, even though he or she did not personally perform them. However, in the hospital setting, hospital staff often perform the administration, and, therefore, the physician should not bill for hospital staff work. For instance, a patient receives chemotherapy in the outpatient hospital setting, and a registered nurse performs the administration under direct physician supervision. The hospital may bill for the administration, but the physician may not.

SUMMARY

- Read applicable (regarding those services in which the facility provides outpatient care) chapters within this book.

- Note how the OCE edits compare to NCCI edits to ensure complete understanding of the differences.

- Refer to the hospital-specific NCCI edits and not the physician NCCI edits.

Definitions and Acronyms Important to Chapter 21

Ambulatory Payment Classification (APC): APCs are Medicare's payment group for the Outpatient Prospective Payment System.

Balanced Budget Act: A congressional act designed to reduce costs in Medicare expenditures.

Balanced Budget Refinement Act: A second congressional act to refine the original Balanced Budget Act.

Diagnosis-Related Group (DRG): The method the Centers for Medicare and Medicaid Services (CMS) uses to reimburse Medicare inpatient facility claims.

medicare severity DRG: CMS updated the methodology of reimbursing inpatient facility claims by adding a level of severity to the calculated groupings. *Current Procedural Terminology (CPT®)*[1] and Healthcare Common Procedure Coding System codes are grouped into APCs for payment purposes.

Outpatient Code Editor[2] **(OCE):** This is a Medicare software editing program that edits a claim for accuracy of the data on that claim. It further serves to assign APCs, status indicators, and payment indicators; compute discounts when appropriate; and package services and edits for National Correct Coding Initiative issues.

Outpatient Prospective Payment System (OPPS): This is Medicare's reimbursement system for outpatient hospital facility services.

CHAPTER EXERCISES

EXERCISE 1

Can an outpatient facility bill for the cast application when a fracture repair is performed?

EXERCISE 2

Can an outpatient facility code for a tetanus immunization administration in addition to an E/M service provided during the encounter?

EXERCISE 3

Can an outpatient facility bill for an anesthesia CPT code in addition to the surgery CPT code?

ANSWERS TO CHAPTER EXERCISES

EXERCISE 1: For facilities and physicians, closure of a surgical site is incidental to the code for the surgery.

EXERCISE 2: Yes. As long as the services are properly documented and medically necessary, both an E/M service and tetanus immunization injection (and the supply) may be coded. However, the tetanus immunization injection cannot be the only service provided—the E/M must be separately documented.

EXERCISE 3: No. Anesthesia may be charged on a separate line item from the surgery, but no CPT code for the anesthesia should be used. These charges package into the surgery reimbursement.

REFERENCES

1. American Medical Association. *Current Procedural Terminology (CPT®) Professional Edition 2009.* Chicago, IL: American Medical Association; 2008.

2. Centers for Medicare and Medicaid Services. Outpatient code editor resource page. www.cms.hhs.gov/OutpatientCodeEdit/. Accessed June 15, 2009.

3. Office of the Federal Register, National Archives and Records Administration. 42 CFR Parts 409, et al. Medicare program; prospective payment system for hospital outpatient services; Final rule. *Federal Register.* 2000;65(68). www.access.gpo.gov/su_docs/fedreg/a000407c.html. Accessed June 15, 2009.

4. Centers for Medicare and Medicaid Services. *Hospital Outpatient PPS.* www.cms.hhs.gov/HospitalOutpatientPPS/. Accessed June 15, 2009.

5. Centers for Medicare and Medicaid Services. "Introduction for National Correct Coding Initiative Policy Manual." In: NCCI Policy Manual for Medicare Services. www.cms.hhs.gov/NationalCorrectCodInitEd/01_overview.asp#TopOfPage. Accessed June 15, 2009.

6. Centers for Medicare and Medicaid Services. "Chapter I General Correct Coding Policies." In: NCCI Policy Manual for Medicare Services. www.cms.hhs.gov/NationalCorrectCodInitEd/01_overview.asp - TopOfPage. Accessed June 15, 2009.

7. Centers for Medicare and Medicaid Services. "Chapter IV Surgery: Musculoskeletal System." In: NCCI Policy Manual for Medicare Services. www.cms.hhs.gov/NationalCorrectCodInitEd/01_overview.asp#TopOfPage. Accessed June 15, 2009.

8. Centers for Medicare and Medicaid Services. "Chapter IX Radiology Services." In: NCCI Policy Manual for Medicare Services. www.cms.hhs.gov/NationalCorrectCodInitEd/01_overview.asp#TopOfPage. Accessed June 15, 2009.

9. Centers for Medicare and Medicaid Services. "Chapter X Pathology/Laboratory Services." In: NCCI Policy Manual for Medicare Services. www.cms.hhs.gov/NationalCorrectCodInitEd/01_overview.asp#TopOfPage. Accessed June 15, 2009.

10. Centers for Medicare and Medicaid Services. "Chapter XI Medicine Evaluation and Management Services." In: NCCI Policy Manual for Medicare Services. www.cms.hhs.gov/NationalCorrectCodInitEd/01_overview.asp#TopOfPage. Accessed June 15, 2009.

Index

C

D

E

F

L

M

N

O

P

T